The Luxury of Time

The Luxury of Time

JANE & MIKE TOMLINSON

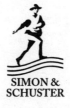

SIMON &
SCHUSTER

London · New York · Sydney · Toronto · Dublin

A VIACOM COMPANY

First published in Great Britain by
Simon & Schuster UK Ltd, 2005
A Viacom Company

1 3 5 7 9 10 8 6 4 2

Simon & Schuster UK Ltd
Africa House
64–78 Kingsway
London WC2B 6AH

www.simonsays.co.uk

Simon & Schuster Australia
Sydney

A CIP catalogue record for this book is available
from the British Library.

ISBN 0-7432-6793-1
EAN 9780743267939

Typeset by M Rules
Printed and bound in Great Britain by
Mackays of Chatham plc

To Suzanne, Rebecca and Steven
You were gifted to us, this is our gift to you
Love Mum and Dad

The Luxury of Time

JANE

December 2002

I still can't quite believe I'm here.

The large studio at the BBC has been turned into a bar and we're sitting in one of the few remaining seats. I can see Virginia Wade and Bobby Charlton over in the corner and Mike points out Steve Backley, the javelin thrower, and Matt Dawson, the rugby player.

'Ben Cohen. Over there.' Mike nudges my arm and I see faces from television greeting each other, laughing and talking over drinks. It's as if I've stumbled into some bizarre local for sporting celebrities.

The letter inviting me here had arrived two months earlier. If I hadn't seen it for myself I would have thought it was someone's idea of a joke, but there it was, in black and white on official headed paper: 'Would I like to spend an evening with my sporting peers at the BBC *Sports Personality of the Year*?' Dumbfounded, I had stood in the hallway and read and re-read the letter.

'What do they mean – "sporting peers"?' I'd said to Mike. As far as I was concerned, you could pluck anyone off the street to do what I do – I'm no Paula Radcliffe.

But here we are, queuing up behind familiar faces whose names I can't recall, nervously waiting to be told what to do next. Mike holds a wide-eyed Steven by the hand as I walk with Suzanne and Rebecca into a huge auditorium with rows of blue plastic seats circling a centre stage. A young, blonde woman approaches and introduces herself as the floor manager. Checking her clipboard, she greets me.

'Hi, Jane,' she says brightly. 'I'll show you to your seat.' I'm amazed she knows who I am – that I am on anybody's list.

She strides purposefully across the centre of the studio. Upturned seats display white labels with more names – Sven Goran Eriksson, George Best. In the middle row I spot my name, Jane Tomlinson. Next to it, Mike Tomlinson. We sit down.

In front of us, a young lad, obviously unused to wearing a suit, fidgets around, pulling his tie to loosen it around his neck. He reminds me of the boys you see at weddings who would rather be anywhere than stuck in such a formal setting. He looks round. It's Wayne Rooney.

The floor manager reappears. 'Can we mike you up, Jane?' she asks.

I shoot Mike a worried glance. He never said anything about being interviewed. I'd been looking forward to this for weeks, thrilled that the children had been invited, but now I know I may have to speak, my stomach is tense, my shoulders tight. Once fitted with the microphone, I clasp my hands tightly on my lap and breathe slowly.

'You're going to enjoy this,' whispers Mike, planting a kiss on my cheek. 'No one deserves it more. Love you.'

I hear someone counting down. The lights change, music booms out from speakers above us. It's beginning. It's live and I still can't believe I'm going to be part of it.

The presenters, Steve Rider, Sue Barker and Gary Linekar, look just as they do on the television at home. On the large screens overhead some of the greatest sporting moments from the year are shown: the Winter Olympics, the famous victory of the British curling team, the success and tears of the Commonwealth Games. As the film finishes, Steve Rider announces the arrival of 'one of the greatest stars of British athletics' and the spotlight falls to the top of a flight of stairs behind the stage.

Paula Radcliffe, looking stunning in a black boned dress appears and smiles at us. She looks every inch a champion. I watch closely as a video of her achievements is played over the screens. The London Marathon, the Commonwealth Games, the European Championships, the Chicago Marathon – I am in complete awe of this amazing woman and watch transfixed as Steve Rider interviews her. I clap loudly when the interview is over.

Steven starts fretting on Mike's knee and I look at my watch. We've been here over an hour – no wonder he's getting grumpy. Mike whispers something into his ear.

The applause dies down and Steve Rider takes centre stage again.

'Another very special triathlon and marathon runner is the recipient of our next award,' he says. 'The Helen Rollason Award, in memory of our late colleague. It recognizes courage and achievement in the face of adversity in sport. That sums up Jane Tomlinson very precisely, especially to those close to her.'

Oh, my God. This can't be real. Completely stunned, I turn to Mike who is beaming at me. He knew. He knew all along. I attempt to smile back but I'm drawn to the huge screen behind the stage.

Images flash up. It's me. Hobbling in the London Marathon, tears pouring down my face. Holding my arms aloft, overjoyed after finishing the London Triathlon. Waving with delight as I beat Mike in the Great North Run. I'm aware that the audience is looking at me, waiting for my reaction as I watch myself on screen but I never take my eyes from the film.

I can hear Mike's voice as it booms around the studio.

'Jane's time is shortened, due to the fact that she has terminal breast cancer, but that does not stop her living life to the full. For this, the children and I are immensely proud.' Goosebumps prickle the skin on my arms and tears roll down my face. The pictures fade and now I see my living room with Mike and the children sitting round in a circle going through a pile of photographs. When on earth did they film this? I look across to Mike and Steven who are both grinning at me. I have been well and truly set up.

On the screen, Steven is holding up a photograph from our holiday in Italy. Mike asks him what he wants to say to me.

'I love her,' he says.

Another snap of Steven and me takes up the full screen. It was taken several years ago, before chemo, my hair is thick, Steven is still a very little boy. The tears drip down over my nose and I wipe them away and stare through them at another snapshot of my life. Rebecca and me on a country walk, wearing woolly hats and fleeces. I know it. It's a picture taken at the top of Mam Tor, a special place in the Peak District where we've spent many a happy time.

'You see my mum as a person who raises money for cancer research,' says Rebecca on the film. 'I see her as a person who, when I am sick, she makes me feel better – even though she's in the same situation every day.'

I turn and smile towards Rebecca and when I return to the screen, I see a photo of Suzanne and me astride a tandem. It's taken outside Mike's parents house in the Yorkshire Dales. Suzanne looks slim and beautiful in her pink T-shirt.

'She has done so much with the time she's had,' she says. 'Other people don't do that and they are fully well. They maybe can, but they don't. They take things for granted.'

She leans forward and says, 'I love you' to the camera. I mouth back, 'Love you' to Suzanne in the audience and return to the screen. Mike reaches for my hand as they show us both smiling in a picture taken from a long past holiday in Cornwall.

'You could not have handled this any better than you have,' says his voice resonating throughout the studio. 'It's been an absolute pleasure. I love you lots.'

The film finishes and I'm stunned. Frozen to my seat, I'm unsure what I'm supposed to do but I watch as Paula Radcliffe joins Steve Rider in the centre of the studio. Between them is the BBC award.

'Paula Radcliffe is here to present the Helen Rollason Award to Jane Tomlinson,' says Steve Rider.

I rise hesitantly from my seat, uncertain how to respond. Walking slowly down the stairs, I watch my footing as my balance is precarious from the chemotherapy. Paula stoops to kiss me on the cheek and congratulates me as she passes me the silver trophy. I look around as the audience applauds. They clap for so long, I don't know where to look. I glance at my family –

all in tears, all clapping. I feel as though I have slipped into a parallel universe as the applause keeps going. What on earth am I going to say in front of all these people?

The clapping eventually dies down and Paula begins to speak. She is slim, tall and beautiful. The comparison between us could not be more stark.

'We both started out doing the London Marathon,' she says. 'But I think what you achieved that day was far greater than anything I did.'

My heart is beating so hard that I fear the camera will see it pounding through the fabric of my dress. My mouth is dry and I'm trembling. I am just an ordinary mum and wife. I never did any of this to win a prize. Paula hands me the trophy and smiles.

'She's a more deserving winner of this award than anyone else will be tonight.'

The audience is applauding again. Nervously I trace out the BBC logo on the trophy and compose myself enough to say a few words. I feel terrified as I focus into the lens pointing at me and I am conscious not to move around too much. I don't want to look like I'm twitching to the people watching at home. As I get to the end of my speech I steel myself, concentrating on articulating the last part.

'A big thank you to Mike, Suzanne, Becca and Steven,' I say, looking over at them and smiling. They all smile back.

The cameras turn away and the longest five minutes of my life are over. I thank Paula again and make my way back to my seat. The cameras are already sweeping round, snakes of wires trailing behind them. I sit down next to Mike and rest my head on his shoulder. I'm exhausted but elated. He puts his arm around me and hugs me, his eyes still damp with tears.

I had wanted to leave my family with happy memories. I had been determined not to spend my last months watching them grieve for me. This was an unforgettable memory – an amazing end to an extraordinary year.

CHAPTER 1

MIKE

1989

The house was perfect – I knew it as soon as I opened the door.

The green-carpeted hallway welcomed me in and I stepped inside to nose around. The patterned wallpaper looked reasonably new and I wandered through, making mental reminders as to what to report back home.

Jane had been clear in her instructions: a house with two bedrooms – three if possible – with a garden and a room where we could all eat as a family. I pushed open the door towards the far end of the hall and found a decent-sized dining room with a large window looking out on to a secluded rear garden. I pictured our pine dining table in the centre of the room and my family, happily sitting around it eating Sunday lunch.

Next door the living room was well decorated but gloomy. Without furniture, it looked huge and barren, but even with our pair of two-seater settees, it would still be pretty roomy. Outside, the lawn needed mowing but it was large enough for the girls to play on. Enclosed by brick walls and an unkempt privet hedge, it meant they would be safe.

I thought Jane would love the kitchen. The fitted, wooden units looked brand new and the modern oven and hob were barely touched, but the room itself felt cosy.

Upstairs, the main bedroom faced out on to the street. This

would be our room. Next door, Suzanne, aged four, and Rebecca, aged one, could share – with bunk beds they'd have enough space. The bathroom was tiny, but I consoled myself with the fact that none of us were particularly big. And the box room – I'd find a use for that.

My search was over.

'Jane, you'll love it,' I said on the phone later that evening. 'Dad came down with Mum, Maurice and Edith and they all liked it. Dad says it's solid, built properly, more substantial than modern ones and there's nothing to do on it, no chain, everything is perfect. I could put an offer in tomorrow—'

'You must be joking,' she said, her voice tense. 'I can't believe your parents have seen it before me – why didn't you ring me?'

'Trust me, you'll love it. Edith and—'

'I am not going to buy a house just because your relatives like it.'

'I don't want to lose it, let me put on offer in. My dad—'

'We'll come up at the weekend and have a look and don't show it to any more of your family, friends or anyone else. You've no idea, no bloody idea.'

It was not the response I had hoped for but I let it go. Slouching on the double bed with the TV on mute and a large mug of tea on the bedside table, I was sick to death of living like this. Ten weeks of living out of a suitcase as a guest of the Kings Arms hotel in Wakefield and at last I thought we were getting somewhere. But I knew it was no use saying anything more – Jane wouldn't budge until she'd seen it for herself.

'Okay, okay,' I said, 'I won't do anything until you've seen it.'

'Good.'

'But honestly, Jane, you're going to like it.'

Friday night eventually arrived and, despite Jane's reservations, I remained confident I had found our new family home. Rushing to the car, the heat of the August sun felt good on my face. After eight hours trapped in a stuffy office, the blue sky, noisy traffic and even the exhaust fumes woke me up.

When my promotion had come through in June, both Jane and I had been overjoyed at the prospect of moving back to Yorkshire, although the two-hour journey from Peterborough to Wakefield was too long to commute daily. Every Monday, I would set off at dawn from our home in Orton, near Peterborough, and make my way up the M1, leaving my girls still sleeping in their beds. On Friday evening, I would find myself making the same journey in reverse. I knew it couldn't go on for ever, but after more than two months, I was desperate to settle down again.

As I pulled off the road on to our estate, I felt the familiar pang of sympathy for Jane mixed with a twinge of guilt. Effectively marooned here, she was unable to drive and was miles away from family and friends with only Suzanne and Rebecca for company. We couldn't even afford a bus trip into town. Still, once she'd seen this new house, I felt sure our situation would improve.

'Hello!' I shouted as I walked into the house. There was no answer.

I padded through the hall peeping into the living room. No sign. As I approached the kitchen I could hear delighted squeals piercing the air through the open patio doors and I made my way to the door and stood unnoticed, watching my family at play in the back garden.

Suzanne and Rebecca were both wearing purple plastic sunglasses and baggy white T-shirts covered their swimming costumes. Rebecca was holding a yellow watering can high above her head, earnestly trying to water the few remaining border plants while Suzanne and Jane were racing through the garden aiming water at each other from empty squeezy bottles. Jane looked stunning in a flowing white cotton dress.

Out of the corner of her eye, Suzanne spotted me.

'Daddy!' She tore over the grass and hugged me while Jane looked at us, smiling.

I was home.

Early next morning, we piled into the car and drove back up to Wakefield so Jane could finally see the house.

'The area's up and coming too,' I said, hearing myself sound like an overzealous estate agent.

'Will you just shut up,' she laughed. 'I'll make up my own mind.'

Entering Lofthouse, we passed what might end up being our new local, the Rose and Crown. The car park was deserted and the windows were boarded up.

'Where the hell have you brought me?' asked Jane.

I didn't answer – I was still confident the house would win her over. Within another minute we were pulling up outside the front gates and I sensed a flicker of a smile on her face as the front garden met with her approval. I knew she had noticed there was little in the way of plants, which would leave her with a clear canvas.

Inside, I could tell she was impressed. She nodded silently, making notes and wandering from room to room. As she went to explore the bedrooms upstairs, Suzanne, Rebecca and I played in the dining room. At either side of the stone fireplace, wooden units were built into the recesses and at the bottom were two cupboards with little doors. In anticipation of Mum's return the girls hid inside them.

After a few minutes, Jane came downstairs.

'Have you seen the girls?' I asked loudly, flashing a wink at the cupboards.

'No, I thought they were with you.'

Never able to sustain a surprise, Suzanne burst out laughing but there was no peep from Rebecca. Eventually, I crawled across the carpeted floor and opened the door on a grinning toddler.

'Come on, Becca.' I stood up smiling. 'It's time to go.' As she shuffled out on her hands and knees, I flipped the door shut but misjudged my timing. There was a sickening crack of wood on bone. Rebecca screamed. I shot down to the floor to pick her up as Jane raced across the room.

'It's okay,' I soothed gently, rubbing her tiny head. Hot tears flowed down her cheeks. I felt sick.

Jane disappeared. I heard the front door go, but a few

minutes later she rushed back with supplies of ice and emergency KitKats. Rebecca's hysterics gradually subsided.

'Keith and Audrey next door,' explained Jane as she applied the cold compress to Rebecca's bump. 'They seem really nice.'

Then she looked up at me and smiled.

'So is the house,' she said.

JANE

1990

We moved in the first week of September. Mike's parents offered to look after the girls for a few days which allowed me some time to unpack our belongings without interruption.

When the girls returned the following week, Suzanne began school in the neighbouring village of Carlton. She only attended reception class in the morning but it meant a good mile walk – there and back – twice a day, in less than four hours. It certainly kept me fit.

We spent most afternoons decorating and making our new house our own. Mike had been right, the house was perfect. I liked the fact we were in a proper village and not just part of a new estate.

It felt so nice to be back in Yorkshire. I was born in Leeds and my family still lived there. I'd missed them while we'd been down south and it was lovely to be able to pop in whenever we liked. Every Sunday morning, Mum, Dad and I would attend mass at St James's Hospital. My dad was undergoing treatment at the hospital for a bone marrow cancer, and the short service was easier for him to sit through without too much pain. Afterwards we'd end up having tea and hot buttery toast back at their house. I think they enjoyed being able to see Suzanne and Rebecca so often.

Although I loved being at home with the children, I was eager to get back to studying. I'd already boosted my A-level grades at night school in Peterborough and, when we moved house, I applied to do a maths degree at Leeds University. Money was tight but I figured if I could get my degree, I could become a maths teacher. Another income would help enormously. I felt I needed some financial independence and although Mike was never selfish with money, the fact that I wasn't earning meant he always had the last word in any financial decision, which led to some inequality – not to mention arguments. Even a night out with friends meant I had to ask Mike for some spending money and the monthly allowance he gave me only just covered the food bills.

My days followed pretty much the same routine. I cared for the girls, cooked our meals and kept our home tidy. It was an average existence, but I was happy.

By February, when we'd been in the house almost six months, the decorating was nearly done. The weather turned bitterly cold and the walk to school was more like an endurance test against the freezing winds. I'd forgotten how bleak Yorkshire winters could be.

One morning, crouching on the chair in the kitchen with my jumper pulled down over my knees to keep me warm, I watched as Mike made his sandwiches for work. Slurping the dregs of his tea, he turned to kiss me.

'What are you up to today?' he asked.

'Not a lot. I thought I might start looking through my reading list for my course.' I gave him a peck on the lips.

'Okay. Well, I'll see you later on' and he was gone. I uncurled my legs and got up from the chair. I walked quietly back through the house – I figured I might just be able to have a quick shower before the children woke. As I tiptoed in, the hot jet of water felt lovely. With a tiny stab of guilt, I turned my back on the cracked grouting in the tiles. I really shouldn't be showering until it was fixed and I was sure Mike would spot the telltale dark circle in the dining room when he came home. I soaped my body and as I ran my hand back over my left breast I felt something. Was that a lump? Was it a rib? At seven stone, I was slim – some people would say skinny – but I had never noticed anything before. It was small but firm and protruded slightly at the top of the tear-shape of my breast. Curious, I ran my hand over the opposite side for something to compare but I couldn't feel anything.

Before I could investigate further, I heard movement from Suzanne and Rebecca's room.

I put my head round the girls' door and could see two pairs of eyes peering out at me. Flicking on the bedroom light, Suzanne – on the top bunk – squinted against the brightness while Rebecca snuggled further down under her quilt below.

'Oh no you don't,' I said, crossing the room to draw the curtains. 'It's time to wake up and get dressed.'

'Come on, you'll be late,' I yelled after breakfast. Seconds later they dashed down. I posted Rebecca into her bright red snowsuit and zipped it up, then fastened Suzanne's coat and pulled a hat down over her ears.

Finally Rebecca was fastened in and we were ready for the walk to school down Cemetery Lane. It was a narrow road which bordered the graveyard and an old railway line.

'Is that where the dead people are?' Rebecca was fascinated by death, and asked the same thing nearly every day.

'Yes, Becca, that's right.'

That night, I climbed into bed and prodded curiously at my breast.

'Do you think that's a rib?' I asked Mike who was already drifting off. 'Mike, look,' I repeated. Reluctantly he turned over.

'What?' he said and I showed him the place where I'd felt the 'rib' that morning. 'Can't feel anything,' he said, after barely brushing the skin. 'It's nothing.'

But it was still there ten days later when my friend Jenny came to visit. 'Do you think I should go to the doctors?' I asked.

'Can't hurt, can it?' she said and offered to sit with Rebecca while I went for the same-day appointment that morning.

Sitting in the waiting room of the local surgery, I felt a bit of a fraud. Around me there were at least half a dozen people who looked genuinely ill. By the time I was called in, I felt sure I would be wasting the doctor's time. I'd never visited him before and, when I sat down, he almost barked.

'What's wrong?'

I told him about the lump and he seemed to take me seriously. He examined both breasts then, as I was dressing, took a seat behind his desk. I sat down.

'It's nothing to worry about,' he said. 'It's quite firm, and mobile, almost certainly a fibro adenoma.'

'What's that?'

'A common, benign, breast lump.' He scribbled in my notes. 'It's sometimes called a mouse. I'll refer you to a specialist, just to be on the safe side.'

'What does benign mean?'

'Don't worry. It's not anything sinister, just another way of saying it isn't cancerous.'

'I saw the doctor today,' I said to Mike as I served tea up that evening.

'What for?' He was winking at Rebecca as she sucked up a piece of spaghetti, splattering her face with the bolognaise sauce. Spaghetti bolognaise was our messy meal and Rebecca and Mike competed to see who could get the most sauce around their faces.

'That lump I told you about. He said it was nothing to worry about, but wants me to see a specialist.' Mike's shirt was covered in red splashes from his sauce.

'So he definitely said that something was there?'

'Yes, of course. I told you.'

'Well, don't worry.' He twirled his fork in front of him, scooping up more spaghetti. 'Steve's sister had a lump out last year and it was fine. You'll be okay.'

MIKE

March 1990

Since the GP had confirmed the actual presence of a lump in Jane's breast, I was more determined than ever to find it for myself. I'd so far failed to locate it, but now I knew it was definitely there, I wasn't going to let the little bastard get the better of me. And besides, I wanted to know what Jane had been harping on about for the last few nights.

She assisted me by moving my finger gently alongside hers, but it was no use. I could still only occasionally feel the squishy bit of gristle, which seemed to have grown to the size of a jelly bean. Sometimes when I prodded it, it buried itself in the fatty part of her breast so I couldn't find it again. I wondered if that was where the lump was hiding, too. Jane was beginning to get annoyed by my incompetence.

'Why can't you feel it?' she said one night as she lay on her back with her left arm above her head. I could tell my heavy-handed examination technique was not being appreciated.

'Ouch, careful,' she winced. 'Watch what you're doing.'

I carried on searching, ignoring her barbed words. I was glad no one else could see me doing this. The bit of gristle moved again as I touched it.

'Does that hurt?' I asked.

'What?'

'There's a lump that just moved – can you feel it when it does that?'

'You felt it?'

I wasn't sure what to say. I'd felt the bit of gristle but not the lump.

'I think so,' I said, not wanting to disappoint her. 'It moves when I touch it.'

'Yes, that's right. What do you think it is?'

I couldn't give her an answer. I had no idea. I'd heard of breast lumps before but I knew that, for someone only twenty-six years old, they were nothing to worry about.

'Is it bigger than yesterday?' Jane asked as we lay in bed one evening. 'What do you think it is? Do you think it's serious?'

I hadn't got a clue. All I did know was that the specialist would be able to put her mind at rest and I could eventually get a peaceful night's kip.

JANE

The brown envelope was on the floor when I returned from walking Suzanne to school. My outpatient's appointment with the specialist at St James's Hospital was scheduled for a week on Tuesday. I was rather relieved. Although everyone had assured me there was nothing to worry about, a passing conversation with one of the mums at the school gate a couple of days earlier had been playing on my mind.

'I had a lump removed last year,' she'd said as we huddled up together, to protect ourselves from the bitter wind. 'I was convinced it was cancer. I even wrote letters to the children the night before the operation – but it was all okay.'

That evening, I waited until the adverts in *Coronation Street* before mentioning the appointment to Mike.

'Do you think Karen would mind coming with me to the specialist?' I said, reaching to turn down the volume on the remote.

'When is it?'

'Week on Tuesday – half two.'

'Yeah, why not – give her a call.'

I looked at him without saying anything.

'I'd be no good,' he said. 'And besides, I've got loads of work on at the moment.'

Karen, my sister-in-law, was only too happy to help. A nurse at St James's, I was reassured when she didn't sound overly concerned.

'Don't worry,' she said on the phone later that evening. 'It's probably just a cyst. You're the right age. I'll check my shifts and take the afternoon off.'

Karen met me at the entrance to the outpatients' building the following week.

'They won't do much today,' she explained. 'Probably a mammogram and maybe a fine needle aspiration.'

She noticed my eyes widen. I was suddenly nervous.

'It's okay, it's just a really fine needle, you won't feel it and they can tell if the lump is a cyst or not.'

The clinic was bustling with activity. Every few minutes nurses would emerge from rooms at either side of the corridor and call out a name.

'Jane Tomlinson!'

I stood up and Karen gave me a reassuring smile. A young nurse took me to a small examination room, where I changed quickly into a gown. I was led to another room just large enough to contain a sink and an examination couch. The consultant, Mr Brennan, a white-haired fatherly looking man came in with a group of student doctors trailing behind him.

'Now, Mrs Tomlinson,' he said, looking up from his notes. 'Let's take a look.'

I eased myself self-consciously out of the gown wondering if I had any say as to whether all these strangers could stand and watch while I got undressed. Mr Brennan prodded and poked both naked breasts.

'Yes, this is a fibro adenoma.' He turned to face his students who were watching the examination intently. 'It's firm, and freely mobile.' He looked back at me.

'Do you mind if the students have a look?'

Did I have much choice? Three student doctors, two male, one female, tentatively pressed my breast and nodded sagely before standing back to take in what their mentor had to say.

'It's what we call a mouse,' he told me. 'We'll just confirm things with an X-ray and see you with the results next week.' As he walked towards the door, he took out a small tape recorder and I heard him speaking my name into it. A nurse came into the room and handed me a sheet of paper.

'Hand this in at the desk,' she said. 'The receptionist will give you an appointment for next week.' She passed me a small yellow card.

'You need to take this downstairs to the X-ray department. They will X-ray your breasts today.'

'How did it go?' asked Karen when I returned to the waiting room.

'I've got to go to X-ray.'

We made our way through the corridor labyrinth to the radiography department, where a white-coated woman showed me into a room with a machine set into the middle of the floor and a small screened area to one side.

'I need you to remove your top and your bra, please, Jane,' she said and I stood naked and embarrassed for the second time that morning.

The following week I returned to the clinic on my own and was shown into Mr Brennan's office.

'Hello, Jane,' he said. 'You'll be pleased to hear the X-rays confirm that it is indeed a fibro adenoma.'

I nodded.

'It's entirely up to you whether or not you want to have it removed,' he said.

'I'm not sure,' I said. I hadn't really considered what to do.'

'Well, go away, and think about it,' he said, moving towards the door to open it for me. 'We'll see you in four weeks' time.'

MIKE

Our finances were never going to stretch to a summer holiday for all of us so when Jane's sister, Anne, offered to take Jane and the girls to visit her relatives in Ayr, she leapt at the chance. Scotland in March didn't hold the same attraction as St Tropez in June, but it was still a chance for Jane to unwind and spend some quality time with her sister.

On Monday evening after work, I drove Jane, Suzanne and Rebecca to Anne's house in Bolton.

When we arrived, Jane took the girls upstairs to get them ready for bed while I stood in the kitchen with Anne as she prepared supper. I knew that I needed to make a quick exit if I was to get back for the eight o'clock kick-off – Chelsea were playing at home – and I noticed that a place had been set for me at the dining table.

'I should be getting back, I've got a long day tomorrow,' I said.

'Are you sure you don't want some tea?'

'No, I'll be fine. What time are you thinking of heading off tomorrow?'

'After breakfast.'

'That'll be mid-afternoon, knowing this lot.'

'Probably,' she laughed. 'Has Jane made any decisions about what she's going to do about that lump? She was telling me she went to see the consultant.'

'I don't know, he said it was her decision. I think she's a bit nattered about it. She probably won't settle until she has it done, you know what she's like.'

'What was that?' Jane appeared behind me.

'I'm just saying I've got to be off, I don't want to be too late back.'

'You mean you don't want to miss the football.'

Anne laughed again. 'Now, now,' she teased. 'Stop bickering, you two, you're not at home now.'

A few minutes later, I was on the motorway heading home. I was glad Jane was getting away for a few days. She'd been tired recently and a change of scenery would do them all good. Plus, it meant I had a free run of the house for a few days.

I wasn't entirely on my own at home. At Christmas our family had increased its numbers by one with the arrival of Podge, the fattest budgie in West Yorkshire. Podge took up stately residence in the dining room. He hadn't flown in years but with some encouragement – especially from Rebecca – he took to flying a few feet across the room. Each time he attempted take off you could see his huge chest expand and contract like a cartoon character. But he never mastered landing and on most occasions he came to a stumbling emergency stop once he'd run out of energy.

By Friday night, however, I'd hardly seen Podge apart from the few seconds every morning when I would check his water. A week of living hard, staying out late after work, had worn me out and made a major dent in our savings. Hopefully Jane would understand. Or at least not ask.

Although I was well aware that they would be back around two o'clock on Saturday afternoon, fifteen minutes before, the house still looked like it had been burgled. I cleared away as much rubbish as I could but figured there was no point getting the Hoover out now – if I let the girls cause as much mayhem as they could when they walked through the door, Jane wouldn't realize what a tip I'd been living in.

Anne's car pulled up outside the house just as I'd sat down to watch the horse racing. The living-room door burst open and Suzanne jumped in.

'Da daaaaaaa!' she sang, followed by Rebecca. 'Did you get our postcard?'

I ran across with my arms outstretched and picked them both up for a cuddle. Only a week had passed but somehow they seemed to have changed, they seemed a lot more grown-up. Suzanne gave me a kiss on the cheek while Rebecca made an attempt to escape, and I put them both down and went through to the kitchen to greet Jane and Anne. Side-by-side, they looked so alike. Anne was five years older and slightly rounder than Jane who had always been thin and tiny, but there was no mistaking they were sisters.

Jane came across and gave me a hug. 'I missed you,' she said.

'I missed you too.' I gave her a little kiss on her forehead. 'Do you want a drink?'

'That would be nice,' said Jane, inspecting the kitchen. 'I see you have been busy. Yep, the same tea towel as last week.'

'I know, but with only me here it doesn't get the use.'

'Michael, it was dirty before we went away.'

'There's some post for you on the table in the living room.' I tried to change the subject. As she walked through to check it, I made a dash to empty the overflowing kitchen bin.

'Look, my appointment for Mr Brennan's clinic has arrived.'

I'd seen the letter with the St James's postmark, but had not wanted to concern Jane while she was away.

'Have you decided what to do?' I asked.

Jane looked at Anne, then at me, giving a short sharp nod.

'Yes,' she said. 'I'm going to ask for it to be removed. What do you think?'

It was clear she had made up her mind and I didn't want to upset her by saying anything to the contrary. Anyway, I couldn't see any reason for not getting rid of it – it was obviously bothering her and we had both noticed it had grown in size.

'I think you're right,' I said.

'What about a scar – won't you mind?'

'Of course I won't,' I answered honestly. 'Are you bothered by it?

'I don't think so.'

Anne interrupted: 'It's the right decision, Jane.'

'Yeah,' said Jane, looking down at the letter. 'It is.'

JANE

The holiday with Anne had been wonderful. It was good to spend time with my big sis and she had been fantastic with the girls. She was expecting her first baby and was thoroughly excited about being pregnant. Despite her morning sickness – and my tiredness – we had some lovely days out.

I missed Mike while we were away and was pleased to be home. Having made the decision to have the lump removed, I was feeling more relaxed and was in a good mood when I returned to the hospital to discuss it with Mr Brennan. Unfortunately, he was unavailable and I was given an appointment with one of his team – a young doctor and one of the many uniformed staff I saw at the hospital whose names and faces seemed to merge into one.

'So what are we seeing you about today?' he said as I sat down. 'I see from your notes that you were here only four weeks ago.'

'I was asked to return to the clinic to decide whether or not I want the lump in my breast removed.'

He asked to look at me and, as I lay back and looked up at the ceiling, he examined both breasts – first the left then the right. After a few seconds, he eased me forward into a sitting position.

'I've decided to have the lump out,' I said, a little hesitantly.

He raised his eyebrows.

'It will leave quite a sizeable scar,' he said. 'Are you sure you want it removed? If it's not causing you any problems there is no real need for surgery.'

'No,' I said, more confidently. 'I've thought about it, and would prefer to have the surgery.'

'Very well.' He went back over to his desk and started writing. 'I'll have to put you on the waiting list. It may be some time before we can fit you in.' He handed me the now familiar appointment form and left the room.

That was that. I was glad I hadn't backed down. I went home feeling somewhat relieved but put the whole thing to the back of my mind as it could be months before my operation.

In the meantime, however, I was becoming a familiar face at St James's Hospital, having been referred there for a completely unrelated problem which dated back to when I gave birth to Rebecca two years ago. This time I was there to see a Mr Lane, the gynaecological surgeon.

Mr Lane was a lovely man – tall and good-looking. I could imagine the nurses swooning in his presence and he seemed genuinely concerned when he was discussing my problem. When he told me I would require surgery to remove a small polyp and gave me a date for the end of June, an idea sprang to mind.

'I'm waiting to have a breast lump removed,' I told him. 'Is there any possibility of having the two operations done at the same time?'

Mr Lane nodded. 'I'm sure that will be fine. Who's your consultant?

'Mr Brennan.'

'I'll contact his team – make sure someone is available.'

It all seemed too easy. I went home and, a few days later, the letter confirming the date of my surgery arrived. It mentioned I should see my GP to tell him about the scheduled operation.

The next day I visited the surgery but the usual doctor was not there. It was a pity – although he had been rather officious, I'd wanted to see what he'd say about the lump doubling in size.

Instead, a new young doctor welcomed me in.

'What can I do for you?' he asked.

'I'm due for some surgery in a few weeks time and I thought I better ask your advice.'

'What is the problem?'

'The lump in my breast seems to have got bigger and I was wondering if I should mention this to the doctors at the hospital.' I shuffled in my seat, feeling a little foolish to be asking for advice. 'Before my operation,' I said.

'I'll take a look if you like, but I haven't seen you before so it will be difficult for me to say if there has been any change in this lump.'

I knew this. His tone of voice made me feel I was wasting his time and I felt uncomfortable as he examined me.

'As I explained, I can't really tell if there has been any change,' he said. 'You seem very concerned. Is there anything else that is troubling you?'

'I've been very tired and I feel sick all the time,' I said. 'I just don't feel very well at all.'

'The tiredness could be an indication that you may be clinically depressed. Have you ever had any depression in the past?'

'No,' I said. I couldn't believe I could be depressed. I rarely got down and upset, I'd just been a little tired and grumpy lately. I wondered if he could be right. Although I wasn't overly concerned about my impending operation, maybe subconsciously it was niggling at me – causing these other symptoms.

When Mike arrived home he'd barely got his coat off before I was telling him about the doctor. The more I had thought about what he had said, the more agitated I'd become.

'I think he thought I was making it up,' I said, as Mike listened patiently. 'Like I wanted some attention or something.'

'It might be just because he hasn't seen you before,' he said calmly.

'But what if he writes in my notes that I'm an anxious patient – I don't want the surgeons thinking I'm some kind of hypochondriac.'

'They won't. Look, take no notice. The lump's coming out and that's the main thing.'

He was right, perhaps I was overreacting a little. But after my frustrating visit with Dr Patel I didn't bother to mention the other symptoms to the doctors at my pre-operative assessment a few weeks later. What was the point?

MIKE

I've never forgiven Chris Waddle. That poor excuse for a penalty in the semis of Italia '90 caused me no end of grief. If he'd scored and put England into the final, Jane might have forgiven me.

My left arm arched over and hit the snooze button on the alarm as if it had a mind of its own. From a gap in the beige curtains I could see the sun wasn't going to be cracking the pavements today.

'We need to get moving,' I said.

'What time is it?' mumbled Jane.

'Six-thirty. Come on, get up.'

'I don't need to be there until nine. They're not going to operate without me.'

'But I have to be at work for eight-thirty.'

'Can't you go in late?'

'No. We've got to close the branch as soon after four as possible.'

Like a surly teenager, she shifted around and perched up on her elbows.

'Bloody football,' she said.

I dropped her outside St James's at seven forty-five and was already aware that I was not in her good books. My few attempts at conversation were met with silence.

'I'll see you about half past five then?'

Jane leant through the car to kiss me.

'Okay.'

'You'll be all right. Good luck, I'll be thinking of you.'

Closing the door, I watched her march off into the hospital, her nightbag hanging from her shoulders. I looked at the clock in the car. Driving off, I went over the mental arithmetic which had been bothering me for days. How could I get from work, visit Jane in hospital and be home by kick off?

I was still grappling with the problem as I walked into the Yorkshire Bank at Westgate in Wakefield forty minutes later. It was a large branch with forty-five staff split over three floors. With a quick 'good morning' to the few already in, I grabbed my daily computer report and was away.

'Morning, Mike. Looking forward to the game tonight?' Frank Fletcher, one of the team managers, was the calmest man in the office. His desk faced the banking hall so he had a panoramic view of what everyone was doing and even when he was looking down at his desk, you knew he saw everything.

'Not sure I'm going to get to see it,' I said. 'Jane's in hospital – nothing serious – but I'm going to have to visit her after work.'

'Don't be so bloody stupid,' said Frank. 'Get off from here at two.'

I needed no more encouragement. At two forty-five I was marching into the hospital like a man with a mission.

The ward was unutterably grim. Jane was lying on her bed halfway up the ward, wearing my vertically striped cotton dressing gown that had been particularly hideous even when new and a pair of ankle-length black socks which left a six-inch gap of sparrow-like leg. I realized how little she and I spent on ourselves.

Seeing me, Jane put down her book and gave me a smile. 'Hello there,' she said brightly as I leant over to kiss her. 'What are you doing here?'

'They let me go early. Frank said it was okay.'

'Oh that's good,' she said. 'I've been bored stupid. Can you stay long?'

I looked at the glass of water and empty vase on her bedside table. I should have brought flowers. The ward was unbearably hot.

'Take your jacket off,' said Jane, noticing how uncomfortable I seemed. 'It is hot in here.'

Her medical chart was hanging at the side of the bed. I dumped my coat on the back of the chair.

'How are you feeling?' I asked, unhooking the chart to have a closer inspection.

'What are you doing?' she snapped.

'Looking at this.'

'Is it yours?' She sounded like my primary teacher. 'No. So put it down.'

Stunned by the speed and venom of the attack, I realized I only had one option – I started to read them.

'Put the fucking chart down, it's mine!' The lady in the next bed looked over. 'I don't read your post.'

I put the chart back.

'Touchy,' I said. 'What have you got to hide?'

'Nothing. But if you want to read my notes, you should ask politely.'

'Please may I read your notes, Jane?'

'No.'

After our initial squabble, Jane was keen to show me her dressings – partly because she knew I was squeamish but also as proof that her ordeal was over. I had expected her to be semi-comatose so that she wouldn't need or want me to stay too long but the lack of a pre-med meant she was alert. The surgeons had said the operation had been easy and Jane seemed pleased that she was not in too much discomfort.

'I told you there was nothing to worry about,' I said.

Forty-five minutes passed incredibly quickly and I was aware of every second. If I left now, it would take five minutes to say goodbye, seven minutes – call it ten – to get to the car and forty minutes to get home. But what if the roads weren't clear? I needed to go. Muttering something about the rush hour, I scraped the plastic bucket seat back across the floor.

'What time will you be back?' she said.

Shit. I slowly returned to the very edge of the seat but I didn't need to say a word.

'I don't believe it,' she stormed. 'You're going to watch the football.'

I knew I'd never be able to reason with her so could see no option.

'I'm really sorry,' I said giving her a tentative hug. 'But I'll see you tomorrow, I promise. I love you.'

'I love you, too,' she said, sounding annoyed.

Within seconds I was out of the ward, feeling an awkward sense of relief. I had known she would not be overjoyed with me, but I had hoped for some kind of blessing. I'd not got it.

But it's not every day England play in the World Cup.

When the game finished I reached disconsolately for the remote control. I felt dirty, alone and a fraud. I thought back to only days before when, during England's quarter final match with Cameroon, the house had been so alive: Jane reading upstairs, Rebecca playing in her bedroom and Suzanne and I watching the game with my mate Steve.

The house was quiet now. The girls were in Settle with my parents and I wondered if Jane was asleep. I glanced at the clock again.

JANE

My friend Jenny picked me up from the hospital and dropped me off at home. It felt odd being alone in an empty house and the kettle sounded too loud as it came to the boil. A letter from Australia, from an old school friend, Amanda, was on the kitchen worktop – Mike must have left it there this morning.

I would love to go back to Australia. Amanda's letters were full of tales from the country I'd lived in for several years in my teens and I often thought I would like to revisit some of my childhood haunts. I would like to show Mike where I used to fish off the jetty in Brighton, just outside Adelaide.

I read the letter, then ran a shallow bath. As I got undressed, I peered at my reflection in the mirror. The dressing was coming away at the edges so I peeled it off, watching the adhesive pull on the skin. My breast was dark and purple and the surrounding area yellow with bruising. A two-inch vertical gash ran down from my armpit. It was held together by neat stitches under the skin which were topped with white beads at either end. My head swam to look at it and I tentatively touched one of the beads. Yes, it was definitely sore.

I got into the bath slowly, careful not to make any splashes. I was under strict instructions not to get the stitches wet so I washed myself slowly and deliberately. The aroma of lavender shower gel washed away the horrid antiseptic hospital smell.

After ten minutes I wrapped myself in a towel and wandered back into the bedroom. I would need a new dressing, so without looking at the wound too closely, I applied a fresh one, given to me by the nursing staff. Covered up, the wound was much easier to cope with.

The pain was becoming a little worse and I eased myself gently into an old baggy T-shirt and snuggled into bed. Tired and sore I dozed for a few hours until Mike came home.

In the ten days following my operation, summer decided to make an appearance. Term was nearly over for Suzanne and this would be the last week I would have to make the school journey for a while.

Arriving at the school gates that morning, Suzanne gave me a quick kiss and disappeared into the squeals and screams of the playground – Rebecca and I forgotten in the excited babble.

'Shall we buy a treat on the way home?' Rebecca nodded, grinning at me. 'We can walk past the giant's house and see if he is there if you like.'

The giant was imaginary. Rebecca would shriek with fake fear as we passed the cottage that had stepping stones set into the lawn at unfeasibly large distances from each other. Only a giant could step up to that doorway.

'Is he there, Mummy?' she cried.

'No, I think we're safe.'

After stopping off at the bakery, we went home and spent a few hours in the garden. After lunch Rebecca was soon fast asleep, curled up in the corner of the sofa.

'Becca,' I called gently when it was three o'clock. 'It's time to wake up to get Suzanne.'

At the top of the hill I could make out Gill and her daughter Judith in the distance. I picked up my pace and hurried on down the hill until I caught up with them as they neared the school gate.

'Hello, Jane,' smiled Gill as I met them and slowed to their speed. 'How are you feeling?'

'Fine, thanks. It's still a bit sore. I've got a checkup on Thursday, and then it's all done and dusted.' The school bell sounded indoors and moments later Suzanne appeared out of her classroom door with Alison, Judith's older sister. The girls trotted over to us.

'Are we going strawberry picking?' Suzanne had noticed the carrier bag I was clutching.

'Yes,' I said. 'I thought we could have some strawberries for pudding.'

Suzanne leapt up in the air and Rebecca bounced her approval in the buggy.

'Yippeeee!' she said and Gill laughed. We said our goodbyes and the girls and I headed off round the corner towards Oldroyd's Farm to get to the strawberry fields.

'Mind the nettles,' I said, setting our basket down and hunting for the ripe red berries. A childish thrill accompanied each delicious find and I couldn't resist popping one of the plumpest in my mouth. The basket was soon half full.

At the house, the girls ran upstairs to change into their swimming costumes and I turned on the water sprinkler for them in the garden. In the kitchen I took out the strawberries to trim them and wash them for pudding. I was just sprinkling sugar on them – the way Mike likes them – when the phone rang.

'I wanted to check what time to pick you up on Thursday?' It was Jenny.

'Hang on, I'll just get my appointment card.' I scrabbled through my handbag and found it, crumpled up. 'Oh, you know what? I think I've missed it.' Although the appointment card had today's date, it was the wrong day. They'd put me down for Thursday, but Mr Brennan's clinic was always on a Tuesday.

'I can't believe it,' I groaned. 'I'm going to have to ring the hospital and get a new appointment.'

Jenny kindly offered to take me again on Friday when I was due my checkup with Mr Lane. As I put the phone down, I heard the drone of the car engine. Mike was pulling into the drive.

He came up behind me while I was elbow deep in warm suds and wrapped his arms round my waist.

'I can't resist you like that,' he smiled and kissed the back of my neck.

I laughed, turned and put my hands to his cheeks, wetting his face.

'Love you,' I said. 'How was your day?'

'Better for being home,' he said.

Jenny was as good as her word and early on Friday morning we dropped Suzanne at school before driving to the hospital for my post-op checkup with Mr Lane.

After a quick examination, he invited me to sit down.

'Everything looks fine, Jane,' he said. 'Have you seen Mr Brennan yet?'

'No.' I explained to him about the mix-up with the appointment and told him I had been given another one for a fortnight's time.

'That's good,' he said. 'And how are you in yourself?'

'I'm okay,' I said.

'Good. I'll see you in six months' time. If you have any problems in the meantime, don't hesitate to contact my secretary.'

I changed and dashed back to the waiting area, eager to get home.

'All done?' asked Jenny.

'Yes. He was very nice. Everything is fine,' I said. 'Just Mr

Brennan to see, and then I won't have to come here again for a while.'

Over the next two weeks the weather got even hotter. On the Tuesday of my hospital appointment with Mr Brennan it was already warm by early morning.

Three weeks had passed since the operation to remove the lump and the wound needed checking. Although Jenny and Mum had both offered to take me, I'd said I could manage on my own.

I wheeled Rebecca's buggy out of the lifts, avoiding the trolleys, and made my way down to the busy outpatient clinic. Grabbing the last remaining chair, I plonked Rebecca and Suzanne on it and passed them a book each to read. When I was called through after just a few minutes, I thought I had queue jumped, but I wasn't about to argue. After changing into the regulation amorphous gown, I was whisked into the doctor's office. I told the girls we wouldn't be long and that they had to be quiet for Mummy.

Mr Brennan arrived and stood before me. He would have looked smart in his white doctor's coat if there hadn't been an ink stain across the breast pocket. I smiled at him but he didn't reciprocate.

'I'm sorry,' he said. 'The lump we removed was a small tumour and you will need some X-ray treatment.'

My stomach lurched and I suddenly felt like a small child sitting on the couch, my legs dangling over the edge. He never said the word 'cancer'. I don't know why, I couldn't take it in. I could hear his voice, see his lips moving, but the sounds didn't seem to have anything to do with me. Surely he couldn't be telling me this with my children sitting only inches away? I opened my mouth, but no words came. What could I say? I just knew I needed Rebecca and Suzanne out of the room.

I managed to ask if there was someone who could look after them, so I could concentrate. Mr Brennan gave a mute nod and went in search of a nurse.

'What's wrong, Mummy?' Suzanne looked at me, puzzled.

'Nothing, sweetheart,' I said, my heart pounding. 'The doctor just wants to tell me something important and a nice nurse is going to look after you. I won't be long and then we'll go to Grandma's.' I crossed the room to give her a hug.

Rebecca hugged me tightly and I swallowed hard, briskly sweeping away a tear from my eye and trying to smile at my beautiful babies. As the nurse ushered the children out, I felt the panic bubble up inside me. It couldn't be true, there must be some mistake. I sat with my arms wrapped around my body, shaking with fear.

I had a tumour. I had cancer. Was I going to die?

CHAPTER 2

JANE

I stared out of the window. My eyes felt bright with tears. A nurse appeared in the doorway, no taller than me, but she looked comfortingly solid and warm. She smiled reassuringly.

'It's Jane, isn't it?' she said.

'Yes.' I nodded.

'And who are these two beautiful girls?'

I patted Suzanne on her head. 'This is Suzanne,' I said. 'And this is Rebecca.'

'Well,' she said, 'you two can come and play with Auntie Avril. Mummy needs to talk to the doctor.'

The girls hesitated, looking to me for permission and I smiled as Avril shepherded them gently out of the way. Mr Brennan came back into the room.

'Right, Jane,' he said. 'Is there anything you need to ask me?'

'Could you look at my wound?' I asked. 'It doesn't seem to be healing properly.'

As he dabbed his fingers firmly across my breast, I felt a swirl of sickness in my stomach. He felt my armpit and frowned.

'Your armpit is quite swollen,' he said. 'How long has it been like that?'

'I've . . . no idea. It was fine before the lumpectomy.'

He drew the edges of my gown back together and stepped

back a little. 'I think the best thing to do is to see you again next week, when you have had time to take everything in.'

'But what about seeing the radiotherapist?' I asked.

'You can see her next week if necessary.'

I sat, my body trembling, silent, unable to form the words to ask all the questions that flashed through my mind.

He opened the door and called for Avril.

'I'll see Jane next week, at two o'clock,' he said before turning back to me. 'I'll leave you to make the appointment.'

I dressed and left the room to find Avril crouching down, listening as Rebecca and Suzanne regaled her with one of their tales.

As I waited for Avril to make my appointment the room began to spin. I felt light-headed and dizzy. Steadying myself on the counter, I gulped in some air. They'd got it wrong, hadn't they? I was only twenty-six years old. I couldn't have breast cancer. What were they talking about? Old ladies have breast cancer. Not me. They cut breasts off to cure them and that couldn't happen to me. It was a mistake. It was a cyst, maybe a fibro adenoma. Certainly not cancer. No way.

I drew another deep breath in. It wasn't the time to fall to pieces. The girls were aware something was wrong, I could tell by their puzzled faces and knew I had to be strong for them. Dependable Mum. Mum who makes everything all right. Avril brought out the buggy.

'Are you all right?' she asked.

'I'll be fine,' I said, my shaking hands revealing I wasn't. 'I just want to go home.'

My mind empty, I was unable to think what to do next . I grabbed hold of the buggy handles tightly, clutching familiarity. At the entrance to outpatients, I bought a small packet of biscuits for the girls to share, a treat to keep them quiet. I poured some loose change from my purse and put it in the payphone in the lobby. It seemed to ring out for ever until Mum finally answered.

'Mum.' I put every effort into sounding as normal as possible. 'I've finished. Is there any chance you can come and collect me?'

'Yes, of course,' she said. 'Where are you?' My mind went blank. 'I don't know.' My words came out hesitantly as I tried to think where in the hospital I was. 'Hang on, it's the Chancellor Wing,' I said, noticing the sign on the wall.

'Okay, I'll be there in twenty minutes.' I could hear the two girls bickering, Suzanne stubbornly refusing to allow Rebecca to share the last biscuit. They sounded further away than from just down by my waist. I closed my eyes, blinking them shut, hoping that it would make a difference.

Opening them again, I shook my head to clear away the words that tumbled round my head over and over. Tumour, X-ray treatment. They were abstract words, unrelated to me.

Looking up I was surprised to see I was waiting outside the hospital, amazed to see that the world was carrying on as if nothing had happened. People still drove their cars in and out of the car park, they still chatted to one another happily, wandering in and out of the building. A wheelchair was slowly lowered from the back of an ambulance and was pulled backwards by a uniformed woman.

The sky was cloudless. I tipped my head back and gazed at the bright seaside blue, forcing back tears which were beginning to surface. The sunlight felt warm on my cheeks and I closed my eyes against the light, trying to shut out the feeling of loss that overwhelmed me. I felt helpless like a small child, lost in the crowds of jostling patients.

'Oh Grace, look at that,' said my gran, lightly grabbing my aunt's arm as they both oohed and aahed over the swathes of fabric in the shop window. I slipped my hand from my gran's, and wandered over to where my brothers Luke and Mark were peering into the fountain. Mark was leaning over, trying to grasp the pennies glinting at the bottom of the water. Luke could only watch and giggle, too little to do more than trail his fingers in the clear water.

'Look at the fishes,' I squealed. They were huge, black, gold, red and silver. I watched as they flickered in and out of the shadows. I turned to the figure in the green dress.

'What love?' she said.

'You're not my gran.' I spun round, searching for the rest of my family – Mum, Dad, Anne, Mary, Mark, Luke. There was no one. I felt cold, the little hairs on my neck prickled and I became hot as panic set in, my face flushed and my plaits stuck against my head. They must be here. I scanned the crowds, turning full circle over and over. Where were they?

A forest of strangers' legs seemed to crowd in around me as I turned from the entrance of the arcade. People jostled past me, ignoring me, my eyes blurry with hot tears.

Through the crowds of skirts and trousers, one enormous black shiny shoe came into view. Another followed, growing larger and larger, until two enormous black trunks and a black-jacketed body with shiny buttons down the front, towered in front of me. Like the policeman from Camberwick Green. My eyes travelled up to his face but the sun shone so brightly behind his black helmet that I couldn't make out his features. I stood there, terrified, as the giant looming over me bowed down.

'What's up, little one?' His voice was strong and friendly and, bent down, he didn't seem quite as large. 'Where's your mum?'

'I don't know,' I whispered. 'I was looking at the fishes. They are very big.'

He smiled and reached down, gently grabbing me round the waist.

'Why don't I lift you up and we'll see if you can spot them,' he said. I sucked on my plait to keep me brave as he hoisted me up on to this shoulder. Perched on this high ledge, I could see the tops of people's heads.

'Can you see anyone you know?' said my friendly giant. I saw my dad across the road, the sun making his hair glint like gold. He looked panicked, his eyes narrowed as he searched for me amidst the crowds.

'It's my dad!' I found my voice. It rang out clearly and my father's head shot up. As his eyes found mine, a smile *spread across his face as he pushed towards me through the people.*

'Jane where did you get to?' he asked as the policeman eased me from his shoulder.

'I was looking at the fishes. They were so big and bright,' I said as my feet touched the ground.

'You be more careful next time, Jane,' said the policeman. I took my father's hand and continued to suck my plait.

I would have given anything for a friendly giant to have put me safely into the hands of my dad, and take away this lost hollow feeling in the pit of my stomach.

The beep of Mum's horn roused me from my dream-like state. I waved and, picking Rebecca out of her buggy, I handed her to Mum while I struggled to collapse it. It refused, jamming and sticking until I could feel anger and frustration whirling up inside me. I kicked it violently and it gave in to my force.

With the children belted in, Mum turned her attention to me.

'Is everything all right?' she asked quietly.

'Let's get home,' I said. 'I'll tell you about it then.'

We made the short journey in silence, the soft mutterings on the radio and the chattering of the girls in the back filling the void. When we pulled into her drive she turned to me again.

'Jane, what's wrong?' she asked.

I breathed in and looked directly at her. 'I've got breast cancer,' I said. Her face turned grey before my eyes and she drew in an audible breath, and turned to look out of the window. I looked away and we sat in silence for several seconds before she grabbed my hand with both of hers and held it firmly. We sat like that for a minute or more. The children were quiet in the back of the car.

'You stay here,' she ordered. 'I'll go in the house and explain to everyone. That way, they won't all be asking the same questions.'

She wasn't gone very long, but those few moments seemed to

last an eternity. What was she saying in there? Were they all right? What was I going to do?

By the time she returned, I felt a little more in control. In the kitchen I was greeted by the sight of Dad's legs poking out from a kitchen unit cupboard, the rest of his body almost hidden. A loose shelf leaned precariously against the cupboard's side.

'I won't be long, Jane,' he called from behind the unit. 'I'll just finish this little job.' I heard the bang of his hammer a couple of times before he poked his head out. He had dust in his brown hair – his curls were tighter after his chemotherapy and the golden crown was now a rich chestnut. He smiled. A smile that reached his eyes, making them crinkle in a way that was so familiar to me, but at the same time he looked tired, his cheeks hollow and gaunt.

'Welcome to the club, love,' he said.

MIKE

'Mike, your mother-in-law is on the phone.'

That sentence alone was odd enough that I immediately questioned its accuracy. Jane's mother never phoned me, especially not at work.

She spoke abruptly. 'Jane would like to speak to you.' The thoughts raced round my head. What the hell's she playing at? Why can't Jane phone herself? What's going on?

Jane came on the phone.

'Mike, Mum collected me from the hospital.' Her voice was edgy, I could tell she was shaking and on the verge of tears. 'The lump's malignant.'

My heart raced, my poor grasp of language thwarting my understanding. What are you talking about, woman? Couldn't this have waited? You know I'm busy at work. Why involve your mum? Sensing I wasn't about to respond, she continued: 'Mike, the lump was cancerous.'

I understood. My legs buckled beneath me and, with my free hand, I grabbed the table to stop my fall. Everything ceased.

Noise. People. Time. I was standing in the machine room – the very guts of the branch that usually buzzed with computers, printers and fax machines – but now it stood silent. Everyone stared. They knew something was wrong. I ignored their worried glances, making every effort to focus on listening to Jane as she told me what had happened.

After a few minutes I knew I couldn't conduct the conversation over the phone. I needed to be with her, holding her, comforting her, loving her.

'I'm coming over,' I said, slamming the phone down. Shaking, I placed both hands to rest on the door frame and breathed in and out, in and out, my head swirling. I focused on my manager's door straight along the corridor deciding I needed to leave, to get to Jane.

'What's up, Mike?' My manager Tony looked up from his desk. I hadn't bothered to knock.

'I have to go,' I blurted. 'Jane. It's cancer.'

He stood up and walked round the desk. 'Go home,' he said calmly. 'Stay with your wife as long she needs you. Your priorities are at home. Take good care of her and be as strong as you can. Are you okay to drive?'

I nodded. Outside, I sprinted to the car. As I got in, my heart was pounding, beads of sweat were trickling down my brow and my glasses had steamed up.

It couldn't be. It just couldn't. The lump was cancer. I started the ignition, a feeling of utter powerlessness flooding over me. Until that moment I'd never considered for one second that there might be a time in my life when Jane wouldn't be there.

Fifty minutes later, I parked the car outside Jane's parents' house and, aware that Jane could be watching from inside, strolled down the path, desperate to exude an air of steady confidence, avoiding the urge to look at the windows.

Paul, my father-in-law, opened the door looking ghastly. His own illness had made him grey and worn, yet he'd always disguised it with his gentle humour and easy-going attitude. Today he just looked broken.

I could hear Suzanne and Rebecca in the living room. I poked my head around the door to say 'hi' but I knew I was needed upstairs. Jane was with her mum in her parents' bedroom. Sitting on the bed, she looked tired and red-eyed. Her world had fallen apart. Our world. Her mum left us and Jane and I stood hugging and sobbing. After several minutes, Jane said: 'You should ring your mum.'

It had been my first thought, too. I'd wanted to hear her comforting tones assuring me that everything would be all right. But this time she couldn't.

'I'll ring them later,' I said. 'I can't face it now.'

We stood looking out of the window on to Paul and Anne's garden. A grey squirrel ran across the lawn.

'Look, Jane!' I whispered. I followed its path as it disappeared into the abundant border plants only for it to appear a few seconds later.

Jane moved closer, twisting me round ensuring she had my full attention, pulling me into the hug again, the warmth of her body relaxing me like a luxurious bath.

'Do you love me, Mike?' she said, quietly.

'Sure,' I replied.

'Sure you're sure?'

'Sure I'm sure.' We smiled, the familiar word game played. She closed her eyes and my hand cradled her head.

The bedroom began to feel a little claustrophobic. Roundhay Park was only up the road so we decided to get some fresh air. Part of me was confident there had been a mistake. It didn't fit together. How could she have cancer? We'd been assured for months that there was nothing to worry about. Jane had even been accused by her GP of being neurotic. The only rational explanation was that Jane had not heard properly, she hadn't understood what he had said.

We strolled hand in hand through the gates at Roundhay and turned on to one of the paths round the playing field. Jane's tears had stopped.

'What did he actually say?' I asked, needing a word-for-word account as to what had happened. She ran through the events of the afternoon but I wanted further proof, the chance to cross-examine.

'Are you sure he said malignant?' I asked.

'Yes.'

'But he didn't say cancer?'

'I don't think so.'

'What you do mean, you don't think so? Did you ever hear him say cancer?'

'He said it was malignant.'

I wondered if she even knew the difference between benign and malignant. She'd clearly not been paying attention. Cross-examining her like an overzealous prosecutor I could sense that she too doubted what she'd heard and I leapt on the hope that she had got it wrong. It was obvious. I wouldn't believe it until a doctor told me otherwise.

JANE

My eyes were streaming when I woke next morning. The house was quiet. Mike lay next to me breathing noisily through his nose. A whimper escaped from my mouth, and I put my hand to my face and groaned quietly. I remembered sitting on the floor in the kitchen in the early hours, the room dark, the floor cold against my thighs. I had been too tired to move and Mike had found me there, helped me up and coaxed me to bed.

As I tried to shake off the impressions of yesterday, Mike grunted and rolled on to his side away from me, taking the duvet with him. How could he sleep so peacefully? I eased myself upright and looked down at him – my momentary flash of annoyance had already passed. I brushed the tears away, but they wouldn't stop.

Mike turned back and looked at me with bleary eyes. Then he opened them wide, memories pulling him from sleep.

'Are you all right?' he said.

I sobbed again for a few more moments.

'Sorry,' he said. 'Stupid question.' Propping himself up on to one elbow, he blinked. 'It's leaked again,' he said.

I glanced down. A yellow and red stain had spread across the floral pattern on my nightdress. Grabbing a jumper from the chair at the side of the bed, I covered the stain. It was only six o'clock, but the curtains were already haloed with the light from the early morning sun. It should have been the perfect start to the summer holiday.

'Do you want a drink?' I asked. He nodded.

I took comfort from the normal: having an early morning pee, washing and drying my hands, noticing that the towel rail still needed fixing. I wandered downstairs, through the dining room and into the kitchen. While the kettle boiled I unlocked the back door and stepped outside. The morning air was fresh, the sky a vivid blue and the sun was already peeping through the birch trees that shaded the kitchen. I went back inside and made black coffee for myself, tea for Mike.

'It's a glorious day again.' I passed him his drink.

We sat in bed, watching our reflections in the dressing-table mirror. I sipped my coffee and cradled its warmth against me. After I'd drained the cup, I lifted my jumper and examined the crusted nightgown, peeling it gently from my breast.

'You need to see the doctor about that,' Mike said. 'You might need some antibiotics.'

'Perhaps I've gone mad,' I said. 'I haven't got cancer; I've just misheard him. He never actually said "cancer". It could all be a mistake.' Mike put his arm around me and kissed me on my cheek.

'We should go and visit the doctor together,' he said. 'He might be able to tell us what to expect.'

We had a long wait at the surgery that afternoon before being ushered through to see Dr Thorpe, who had been the doctor I'd first seen about the lump. He flicked open my notes.

'Mr Brennan telephoned last night to say that he had seen you in clinic,' he said. 'If you have any questions I will try to answer them. If there is any other way I can help I will try.'

Finally, someone to talk to. We bombarded him with questions: would I die? Did I need more surgery? What about chemotherapy? The questions came thick and fast and he answered them as fully and as openly as possible, but we still felt we were left with no definite answers. Apparently Mr Brennan was concerned about the fullness in my armpit.

'He has his own team of pathologists,' explained Dr Thorpe. 'He'll want them to take a good look at the tissue that has been removed from your breast. This will give him a clearer idea of what sort of cancer you have and what treatment you will need.'

There was talk of chemotherapy, of drugs and of operations. It was possible that I would need to have a mastectomy, that my breast might have to be removed. Mike and I left the surgery in no doubt that I had cancer but with every doubt as to what would happen next. As we returned home, the telephone rang.

'Hi chuck.' It was my good friend, Michelle. 'Just wanted to know how you got on yesterday at the hospital.'

'Hi,' I said, then paused. What on earth could I say next? I started to shake. 'Michelle, I've got cancer.' There was no response, just silence that echoed down the line following my bombshell. I started to sob uncontrollably and only managed to say, 'I'll ring you in a couple of days. When I know what's happening.'

As I put the phone down, I realized just how many people I would have to tell. It was a sobering thought. Michelle's reaction had been tearful, mirroring my own emotions, but I couldn't cope with that every time. If I was to break the news to others, I needed a few days to become strong.

Several days passed, with no further news. The prospect of having my breast removed seemed so imminent and daunting, I wasn't sure how I would cope. When I discussed it, most people tried to be positive, reassuring me that I might not need further surgery; that I might get away with having some radiotherapy instead. But I had my doubts. My breast was redder and more sore each day and while I wasn't sure if that was significant, there was no one to tell me any different.

Mary, my older sister, knew how isolated I was feeling. Her

answer to my woes was just the tonic I needed. Calling round one sunny morning, we loaded the car with picnic goodies, and strapped Suzanne and Rebecca into the back of her old Citroen 2CV. Taking the top down, we roared off down the road. My hair whipped at my face and for the first time in days I felt alive. I had no idea what the future held, but today I could believe that even if I had to have surgery, it wouldn't stop these moments.

'I'm hungry,' said Suzanne, when we arrived at the farmyard in Temple Newsam, her eyes round with the anticipation of picnic treats.

'We better go and get the goodies then,' said Mary. The morning had been getting cooler. Rebecca shivered as we walked back towards the car park. Heavy drops of rain were splashing on to the dusty ground. Laughing, I turned my face upwards and let the cold water bounce on my skin before hurrying after the three figures racing to the car. We sat in the steamy interior watching tiny rivers of water joining up to meet at the bottom of the windscreen.

'This isn't much good,' said Mary, 'what shall we do about our picnic now?'

Suzanne's face dropped at the thought of chocolate biscuits left untasted.

'Don't worry about it,' I said, 'we'll think of something.'

Mary drove home through heavy rain, the windscreen wipers thudding across the screen, keeping the water at bay.

Suzanne and Rebecca watched as I draped a large white sheet over the kitchen table.

'What's that for?' Suzanne asked.

'It's our special picnic bench,' I replied. Two faces looked back at me distinctly unimpressed.

'Where's our picnic?' Rebecca asked, looking around for the crisps.

'Under here,' I said and lifted the corner of the sheet to show them. They giggled as they crawled under to start their feast. Mary joined us and with the sheet hiding the room we could pretend to be anywhere we wanted. Ignoring the sound of the rain lashing against the windows, we enjoyed our lunch in our den, a secret sunny picnic spot no one else had found.

Mike and I only had to wait a week to see Mr Brennan but it felt like a month. Returning to the clinic and sitting in the same grey waiting room, a tight knot of anger began to form in my chest. How could they tell someone she has cancer and then leave her to it? No information. No support. Did that happen to everyone? Were there other women who had to leave the hospital, on their own – perhaps with *their* children in tow – who were then set adrift to get on with dealing with a deadly disease? There must be better ways of giving bad news to people.

Mike was fidgety, fed up with waiting. He scowled at nurses as they passed him and hardly spoke a word. The minutes dragged by. Eventually Mr Brennan swept into clinic and disappeared into his office. Seconds later my name was called and we were shown into his room.

'This report shows you have invasive ductal carcinoma,' he said. My notes were open on the desk in front of him and he raised his eyebrows. 'That's unusual for such a young woman. I think we need to carry out some investigations before we consider surgery. If all the tests are clear, I can perform a mastectomy. That will give you your best chance of survival.'

'What if I don't want an operation?' I asked.

'A mastectomy will give you a fifty per cent better five-year survival rate,' he said, before adding: 'But we are getting ahead of ourselves. I need to check if the cancer has spread beyond your breast, before we can consider further surgery.' He stood to leave the room. 'If you'll excuse me a moment, I'll try to arrange some scans.'

In the chair next to me, Mike reached for my hand. The room was silent, apprehension took away our voices, and through the open door we could hear Mr Brennan, his voice raised and agitated as he spoke on the phone.

'This patient can't wait that long,' he said. 'She could be dying.'

I felt Mike's grip tighten round my fingers.

'Oh shit,' I whispered. 'That's me he's talking about.'

'I know.' Mike's face was pale with the strain. I felt sick. Suddenly, it wasn't simply a question of surgery – whether I wanted it or not. I might not even be offered surgery. I might be dying.

MIKE

Our bedroom door groaned as I eased it open. Jane was perched up in bed, her eyes shining like two diamonds.

'You're up early,' she said, surprised.

'I need to be at work early. Is there a problem with that?' I replied. I felt a twinge of guilt at my tetchiness.

'No, of course not. I just wondered if you were all right?'

'Do you fancy eating out tonight?' I asked.

'Mmmm that would be lovely. You choose. I decide every night.'

I stooped down to give her a kiss and headed off to work. I'd lied. My early departure had nothing to do with work. I wanted to go to Mass. I had never figured out why anyone would want to go to church more than once a week but since Jane's diagnosis I'd occasionally attended daily services before work. Desperate times called for desperate measures.

St Austin's Church in Wakefield was a most unlikely looking church; with a wooden door, with none of the ornate handles that normally adorn church doors, and dull, faded paintwork – it looked more like a youth club from the sixties.

Remarkably, for a Monday morning, there were some thirty other people dotted throughout the pews. Were they, I wondered, here like me, out of desperation? Or was this part of their daily routine?

I barely listened to the half-hour service, but found it gave me time to reflect. My world had been turned inside out and just sitting there, on my own, surrounded by strangers, gave me the chance to piece together all the information that we had been bombarded with since the diagnosis. Jane had brought home a leaflet which explained the different stages of treatment, but it was complicated and every case had to be treated individually. I couldn't get my head around a lot of it.

I hadn't realized that there were different types of breast cancer; it could be invasive or evasive or hormone receptive. I had assumed there was just one type of breast cancer – one to cover all occasions. More worryingly, we discovered that the younger the patient, the more aggressive the cancer was likely to be.

So far, Jane had had a bone scan and a CT scan, which would indicate whether or not the cancer had spread to other parts of her body. If the scans were clear, Jane would have her left breast removed and the lymph nodes would be taken away from under her arm. Pathology tests on the nodes would show if they were cancerous and whether the disease may have spread. If so, Jane would require further treatment such as chemotherapy but if clear, she would be cured.

If the bone scans showed the cancer had already spread there would be little point in a mastectomy – I didn't want to even think about what the consequences would be if that were the case.

Sitting in the pew, I was consumed with anxiety. Inadequate and unqualified – how could I be a mother to two small girls? I couldn't wash or iron clothes, I'd never had to clean the house let alone give the emotional support that only Jane could provide. I had zero motherly instincts and, in truth, my fatherly ones were well hidden. Jane was the main parent, I was merely standing on the sidelines watching her in awe.

My hands were trembling as I sat, head bowed, listening to the prayers. I removed my wedding ring from my finger and twiddled it between my forefinger and thumb before sliding it back on. It was a habit I'd developed recently, I wasn't sure why. Deep down I felt there was something symbolic about it, that I was controlling the longevity of my marriage and, in turn, Jane's life. It was rubbish, of course. As a child I'd had superstitions when I watched Chelsea playing football. They hadn't helped Chelsea win then and I knew they weren't going to help Jane now. But it helped me in some way.

After Mass I walked slowly to work, still thinking about the results of the scans, which were due the following day. I knew there was nothing I could do, but the praying and the superstitions provided me with a sort of emotional crutch. Despite my slow pace, I arrived at the office at my usual time of eight thirty. Waiting to be let in, I was miles away in thought when I realized someone was speaking to me.

'Why are you here, Mike?' It was Tony, my manager. 'I told you I don't want see you until it's clear what's happening with Jane.'

'I'd only mope about at home,' I said.

'You are out of the branch at two,' he ordered, clearly in no mood for negotiation.

I had asked Frank Fletcher to advise everyone of Jane's illness while I accompanied her to her bone scan. It avoided embarrassing questions such as 'Where were you yesterday?' or 'Skiving again?' and meant I didn't have to tell the same gloomy story over and over again. There had been a mixed reaction when I returned the next day. Some people tried to avoid me, some overcompensated by asking intrusive questions, but the vast majority were fantastically supportive. I knew the best policy was to be open about Jane's illness. Regularly leaving early would have built up resentment and the last thing I needed right now was a sense of unease in the office.

It was a relief that the following afternoon we seemed to be fast-tracked through the clinic. Spirited to a room, we sat alone for thirty seconds looking at each other before Mr Brennan arrived. He came across and forcefully shook our hands.

'Hello, Jane. The news is good. The scans are clear,' he said. He was perched on the front of his desk, Jane's notes in his hands. 'I've put you on my list at Seacroft on Friday morning, you'll need to come in on Thursday for tests. Once we've done the mastectomy and it's healed we'll talk over options for reconstruction.'

The pressure on my brain seemed to lift. My vice-like grip on the chair weakened as my body relaxed with relief. Jane sat nonplussed, with barely a flicker of emotion on her face as she said a quick thank-you.

'I'll see you Friday, then.' Mr Brennan left the room, allowing Jane and me to collect our thoughts before heading out. We stood and I held her tight. The death sentence had been commuted and for the first time since the diagnosis there was some hope.

'We should ring your mum and dad,' I jabbered, 'and the kids. They are going to be so pleased.'

Jane nodded mutely and forced a shallow smile. I couldn't understand why she looked so deflated.

'What's up?' I asked.

'Nothing. I just want to be on my own for a minute,' she said. I watched her cross the road and head for the chapel. I didn't get it. Didn't she realize this gave us some real hope? Whatever happened now we had some weapons to fight this disease – chemotherapy and radiotherapy. Even if the lymph nodes were affected, we had a chance. Couldn't she see that?

JANE

As I began to feel more and more panicky and hopelessly adrift in this strange new world of hospitals, it was Dad who suggested I might want to get some prayerful help. When he'd undergone his own chemotherapy, he'd had the sacraments of the sick and he'd explained about how it helped him stay calm and made him feel more prepared.

I telephoned the sacristy of St Mary's, my local church. Father John said he would call round later that day. I had no idea what to expect, but hoped it might help bring a sense of acceptance about my situation. It just might help me feel more at ease with the loss of control I was experiencing.

We sat in the living room, and Father John kissed his stole before placing it round his neck. He brought out a small wooden box from beneath his vestments and placed it on the table near us. Reaching his hand in again he brought out a small, rounded, silver container, which I knew contained the host, for us to share.

Father John blessed me as he anointed my forehead with scented oil from the box, and I joined him in prayers. I've always liked the 'Hail Mary'; the thought of another mother looking down on me and my family was comforting. I prayed for a way to cope with my illness. Father John asked me if I wanted to make confession, I declined, and he made the sign of the cross over my head, absolving me of my sins. We shared a host, the blessed bread of the Eucharist, and then there was a final blessing.

Afterwards, I did feel a sense of calm. I was more relaxed about the future. I had stopped struggling to make sense of what was happening. I accepted that I had cancer, and prayed for my family and myself, that we would all be given courage over the next few weeks. I felt I had been given some respite and slept more easily, having placed my faith in God.

The calmness stayed with me over the next few days, until the day came for my pre-operative assessment. The ward was old-fashioned and dreary with twelve beds lining the walls. There was little natural light and the glare of the fluorescent tubes made the ward look stark and uninviting.

I was shown to my bed at the furthest end and as we walked I glanced at the other patients. Some sat in chairs alongside their beds, others were too frail and sat, supported by mounds of pillows, in their beds. There were drip stands, oxygen cylinders, wheelchairs. I had been trying all week to be positive. Now, the awful reality of my situation was all too clear. My faith faltered and I sat on the bed with tears in my eyes.

'You'll be all right,' whispered Mike, holding my hand tightly. 'Come on. You can do this.'

'I know.' I said, biting my lip. 'It's just . . . I didn't expect this . . . I'm frightened. I don't want to be ill.'

A dark-haired woman in a white coat approached us carrying a clipboard and some papers. She called my name and, when I raised my hand, she smiled and pulled up a chair beside the bed.

'Hi, Jane, I'm Dr Carr, one of the junior doctors. Can I just check a few details?'

I nodded.

'What are you in for?' she asked, scribbling furiously in her notes.

'A mastectomy.'

That made her look up.

'How old are you?' she asked.

'Twenty-six.'

'Oh,' she said. I could see she was flummoxed. After some time she asked, 'Is there a history of breast cancer in your family?'

'No.'

'You're so young. Only the same age as me.'

I shrugged. What could I say to that?

When she'd finished her questionnaire, she took blood samples in case I needed a transfusion in theatre the next day.

A nurse, Carol, came over to go through my operation with me. Chatty and cheerful, she put me at ease after my visit from the junior doctor. I liked her.

'This is what the surgeon will be inserting into the breast.' She placed a piece of jelly-like substance in my hands. It felt like a stress toy. I squeezed it with my fingers. It was rubbery and pliable, but I felt queasy thinking that this would be part of me tomorrow.

'You can expect there to be some tubes in your chest to drain the wounds,' she warned. 'And you'll also have a drip in your hand. You might need an oxygen mask. But don't worry, it's all very normal and the nurses will make sure you're not in any pain.

After a couple of hours I had as much information as I could cope with. My checks done, we returned home, promising to be on the ward for seven-thirty the following morning.

My last night as a whole woman. Mike joked about asking for a bigger bust but his light-hearted comments couldn't disguise his fears or abate the horror I felt at the prospect of the mutilating surgery. The next day loomed large in unspoken words. We were both nervous of how we would cope; my main worry was the pain and what they might find when they operated.

I slept badly and rose early, anxious to be on the ward on time. When we arrived the nurses were ready and waiting – it was all systems go. The nurse checked me for theatre and gave me my pre-medication. It was only after I had taken the two white tablets that she remembered something.

'Jane, did you shave your armpits?'

Woozy and wobbly, I found myself minutes later in the ward bathroom clutching the sink unit with one hand and holding a scratchy blue razor in the other. 'What must this look like?' I wondered as I depilated my armpits, feeling and no doubt looking like I'd had one too many beers.

Freshly shaved, I stumbled back to the ward where the porter was waiting next to the trolley.

'Your chariot awaits,' he said, indicating my trolley with a flourish of his hand. My stomach tightened, there was no going back. I climbed on to the trolley and drew the thick, taupe blanket over me. I had just enough time to give Mike a hug and a kiss.

'I love you,' I whispered, tears in my eyes. 'I'll be okay. See you later.'

Mike's lips tightened and he nodded silently, crushed.

Mr Brennan was waiting for me in the operating theatre. He looked different in his surgical guise, but his voice was as reassuringly authoritative as always.

'You know what we're going to be doing here today, Jane?' he asked.

'Yes,' I replied. 'It was all explained yesterday.'

'Good,' he said, backing away to allow the anaesthetist to jab the back of my hand with a needle.

'Okay, Jane, I'd like you to start counting back from ten, please,' she said.

'Ten, nine, eight . . .'

MIKE

Spots of rain hit my face as I returned to the car. The water on my cheeks made my face cold. It was supposed to be the middle of summer but it felt more like March – somehow though it felt strangely fitting.

Jane had been bubbly all morning. Had that been for my benefit? My heart slumped as I imagined what was happening to her at that precise moment.

I resolved not to phone the ward until eleven o'clock and, when I did, Jane was still in surgery. Fridays were always busy at work and today was no exception. At least the constant flow of customers meant my mind was occupied. By two o'clock I knew the ward's telephone number off by heart, but the message was still the same. I became more and more anxious and the gaps between the calls lessened.

At around 2.30 p.m., I telephoned my parents to speak to the girls.

'Hello, Daddy, we have been bowling.' Suzanne seemed cheerful and it was a delight to hear her soft little voice. Mum and Dad had done their best to keep them busy but, even so, Suzanne was aware of the seriousness of the situation.

'Is Mummy all right?' she asked.

'She's having the operation,' I said.

'When will she be finished?'

'I don't know. Not long now, I think.'

'What are they doing?'

At only five years old, Suzanne's inquisitive mind meant we could keep nothing from her for long and we didn't want to scare her by pretending everything was all right when clearly it wasn't.

Jane and I had agreed from the outset that it was best to keep the children in the picture. When I was eleven, my grandmother's own breast cancer had been kept secret from me and the other grandchildren. But we knew something was going on and found the hushed conversations and parental tears, not to mention the lack of honesty, unsettling. Jane's family had dealt with her father's cancer in a similar fashion – all families have their own ideas on how to deal with such a situation – Jane and I decided to be as honest as we could. Rebecca understood that Mummy was poorly and needed some medicine to make her better but Suzanne was always the one with the questions.

'Is Mummy better now?' she asked and I felt my heart constrict.

'I hope so. I'll ring you tonight after I've seen her,' I said. 'Love you.'

I knew that Jane's surgery would take a while but, as each hour slowly ticked away, my nerves were in shreds. I felt sick with worry. I resolved to leave at three o'clock whether Jane was back from theatre or not. I was of no use to anyone in this state at work.

Bang on three, still with no news from the hospital, I made my way to Seacroft. I knew there was no sense in hurrying. Arriving early would only mean more time to pace up and down the ward so I made a conscious effort to take everything at a leisurely pace. When I arrived at the reception desk an hour later, two nurses were wrapped up in conversation, too engrossed to acknowledge me. Then one of them looked up. 'Can I help?' she said.

'Yes, I'm here to see Jane Tomlinson. I'm her husband.'

'She's been back about fifteen minutes. She's sleeping at the moment but everything is normal. She's in the first bed on the right.'

I turned and entered the ward. The face in the bed they had directed me to wasn't Jane. I looked closer.

'Fucking hell!' It was Jane. Lying in the bed, a drip to each side and a black oxygen cylinder next to her. She looked half dead, her skin a grey ghastly colour with a tinge of jaundiced yellow. I'd left her that morning, smiling and chatting; there'd been no tangible evidence of illness. I wasn't prepared for this sudden deterioration of her appearance.

I approached the bed carefully, trying not to display my alarm. I wanted to reach across and hold her hand but decided against it, worried I might disturb the drains. Her small frame made the narrow hospital bed seem king-size. Staring at her frail body, for the first time, she suddenly seemed so mortal.

'Mike?' She was beginning to stir.

'It's okay, love, I'm here. Do you need anything?'

A nurse's radar picked up the fact that Jane was rousing and she came over.

'You're on the ward, Jane, everything is fine,' she soothed as Jane drifted back to sleep. The nurse turned to me.

'She'll be very tired,' she said. 'It was a long operation. Don't be alarmed. It is normal in the circumstances. Do you want a drink?'

'Yes, please,' I replied. 'I'll be back in a minute. I'm just going to get some fresh air.'

The cold air hit me as soon as the door opened and I took huge lungfuls, looking up at the grey sky and down at the tarmac, trying to breathe normally. I wandered down the side of the building and then stopped, resting my back against the rough brick wall.

Jane had been realistic about what she had to face. She knew the enormity of what the illness meant, what it could do to her and to us, her family. Meanwhile, I had confidently dismissed the surgery as a stepping stone to recovery.

I knew there and then that it wasn't going to be that simple.

JANE

The curtain railings came into focus. I was back on the ward. Drowsy and dry-mouthed, my right hand was sore. I held it up. I could see a drip in the back of it. I felt sure that they had put it in the other hand.

Sound seemed to come in bubbles. Round, noisy moments which then burst into silence. The effort of focusing became too much and I closed my eyes, listening for something familiar. I could hear a low, chugging, hissing sound, which seemed to puff around my face. I reached out with my hand, trying to understand what I could feel.

'Jane. Jane. Leave that. It's just an oxygen mask. You need to leave that on.' The disembodied voice seemed to come from a huge distance away. My chest hurt and I couldn't move. A sharp pain pinned me to the bed. I looked down to where the pain was coming from. Plastic tubes curled out from under a bloodied gown. I felt a tightness around my other arm, and saw a blue cuff wrapped round it.

'It's just the blood-pressure monitor,' said the nurse who had come to check it. Mike was sitting beside the bed. His brows furrowed; the red mark of tiredness between them stood out against the white of his skin. I smiled at him and his eyes opened a little wider, the creased brow smoothed as he smiled back at me.

I drifted in and out of consciousness. My full bladder woke me and I used the call button that someone had placed by my pillow to summon help. Unable to get out of bed, the nurses brought me a bedpan. They eased me forward, and as I sat upright it felt like my left side had been torn from me and left on the pillow. The searing, red-hot stabbing pain brought tears to my eyes.

'I'm a bit sore,' I mumbled. Easing me back down, they placed pillows under my head and shoulders to make me comfortable. The room slipped and I felt like I was falling, then spinning, the motion making me sick. I pushed myself upright, and found the bowl left for me. As my stomach heaved, a nurse came to support me and, when the retching had finished, she wiped my forehead with a damp cloth and helped me to lie back down. I could hear voices on the ward, the lights too dim to make out who was talking. I felt a sharp scratch on my thigh.

'That should help with the sickness,' the nurse said quietly to me. I murmured a faint 'Thank-you' and drifted back into darkness.

The quiet whisperings of the night were replaced with the business of the morning. Waking, I could see dark blood-red tubes appearing from the bandages that surrounded my chest. They were tied to the edge of the bed so I could not accidentally dislodge them, I guessed. The urgent, sharp, tearing pain in my breast had faded and was replaced by a dull, throbbing ache. I looked down at where my breast had been. There was still a breast shape, but it was covered in bandages. It didn't look very different but it didn't feel like it belonged to me. My left shoulder was sore and I could only move my arm by pulling it around with my right.

'How is the pain?' a nurse asked as she took my temperature.

'It hurts,' I said. 'I feel better though. At least I've stopped being sick.'

I was given two options to help me deal with the pain: injections, like the ones I had been having since I woke up, which left me feeling confused and disoriented, or tablets, which would leave me feeling less woozy. It was a clear choice. As the day went on, I found I could gently ease myself out of bed with some help from the nursing staff. Just that little bit of independence felt rewarding.

Carol, the nurse who had talked me through the operation the day before, brought a bowl to my bedside to bathe me. Gently, she soaped my arms, back and chest and rinsed them clean. The roughness of the towel as she dried me felt refreshing. She eased my left arm into my own nightgown, but even the slightest movement left me feeling raw.

By the time we had finished I was exhausted and queasy. Carol helped me into the chair at the side of my bed and put a pillow behind my head

'It looks really good,' she said, pointing at my breast. 'They've managed to put in your implant, and your notes say that they've saved your nipple.'

That wasn't much comfort. It seemed strange to be talking about my breast, which no longer felt like it was a part of me. I was relieved that the bandages covered everything. I wasn't prepared to see it yet.

I sat dozing. The tension I had felt that morning was gone. I had survived and I felt like an enormous weight had lifted from me.

I was still in the chair when Mike visited. After leaving me so ill and confused the night before, he was surprised at my transformation. We sat in companionable silence until a nurse came to say that my mum had phoned.

'You can tell her I am up and about a little,' I said with a smile. 'The pain's not so bad, but the food is terrible.'

Mike picked up a copy of *Vogue* from the side of my bed. He muttered to himself as he read through the contents.

'I thought you came to see me. You can read the magazines when I get home,' I said to him.

'I can tell you're feeling better.' His face closed in, his eyes became small, his mouth pinched. 'Just like you to give me a hard time. I've made the effort to come to see you, and all you can do is moan.'

'Lighten up,' I said. 'I was only joking, don't get mad. You're just jealous you haven't got a body like that.' I pointed at a picture of a well-built, oiled young man on one of the pages. Mike smirked and tossed the magazine to one side.

The lunch trolley's arrival was a signal for him to leave.

'You've been so brave,' he said, leaning over to kiss me. 'It's good to see you smile. I'll be back later. The kids want to visit tomorrow. Will you be up to that?'

'I'll make sure I am,' I said. I couldn't wait to see them. 'Say "Hi!" from me, and give them a kiss each.'

I ate lunch, determined to be fit to leave the ward as soon as possible and, by the end of the day, I could move around with much more ease. I could even visit the toilet without assistance. The previous night seemed a distant memory; hopefully this was a good sign.

Sunday morning arrived. I had managed some sleep. I awoke as the breakfast trolley rattled on to the ward. I felt groggy, my side hurt, despite the numerous pillows I had used to prop myself comfortably in bed. I hadn't managed a proper wash since Thursday night so begged Carol to help me into the bath.

I looked at myself in the water. It wasn't so bad. A huge white dressing swathed me from my left side across to the other breast. I could see the stitches that held the drains in place; they itched and I longed to scratch. I could see where my flesh was bruised at the very edges of the dressing. Dark green and swollen, I touched it gently. It felt hard and lumpy. I shuddered. I couldn't feel my hand on my breast. It was a strange sensation and made a shiver run over my body.

I was a squeaky clean mum for my two gorgeous girls. They jumped on the bed and I put my right arm around them in turn.

'Have you been good for Daddy?' I asked.

'Yes, Mummy,' they chorused.

'When are you coming home?' Suzanne asked.

'I had an ice cream today,' Rebecca told me.

'Mum has to be careful not to hurt herself. Come and sit on my knee instead,' Mike urged before I could open my mouth.

'Come on,' I said, pulling Rebecca on to my knee. I ignored Mike's hard stare. She snuggled into my side.

We sat quietly together, each of us with our own thoughts, the children calm and a little bemused by the ward setting. Mum bustled in not long afterwards.

'How's things?' she asked, as she stood back to have a proper look at me.

'I'm okay. Still sore, but managing to do my exercises.' I eased my arm up to show her how much mobility I had managed to achieve.

'Dad's outside in the car park,' she said. 'He's got a nasty cough and doesn't want to pass it on to to you. He's waiting to give you a wave.'

I eased Rebecca off my lap and Suzanne climbed down off the bed.

Dad noticed us immediately as we looked out of the window of the day room. He looked uncomfortable, his eyes hooded with pain. My heart sank as I took in how ill he was. I wanted to be able to speak to him, to let him know I would be okay but knew he would be upset if I tried.

Mum spoke. 'Right, I'll be off then. Behave yourself, and don't be doing too much.' With that she rummaged in her bag for the car keys and gave me a farewell kiss.

'Bye, Mum, thanks for coming. Give Dad a hug from me.' I stood to walk her to the door.

'No. No. You stay here,' she said forcefully. 'I'll call by and see you tomorrow. Behave yourself, girl.' I smiled at her, and she marched down the ward towards the exit.

'Come on, you two, we better leave Mum now, she's looking

a bit tired.' Mike was right. I was exhausted and could feel the pain in my breast increasing, the tightness under my armpit pulling on my shoulder. Hugging me and giving me a kiss in turn, the girls turned to leave, chatting and giggling as Mike ushered them out. I watched them as they skipped down the ward two blonde heads either side of Mike, small hands clasped in his. They turned while their dad opened the door, waving at me still standing, watching them, blowing them a kiss as they disappeared down the corridor.

I felt empty watching them go. I ached at the emptiness of the space round my bed left by my family. It was so hard being grown-up when I felt in need of comfort and reassurance myself. I eased my aching arm out of my dressing gown and lay down letting the wave of tiredness wash over me.

MIKE

Jane was lying back in bed still attached to the drains, which accompanied her everywhere. In just a few days she had become accustomed to them and barely noticed them as she wandered down the ward or climbed into bed. I, on the other hand, never got used to seeing her attached to so many wires and tubes.

'What time did they say that they'd be round?' I asked, looking over my shoulder towards the nursing station at the top of the corridor.

'They didn't, but it won't be too long,' she replied.

I checked my watch. 'I'm going to the loo,' I said.

'Again?'

'Yeah, why, am I being rationed?'

I was off before getting her response. Rushing down the ward, I suspected my toilet trips were the result of nerves. The mounting tension had been palpable for weeks and D-day was upon us. The whole family had lurched from one test result to another but this could – and hopefully would – be the last. If the cancer wasn't present in the lymph nodes, there was a good chance it would be restricted to the breast. If not, we were back to stage one – more treatment and a future which was uncertain. The stakes were higher than ever – we were so close, so very close. My armpits were sticky with sweat, but I didn't want to appear so scared in front of Jane. I went to the toilet, ran my hands under the cold water to calm myself down and made my way slowly back to the ward where I could see Jane following my every step.

'Still working is it?'

'What?'

'I thought there must be something wrong with the plumbing.'

'Oh piss off,' I said. 'You're just jealous – at least I can bath myself.'

She pulled a face at me. I knew she was putting on a brave act but I could see through the mask. I sat on the bed.

'Mike! Are you trying to squash me?' she screeched.

'Sorry,' I said, adjusting my position.

'Mr Brennan's here.'

I jumped up from the bed like a guilty child. Mr Brennan moved unnaturally quickly for a man so stout and was soon upon us.

'Jane, you'll be pleased to know your lymph nodes are clear,' he said. He was not given to showing emotion in front of patients but was clearly enjoying giving us the news. I felt tears in my eyes. When I looked at Jane she was also welling up.

'Now, Jane,' Mr Brennan continued, 'while we had you in theatre, we took the liberty of reconstructing the breast with a silicon implant. For someone of your age we felt you could stand the rigours of longer surgery and a quick reconstruction will help you recover. One further bonus is we've saved your nipple and it's on your breast.'

The smile melted from my face and I felt myself leaning in towards him a little to catch those words again. What did he just say? The nipple has been saved? When was it ever in any danger? Where did it go? After a few seconds I began to wonder. If they'd not performed a reconstruction, what would have happened to the errant nipple? Would it be on Jane's shoulder? Her midriff? Under her arm? How many people, I pondered, were going round without a nipple? Where did they put all the spare ones?

Mr Brennan was still speaking and I quickly gathered my thoughts, aware that now was not the time or place for such questions. This was my wife's breast we were discussing, silicon implants, flaps, misplaced nipples and reconstructions. It felt surreal.

I looked at Jane, sensing that she was about to dissolve into tears of relief. I moved gingerly forward, just close enough to kiss her forehead.

'It's okay, Jane, it's over,' I whispered. 'The cancer's gone.'

'That's right, Jane,' said Mr Brennan. 'You shouldn't require any further treatment – radiotherapy or chemotherapy. Forget about this awful episode. Go and get on with your life.'

JANE

I felt the knots in my stomach release. I hadn't really realized how tense I had been, waiting for the results, but on hearing those words I felt awash with relief.

'Will I be able to start my degree course in October?' I asked. 'I've got a place at Leeds Uni to study maths.'

'Yes, you should be ready,' he replied.

Great. I had coped with the surgery and just needed to get myself fit. I couldn't wait to get back home, to pick up the pieces and start some training.

Mike turned to me, and we hugged each other tightly.

'I knew you'd be okay.'

I hadn't been so sure, but could feel my stomach unclenching, my muscles relaxing. I smiled. We had a future to work towards.

'Why don't we go across to the radiography school and pick up an application form?' Mike squeezed my hand reassuringly.

'What, now?'

I looked down at my pyjamas, the drains from my wounds in a plastic bag beside the chair. It seemed a ludicrous idea.

'Yes, now. It's what you want to do, isn't it?' he asked.

'Well, yes,' I said. 'But . . .'

'No buts. There's no time like the present. Come on. It's only a short walk across the lawn to the school. It can't hurt to speak to someone.'

I had been having second thoughts about studying maths. During my scans, I had become interested in radiography and had asked the radiographer what qualifications I would require if I were to study it. He told me I'd need A levels in sciences. I had A levels in maths, physics, chemistry and biology.

Before my operation, I'd rung the two radiography schools in Leeds and explained my situation. The heads were both enthusiastic that I should apply if all went well with my surgery.

'Let's go then,' I said to Mike, and we headed down the ward. 'I'm just off for a little wander in the grounds,' I told Carol as we passed the nurses desk.

She looked quizzically at me. 'Don't go too far,' she said. 'You'll be more tired than you think.'

We left the ward and headed down the corridor that led to the large expanse of lawn. Supporting my arm so it didn't jog my breast, I walked slowly.

'Slow down a bit, will you?' I said. Mike was striding purposefully on ahead and I wasn't able to match his pace. It was great to be away from the ward. I had been able to sit outside in the warmth but this seemed like a huge step to be taking. The colours in the sunlight seemed enhanced. The outside world seemed to zing. Everything felt so positive.

'Why don't you fill that out this afternoon?' Mike said when we had picked up the form. 'It's best to strike while the iron is hot.'

'I don't know,' I said a little hesitantly. 'I doubt if I'll get a place this year anyway.'

'You'll never find that out if you don't put the form in,' he shot back.

I struggled with the form after lunch. The first parts were straightforward: qualifications, previous work experience. The area that was more difficult was providing other relevant experience to back up the application. I wrote down why I thought I would make a good radiographer: good communication skills, ability to learn technical skills. But more important, I thought, was my ability to empathize with patients having just gone through my own experiences.

The next morning Jocelyn, who had given me the form the day before, was on the telephone.

'Can she come and interview you this afternoon?' the ward clerk said. 'Are you up to it? Or shall I tell her you'll phone her when you are well enough?'

I hesitated for a moment.

'No, that's fine. When does she want to come over? I need some time to make myself decent.'

'Two-thirty this afternoon,' she said. 'Jocelyn said to let you know that she and a senior tutor called Anne will be coming to interview you.'

I managed, with some degree of difficulty, to wash my hair by kneeling up in the bath and rinsing the shampoo out using the shower with one hand. I put on clean pyjamas and tidied the drains from my breast wound back into the plastic carrier. I sat nervously on a chair beside my bed.

Jocelyn approached, said a hearty hello, and introduced Anne. I was relieved to see her give me a warm smile. I assured them I was fine and fit for the interview.

Formalities regarding qualifications were over very quickly. I more than fulfilled the minimum educational standards required. Neither of them seemed particularly interested in my previous work experience, but they were curious as to why I thought my illness could be an advantage.

'I can see the patient's point of view,' I said. 'I know what sort of fears they have.'

The interview didn't seem to last long but when I glanced at the clock we had been chatting for forty-five minutes. I was astounded to hear Jocelyn tell me that there was a place available in September, as long as I was declared fit for work. I was overjoyed. This was the extra impetus I needed to get fit and well as soon as possible. I couldn't wait to tell Mike. I had just six weeks time to get myself into shape.

MIKE

Tomorrow the bandages were coming off. Since Tuesday night I'd thought of nothing else. Terrified of what lurked beneath, I imagined the bandages being slowly unwound – like on an Egyptian mummy in a crap 'B' movie – and in my mind I'd rehearsed the smile in the bathroom mirror, naked from the waist up, carefully repositioning my man breasts. 'That looks great!' pushing them up further. 'What an improvement', covering one up. 'You can hardly tell' – no, that doesn't work. 'Who needs two when you've got one like yours?' No, no, no. 'They've done a good job, Jane', letting go. 'You look as beautiful as ever.'

I knew Jane wouldn't be fooled. She would be monitoring my reaction intensely, gauging whether or not I was being sincere. I was scared my facial expressions would give me away, that Jane would see through me and I'd lose her because the damage would be done.

When my grandmother had had her breast removed, I remembered thinking how my grandfather had coped so admirably. He had been so strong, so brave. As a boy, I'd found the thought of a one-breasted woman entirely repulsive and now here I was as a 29-year-old man, ashamed to admit I still felt repulsed.

I paced up and down the living room and kicked the sofa.

'Oh shit!'

I closed my eyes and pictured Jane on our wedding day, walking down the aisle escorted by her dad. Her slender frame and physique looked stunning inside an ivory dress. I remembered thinking, as I stood there waiting at the altar: 'How did I get this lucky?'

I hated the fact that now I felt like one of those shallow blokes who labelled themselves 'breast-men'. Because I wasn't.

I was different. I knew I would always love Jane no matter how she looked. But at the same time, I couldn't imagine a lifetime of being married to a woman with only one breast.

'It doesn't matter,' I told myself, over and over again. But no matter how often I said it, the tiny gremlin inside my head argued differently.

Jane needed my support and a lot of love. She was losing part of her femininity and confidence, she needed me to be there for her, to be strong and brave like my granddad, not wincing at the bedside in disgust.

The next day was mapped out: hospital for the bandages to be removed, then work, Suzanne and Rebecca would come home with my parents, then I would collect Jane. The girls were primed not to hug or jump on their mum and they had to promise to try to be quiet at home. I'd noticed how everyone's mood had lightened as each piece of good news had come in and, today, the house was filled with almost a carnival atmosphere to welcome Jane home.

As I arrived at the hospital, I knew what was required of me but I was not convinced that I could pull it off. A young nurse at her bedside looked across at me and smiled.

'You're just in time for the bandages being removed,' she said.

Great. Where was the traffic jam when I needed it? A second nurse appeared with a screen to shield Jane from the other patients and my heart sank.

'Hi, gorgeous,' Jane whispered. 'It's really good to see you.'

'I can't wait for you to come home. The kids sound so excited.' I focused on her eyes and tried desperately not to look down.

'They're going to take the bandages off,' she said. 'You don't have to watch.'

But as I turned, a nurse flashed me a definite don't-you-dare-look-away-you-gutless-wonder look. I had no intention of going anywhere. I was squeamish at all things medical, but I was well aware that Jane needed support now.

'Of course I'm staying.'

I braced myself for the worst. One of the nurses moved in between us, obscuring my view. I was delighted, but – as if she could sense my relief – she moved to the left and I could see Jane's chest area easily. I tried a smile as the first bandage began to unravel, but I suspected I looked like a toothless old man sucking on a sherbet lemon.

CHAPTER 3

MIKE

Allowing my eyes to skirt over Jane's breast, I saw that a skin-tight second bandage hugged her new contours. I let out a barely audible sigh and allowed my eyes to study her new appearance in detail. The bruising seemed extensive. I flashed Jane a smile and mouthed 'I love you.' She mouthed it back, then I saw her grimace as she elevated her elbow to allow the nurse easier access to the dressing. As the second bandage came off, I noticed that the area under Jane's arm looked like it had been quarried.

Within seconds the last bandage was removed and Jane's new breast was exposed. The nipple looked like a burnt currant, flattened and shapeless sitting on skin badly discoloured from week-old bruising. It still had a feminine curve yet it didn't look like a breast at all, the bounce and natural movement had gone.

I looked at Jane, trying to gauge her reaction.

'It looks fantastic,' I said. 'When can we get the other one done?'

Jane stood silent, her feet rooted to the spot. Gingerly she began to examine her new body and it was at that second I realized I hadn't been alone in fearing this moment.

'We're just going to clean the wounds up,' said the nurse, 'then we'll apply a smaller dressing.'

Sensing it was a suitable opportunity to escape, I made my

excuses, and left the enclosed area so that Jane could get dressed. Fully clothed, she seemed herself again; the traces of her hospital self had vanished. Already it seemed that some elements of normality were returning.

'I'll get to work now. I'll be back at two,' I said. 'I can't wait for you to come home. I love you, Jane.'

When I arrived back at the hospital later that day, Jane was sitting by her bed reading. For the first time in a while she looked totally at ease, the tension disappeared from her face. Her bags were packed neatly and she was beaming a smile.

The other patients on the ward were older than Jane and they had shared concerns at watching a young person being so ill. They had all expressed their relief to Jane throughout the last couple of days.

As Jane moved, her face contorted from the pain and became ghostly pale. She soon lagged behind and I was obliged to wait every few seconds to allow her to catch up.

'Mike, please will you slow down. I can't walk that fast.' I wasn't trying to irritate her but it was hard to walk so slowly. 'Shit, that hurts, Mike,' she said as we drove down the uneven road from the hospital.

She winced whenever I changed gear and by the time we neared home, the microscopic attention she'd given to each manoeuvre made it feel like I was repeating my driving test. Each pothole seemed to act like a magnet for the car, causing her to groan in agony.

As I finally pulled up at home, in my eagerness to get out of the car, I accidentally let out the clutch before turning the engine off.

'Mike!' Jane shouted as the car lurched forward to a halt.

JANE

It was a relief when Mike finally pulled up into the drive. I'd spent only a week on the ward, but suddenly the outside world seemed to have speeded up to an unbearably fast pace.

'It's good to have you home,' he said.

'It's good to be here,' I replied. 'I can't wait to see the kids.'

The sight that greeted me when I got into the house made my heart leap. Suzanne and Rebecca were sitting side by side on the back door step, blonde heads close together, eating ice cream and carefully catching the drips.

'Hello, you two,' I called.

'Mummy,' they chorused, jumping up.

'Can I have a lick of your ice cream?' I asked.

'Grandma made them for us,' said Suzanne.

The house was almost as I had left it. Well, not quite. My mother-in-law's presence was noticeable in lots of little ways. The mail was piled in an unfamiliar place – a tidy pile on the piano rather than strewn across the kitchen worktop. It looked much more orderly and I was grateful to Alice for the help. But I knew it would feel more normal when we were back to our chaotic household.

Alice fussed all day and it was good to be looked after, but there were only so many times I could tell her I was fine. She was surprised I didn't need to lie down and, although I needed a rest, I was too excited at being home. But by early evening, my shoulder and arm ached and I was ready to lie down.

I lay nervously, the smallest movement giving me deep pain in my armpit. My shoulder felt as tight as an overstrung violin, screaming discordantly as I turned slowly. Exhausted by the physical effort of my homecoming, I longed for sleep but, instead, fidgeted uncomfortably.

Ignoring the twinges and stabs, I closed my eyes and tried to relax. I could hear the noises of my family, the television rumbling away and Mike's voice as he chatted to his mum and then admonished my two unseen angels.

'Quiet, your mum's resting.'

The door to the living room opened and I could hear Rebecca and Suzanne climbing the stairs whispering and giggling.

'Quietly now,' Mike said.

But it was impossible for them to be silent and I smiled to myself. With sleep eluding me, I admitted defeat and gently rolled out of bed. I pulled my dressing gown on and went to stand in the doorway of Rebecca and Suzanne's bedroom. I watched them through the mirror as they hunted for their night-clothes.

'Do you want some help?' I whispered.

'Yes please, Mummy.' Rebecca smiled.

Suzanne looked horrified.

'Did we wake you up?' she said.

'No, don't worry. I couldn't sleep. I thought it would be nice to tuck you in tonight.'

Suzanne undressed herself and I helped Rebecca in an awkward one-handed fashion into her pyjamas.

'Downstairs for some milk and biscuits,' I said, stiff from kneeling down, and I cringed as I got back to my feet. It took some effort to get upright.

Suzanne and Rebecca flew through the living room door.

'Da-daaaaah,' beamed Suzanne. 'Mum helped us.'

Mike raised his eyebrows about to say something but then noticed me.

'I couldn't sleep,' I told him. 'You could get these two some milk and biscuits.'

I gave them a head start before following them back upstairs for bed. Suzanne was rinsing her toothbrush and Rebecca was already tucked in.

'Prayers,' I said.

'I love Mummy. I love Daddy. I love Grandma and Granddad. I love everybody and I love you,' they both joined in. We made the sign of the cross together as we finished, but Suzanne continued: 'Please God. Look after my Mum and help her get better soon.'

'Thank you,' I said and blew them both a kiss, pulling the curtains to, just leaving a chink where the late summer sun shone through.

'Sleep tight,' I said. 'It's good to be home.'

MIKE

'Bog Trotter!' I announced as we drove towards Keswick.

'What?' said Jane, looking across from the passenger seat.

'In the race.' I nodded towards the car radio.

'Like I care.' Jane wasn't interested in most sports. I loved horse racing. The Champagne Stakes at Doncaster was the Friday highlight of the St Leger meeting and, as a child, the family had always spent 'Leger' week at my maternal grand-parents' in South Elmsall to attend the races.

With Thirlmere Lake resplendent on our left and the steep Lakeland fells on the right, it was impossible not to feel uplifted. This was our first trip away, just the two of us, since our hon-eymoon. My parents had offered to look after the children to give us some quality time before Jane started her course.

Even with a pillow under her left arm, it was clear that the meandering roads were causing Jane some discomfort. The views of the lush green valleys and wide stretches of water were a welcome distraction and she'd been chatty most of the way, but two hours into the journey, it was obvious she was in more distress. It was a relief for both of us when we pulled up to the budget B&B we'd booked earlier that week.

Our room was basic, a double bed, a dressing table near a window overlooking the street and two bedside tables with lamps. The bulb had gone on my side. Jane gently lowered her-self on to the bed, where she rested for an hour before we set out for a meal.

On Saturday morning, the weather was dry and mild. We woke early after a disturbed night. Jane, though, was adamant that she wasn't too tired. We set off to walk the banks of Derwent Water. We wrapped up appropriately, knowing how quickly the elements could change in this part of the world, and headed out of the door. I watched as Jane made her way down the hallway. Never one to shy away from unconventional fash-ion, today she was wearing 'paint-splatter' leggings and a black woollen jumper with patterns that looked like a nursery group had been let loose with crayons.

An hour into the walk, our pace slowed to a dawdle. I tried my best to stay level with Jane, but each time my concentration wavered I would stroll on ahead only to look back and find her twenty yards behind. It soon became clear we would only reach the falls which were four miles away if we extended our weekend until Tuesday.

'Shall we go back?' I suggested. Jane nodded. She looked pale, but I had seen her looking worse and felt confident she could make it back. After only a short while she stopped, looked down at the ground and leant against a drystone wall.

'I don't think I can make it back,' she said. I stood watching her grimace. I looked around, feeling like a spare part. She would be all right in just a few minutes.

'Where does it hurt?' I asked.

'My shoulder, boob, arm, pretty much all my left side.'

'What have you taken?'

'Some Coproximal an hour ago. I can't take any more until six.'

'Are you okay to go on?' I asked. Her body was slumped against the wall like a boxer against the ropes. She nodded and we set off again but she'd have been quicker with a zimmer frame; walk fifty yards, stop, walk another fifty. I was beginning to get nervous. We'd only seen four other walkers along this section in twenty minutes and one car, which had sped by so quickly we'd hardly had time to see its colour.

'I'll run ahead for the car,' I said. 'It'll only take about forty-five minutes.'

'No,' Jane sounded alarmed. 'I'm too poorly, stay with me.'

We continued for another ten minutes, but barely covered a quarter of a mile. At each opportunity we sat down, Jane barely able to move. I glanced at my watch. I'd definitely miss the St Leger. It looked like the football results were out of the question, too.

'I'm going to get the car,' I said, standing up. 'I promise I won't be long. You can't go on like this. Will you be okay?'

She nodded and I was a little surprised. I'd assumed that by taking this stance, it would have prompted her into getting up and forcing herself onwards. I knew she didn't want me to go but if she was willing to be left alone on a deserted road in the middle of nowhere, it must be serious. I was suddenly a bit frightened.

I turned and started jogging back to the car, looking back every so often to check she was okay. After a few minutes she was out of sight and that's when I began to run faster. It seemed to take for ever to reach the B&B but I didn't have time to catch my breath. I looked at the clock in the car, I'd been gone half an hour. It was a relief to spot her in the distance, still sitting in the same spot, waving as she saw the car approach.

'Taxi for the jibber,' I said, leaning over to open the door.

'My feet are like ice,' she said, climbing in and turning up the heating two notches. Within minutes we were back at Bleak House. Up in the room, I turned up the radiator but soon discovered the owner's heating policy: never to turn it on.

'I'm sorry, Mike'

'What for?'

'Not being able to finish.'

'There's nothing to apologize for, I'm just glad you're okay.'

'If I get rested, can we go swimming tomorrow? I know you won't want to, but I'd quite like to.'

'Yes, of course.'

Swimming seemed like a good idea at the time. There's little to do in Keswick on a damp Sunday morning. We could have gone to Mass but our Catholic consciences didn't guilt trip us on holidays. It would be Jane's first time in a swimming costume in public since her mastectomy.

The pool was like no other I'd ever seen – a large triangular expanse of chlorinated blue with a huge tubular water slide spiralling above. I stood transfixed.

'It's a fun pool, Mike,' said Jane as she plopped into the water. 'Come on, you miserable sod.'

A fun pool – there was a misnomer. I hated water. I am a weak swimmer who can't even master breaststroke.

In her blue, patterned all-in-one swimsuit, Jane's figure

looked perfectly normal. As she emerged from the changing rooms, I studied people's faces as they saw her, but no one took the slightest notice.

'You look beautiful,' I said.

'No, I don't.' She smiled and was off.

A couple of minutes later, I slid into the shallow end and sat kicking my legs. Jane was swimming in what was obviously the deepest part of the pool. A siren blared out, vibrating and echoing off the walls. I looked around – no one appeared to be evacuating the building.

Swimming gingerly over to Jane, waves slowly started rippling through the pool. We positioned ourselves at the epicentre of the current and for a few seconds enjoyed the gentle undulation of the water. Steadily the waves became more intense and I could see Jane was starting to struggle. Where we could once stand safely with our feet firmly on the floor, now the waves were crashing over her head. I tried to reach her, my legs paddling under the water, but the force of the tide kept pushing me back. Jane disappeared under another wave and popped up, clearly gasping for breath. She was clutching her left arm tightly to her body. I spun around to see if I could attract the lifeguard's attention. Somehow Jane began moving to the side of the pool and I tried to do the same. Clinging on to the wall, rising and falling with the water, she was in obvious distress and I couldn't reach her.

The waves died down after three long minutes and I waded out as quickly as I could to where she was standing.

'You okay?' I said and she nodded.

'I think I'll get out,' she said.

We left Keswick early and headed to Mum and Dad's to pick up the girls. On the journey back home, Jane slept like a child. She looked frail and vulnerable, not the same person I'd set off with on Friday towards the Lakes. I turned the car heater up and the radio down.

As I drove through Kirby Lonsdale towards home, I began to wonder how, if a relaxing weekend away could exhaust her, would she be able to start her diploma? I would never have dreamt of saying as much but I couldn't help but wonder how on earth she was going to do it.

JANE

My first day as a student radiographer arrived. The school was on the top floor of Leeds General Infirmary and the lift took ages to arrive. As I stepped inside, butterflies began to flutter in my stomach.

The lift opened on to a darkened corridor. I followed the arrow to the principal's office. A classroom door was open and, hearing voices, I peered in. There were about ten people ranging in age from about eighteen to forty, an even spread of both men and women.

'Is this the right place for the induction course for radiography?' I asked one of the older male students.

'Yes,' he said. He was tall and lanky. 'I'm Trevor. Who are you?'

'Jane,' I said. 'I'm really nervous.'

'You'll be fine,' Trevor laughed. 'Besides, there's no time to escape now.'

I sat next to Trevor. Thumbing through the introductory booklet, I struggled to take in all the information but made a few rudimentary notes. An hour later, we were being taken on a tour of the hospital.

It was like a rabbit warren. As we marched up the spiral staircase, past the staffroom, along a corridor and down another flight of stairs, I began to lose my bearings. Would I ever be able to find my way around? We were given film badges, which would record any accidental exposure to radiation. We were responsible for changing it monthly and were required to wear it at all times. We were handed metal markers, a small but essential piece of equipment, we were informed, to permanently mark films to show which side had been X-rayed.

Over the next few days, the building became less alien and I had managed to remember the names of most of my fellow students. Trevor, Alan and Cathy were all mature students, like me, all from different walks of life. I was the youngest. The group seemed to split into school leavers and those older. At twenty-six I was definitely not welcome in the younger group.

The days turned into weeks and I began to settle into a routine at home and work. In the morning Mike dropped Rebecca off at nursery while I would walk Suzanne to a friend's house before catching the bus into Leeds. In the evenings it was the reverse and after putting the girls to bed I would continue studying, spreading my books across my bed.

The actual study wasn't too intense, just very unfamiliar and demanding a great deal of my attention. There was physics, with electromagnetic waves and atomic structure. Anatomy I found the most difficult, we were constantly studying anatomical landmarks on the body to put to use when X-raying patients. We were taught how to study the X-rays themselves and were tested regularly on our knowledge of the skeleton.

I read and reread, learning by rote. We were given mnemonics to aid us in remembering the foramina of the skull, where the nerves and the blood vessels traversed through them. I enjoyed the work and sometimes my own experiences of surgery felt more immediate after reading one of the textbooks.

On my first day in the orthopaedic department, Ruth Porter was my supervising staff member.

'There's a dynamic hip screw taking place in theatre. Have you seen any hip surgery?' she barked at me.

'No.' I hesitated. 'I haven't been to theatre at all yet.'

'Follow me, then.' She marched swiftly out of the department and I followed behind, keen not to lose sight of her. Ruth had a reputation for being intolerant and the last thing I wanted was to incur her wrath.

She pushed open the swing doors to the operating theatres and I stepped forward to follow her, the clean antiseptic smell hitting me in the face. Memories of my own operation, lying there anxiously on the table, suddenly washed over me. I froze. Around me, people were busy at work, patients were wheeled past me. I collected myself and realized Ruth had continued down the corridor without me. She turned, beckoning me dramatically.

'This way, Jane,' she hissed.

I entered the female changing area, where she thrust a blue gown into my hands. I changed out of my uniform and grabbed a pen and my film badge. I pulled plastic overshoes on my feet and put on a surgical cap. Then we were back in the corridor, where she gave me a mask. We put them on, making us as featureless as everyone else in the theatre.

As we pushed the heavy image intensifier and screen into the theatre, Ruth turned to me.

'Don't touch anything,' she warned. 'Watch me and I'll try to explain. But you must be quiet.'

I nodded obediently and, following her lead, donning a leaded apron. Standing in theatre I felt nervous, the sound of saw biting into bone and the smell of burning flesh all made me lightheaded. If I concentrated on the technical side – where the machine was positioned, how Ruth swung it deftly around and through so the surgeon could see two views of the hip – the fuzziness disappeared. I even began to understand what we were looking at. The hip bone was lying horizontally across the screen and as the surgeon drilled, he would ask us to produce an X-ray image to show how far the drill bit had been driven into the bone. Then he needed to double-check by looking at the other angle of the hip, which required us to move the heavy equipment about ninety degrees.

Eventually, with the plate screwed into place, the fracture site was stabilized by the long pin. The surgeon started to close the incision and we were dismissed, but had to remove the heavy machinery from the room.

By the time we got back to the department I was feeling elated; my first theatre case and I hadn't put a foot wrong. Ruth was quick to bring me back down to earth, handing me my film badge which I was supposed to remove with my theatre gown.

'This is yours, I believe,' she said tersely. 'I found it in the laundry bag.'

MIKE

I'd been sitting at my desk barely more than five minutes when Frank Fletcher approached.

'Lazarus is coming this afternoon,' he said. 'He'll want to speak to you.'

'Who?'

'Lazarus, staff welfare to thee and me.'

'Lazarus?'

'Because he'll make all your troubles disappear.'

I rolled my eyes and sat back in my chair. It was the last thing I needed. The shortening daylight hours and the colder, wetter days were doing little to help my flagging spirits. Jane's dad was becoming increasingly ill and Jane was struggling to cope with the stress. I didn't want to see what was effectively the bank's social worker. I gave Frank a do-I-have-to? look.

'I'll only get nagged, Mike. Can't do any harm, can it? He's on a routine visit, but he's going to ask to see you.'

Lazarus arrived, looking like Nobby Stiles with girth. We headed off to the most private interview room in the building. Our conversation wandered for about thirty minutes. He asked after Jane, asked how my job was going, all pretty pointless until we neared the end.

'Any questions, Mike?'

'Only one,' I said. 'If Jane dies and I can't afford the mortgage and childcare, will the bank be sympathetic?'

'I'm sure they will,' he said flatly. It was the response I had expected.

'My dad's offered to help out as well if I'm stuck.'

'Well, I notice you are taking a £10,000 equity release to repay your dad,' he said. 'I'm not sure the bank would approve of that. Can you leave the £10,000 and reduce your mortgage?'

I looked at him and half smiled. He was joking, wasn't he? When the bank had moved me to Peterborough in 1986, we had been unable to afford to buy even the cheapest of houses with the mortgage that the bank had arranged, so my parents agreed to invest £10,000 as a favour. As a result, my dad was a third owner on the deeds. We bought a semi for £36,500 in 1987 and the following year next door had sold for £68,000. By 1990 it had fallen back to £50,000. Meanwhile the price of the property in Leeds we'd bought a year ago for £63,000 had fallen to £55,000. Each time the price of the house in Peterborough fell, it added to our residual mortgage. Of more concern was that it had been empty for over a year and the onset of another winter was due. The estate agent had already told us that the chances of finding a buyer were minimal.

'It's not an equity release,' I said. 'He owns a third of the property. It's a legal entitlement.' I knew where the conversation was heading and I could hear my voice straining with frustration.

'Well, it appears you are repaying your dad. You borrow the £10,000 increase on your mortgage at five per cent. Your dad gives the £10,000 to you, which you can invest at nine per cent, which means you'll make a profit. The bank would take a dim view of such a transaction.'

I couldn't believe what I was hearing. I sat forward in my chair, almost spitting my words.

'Only if Jane dies,' I said. 'In any event it's my dad's money, he can do what the hell he likes with it.'

'Failure to make the payments on your mortgage could result in you having to sell the property.' He suddenly sounded like a banker. 'I'll check with personnel to see where we stand.'

I couldn't see the point in arguing further so we said goodbye and I returned to my desk.

'How did it go with Lazarus?' asked Frank when he phoned later.

'Fucking fantastic.'

Jane sat opposite me in the dining room after supper.

'Well, what did personnel say?' she asked as she started to clear the plates.

'Just the same as Lazarus, only they were more officious. I lost it big style. They just don't want to listen.'

'If they'll let your dad get his money back, where's the problem?'

'They were saying if you died and I borrowed money off my dad, I could be disciplined.'

'How on earth does that work?'

'Because it's perceived as fraud.'

'What?'

'Well, they think Dad may be getting his money out of the property, giving it to me and making money on the interest rate hedge.'

'Hedge?'

'Difference between high saving rates and the bank's subsidized staff mortgage rate.'

'But it's your dad's money, what's it got to do with the bank?'

'Exactly. We wouldn't be in this mess if they hadn't moved me to Peterborough. Anyway, it turned into a slanging match, I slammed the phone down and walked out.'

'Walked out, what do you mean?' I could see Jane was concerned.

'Don't worry, it was about lunchtime.'

She didn't say anything. She picked up the plates and took them through to the kitchen.

'Well, what's the fucking point,' I carried on ranting. 'If you die I can't repay the mortgage, I'll have to sell up. Even when the house sells it won't clear the debts because we have negative equity. If I borrow money off dad I could get sacked. I thought fuck 'em, who needs it.'

'Mike.'

'It's all right, don't panic. I sat on a bench by the cathedral for an hour.'

Jane caught me looking at her and pulled a face.

'Resigning would be pointless,' I said. 'It'd be easier to get another job while working and we can't afford to lose the wage.'

'Mike, can't we just have one part of our life settled? I'm all right. I'm not going to die, it won't be a problem.'

'That's not the point.'

'It is, Mike. We've got to have somewhere to live.'

'Let me finish.'

'I thought you had.'

'I let the boss know the problem, he went absolutely ballistic. He phoned personnel and whatever happens there'll be no disciplinary action. If you die they'll help for a short time by making the mortgage interest only.'

'So what's the problem?'

'Isn't it obvious?'

'Not really, no.'

'I just think it's big of them to be so gracious not to discipline me over something legal.'

Jane shook her head and turned the tap off.

'Get over it, Mike, and move on. They're being reasonable.'

The television suddenly blared out in the next room. 'Suzanne, turn it down,' I bellowed.

'It's not their fault, Mike. It's not the bank's either.'

'I'm just so pissed off.'

'It's two people, not the bank as a whole. Keep things in perspective.'

'But I'm really mad.'

'I know but they are being fair. There's no need for you to be vitriolic, it's not important.'

'But—'

'Look, they've sorted it out, just leave it.'

As she turned her back to me, she stared out of the window into the night-time. I flicked her the Vs with both hands.

'Don't think I can't see that,' she said.

JANE

As autumn drifted into early winter, the cold weather and a clumsy fall while I'd been gardening set my recovery back several weeks. I had increasing discomfort in my left arm and a constant buzzing cramp in my wrist that continued down towards my fingers and never seemed to ease. Holding it, to try to rid myself of the unpleasant sensation, caused further pain in my shoulder, causing it to stiffen. I was beginning to lose mobility and could no longer put my arm above my head as I could only a matter of weeks ago.

I desperately wanted to be well, not only so I could continue with my course, but so I could visit my dad. Over the summer, his health had deteriorated. Every time I visited him he seemed more frail.

He had been admitted to hospital on several occasions and visiting him was a laborious exercise. I would catch the bus home after college, peering out of the grimy window into the grey damp outside, willing the bus forward with greater speed up the hill and home to Rothwell. Tired and fractious, I would push through the grumpy bodies at my stop and pick up Suzanne from her friend's house. I would listen to her chattering as we made our way across the road. Then there was tea to make and, if I had time, I would take a quick soak in the bath to try to alleviate some of the tension in my shoulders and relax my fuzzy arm. Leaving Mike to settle the children for the night, I would head back out into the cold night to catch the bus to Leeds and then another to St James's Hospital. It was always a long cold wait and the whole journey took nearly an hour.

Each time I arrived on the ward, Dad looked more gaunt. But he never complained; it wasn't in his nature.

As his disease progressed, Dad's treatment and options came to an end. The doctors discharged him from the hospital so he could come home to spend some time with his family. Although the cancer was eroding his spine and he was in much pain, he was stable enough to leave hospital. But I knew he didn't have long, which is why the hour-long journey to see him didn't matter to me at all.

Whenever I entered the room where Dad was sitting, he would visibly perk up. He always managed a smile, always asked how I was, it was just his way to ensure others around him were happy. We didn't talk about illness or death, but about family. It was obvious to me how ill he was but he never showed it outwardly and I knew exactly what he was doing – showing his daughter she had nothing to fear from her own disease.

The sorrow of seeing my caring dad in so much pain was like

the pall of grey fog that dominated every day in November, never lifting. This gentle, patient man I had known and loved all my life was gradually fading away. He grew more tired, sleeping most of the time. Sometimes he would wake suddenly, disoriented, and it would take him a while to gather the strength to ask where he was.

One night he called out for Suzanne and Rebecca, so the following day Mike drove us all to the house to see him. He was gravely ill and unconscious for most of the time we sat with him. Sitting with the girls on my knee, we watched over him. His eyes opened and focused on us, and he smiled at his two grandchildren before tiredness overtook his body and he fell asleep once more.

I carried on working, visiting my mum and dad as often as possible but I was at work when Mum phoned to tell me that Dad had died and she wanted me and my brothers and sisters by her side. Even though I'd known how ill he was and had watched his physical deterioration, it was still a shock to hear he'd gone. The thought that he would not be suffering pain any more did not give me any solace and I was numbed and tearful.

Several days passed, my sadness unabated. Visiting my parents' house, I explained to Suzanne and Rebecca that their granddad had gone to heaven. Rebecca couldn't understand where he was, looking under the beds to see if he was hiding. It was horrible losing him, such a kind, gentle father. Dad had always taught me that holding on to the good things in life was important. I missed him and ached with grief for him, but knew I would see him again one day.

The following week, I sat at home and hugged Suzanne and Rebecca as we prepared to go to his funeral. Dressed in sombre clothes, I looked down at my skirt and picked at the soft fabric. My thoughts wandered to another day, a different chair, when I was picking at the light towelling dressing gown I was wearing. A nurse had appeared at my bedside.

'You've got a visitor,' she said quietly. 'He's in the day room.'

I walked slowly down the ward, still feeling pain from the night before, and in the day room I saw a familiar face, nearly lost behind a bunch of heavy bloomed flowers. My dad looked tired, a little anxious, but when he saw me his face lit up and his eyes crinkled up at the corners as he smiled.

'Hello there,' he said. 'I brought you these.' Placing the bouquet in my arms, he whispered, 'Well done, Jane.'

The flowers were almost crushed between us as he hugged me. After a few seconds he released me and said: 'I can't stay long, I've got to get back to work.'

'Come and see, Dad,' I said, placing my hand in his as we made our way back to my hospital bed. Dad stood over the cot where a small figure with black hair, some stuck to her head with reddy brown mucus from her arrival late last night, lay fast asleep.

As Dad leant over, her little strawberry-red tongue peeped out of her tiny lips and her heavy lashed eyelids opened. Dad looked across at me, amazed.

'Give Suzanne a cuddle then,' I said. He lifted the white feathery bundle out and held her with the confidence of a dad many times over. Looking down at her, their eyes met and I heard him gently whisper.

'Welcome to the world, little one.'

CHAPTER 4

MIKE

The dining room was transformed, the table fully extended and relocated to the centre of the room. A tablecloth covered plates of sandwiches, crisps and chocolate treats.

'Hi, Mike.' Michelle, Jane's school friend, walked in with a present under her arm. 'Where's the birthday girl?'

'Becca,' I yelled. Suzanne echoed the call upstairs, there were heavy thuds on the stairs followed by the door swinging open and Rebecca bursting through. She ran over to Michelle, who picked her up and gave her a hug. Then came Suzanne, followed by Jane's sister Sara who, at thirteen, was closer in age to Suzanne.

I went through to the living room where Jane's mother and mine were deep in conversation. My dad sat watching the horse racing.

'Do you have a paper, Michael?'

'No.'

'All I can find are these holiday brochures. How many do you need? Is tha' going on holiday?'

'Oh, Jack,' Mum interrupted. 'Don't you listen? They're going to Ireland. Whereabouts again, Michael?'

'Just across the Irish Sea, Mum.'

She laughed. 'No, you daft so and so, the town where you are staying.'

'Cork.'

'You've never said anything, Alice,' said Dad.

'I have.'

'Not to me.' My dad pondered the situation, his mouth looking as though he was going to say something. 'What's possessing you to go over there?'

'It's somewhere different.'

'Nay, I'd've thought you'd have gone somewhere o'er 'ere. Especially with that car of yours. You'd have been better off spending your money on a newer one, not on a holiday.'

'Jack, they need a break,' said Mum. 'They've never had a holiday together as a family.'

Since Jane's diagnosis many people had said we should get away on foreign holidays, spend rather than save. For us the opposite was true. We craved security rather than the desire to travel. A cheap break in Ireland was a compromise – we needed some time, cocooned together as a family.

I moved to sit by the window although the draught from the damp March day made me a little uncomfortable. Rebecca bounded in.

'Look, Grandma,' she said, showing her newly unwrapped present from Michelle.

'How's your new job?' asked Mum.

'I'm enjoying it.'

'I didn't know you'd changed jobs, Michael,' said Anne.

'I'm still at the bank but I've moved to head office to work in the debt recovery department. There's been an increase in their work because of the recession. It's working out quite well as I can give Jane a lift most days which is shortening her day.'

'Party time,' Jane shouted from the kitchen.

'I'll just watch this race, Alice,' said Dad. Mum scowled, before tutting and leaving him to it.

Walking slowly down the steep steps, one hand on the rail, the other carrying Rebecca, I carefully made my way to the vehicle hold of the ferry. Peering down upon the wide collection of vehicles, our red Polo looked tiny at the end of a long line.

Because the boot was full, Jane had strategically packed the remaining luggage around the child seats. Rebecca and Suzanne were strangely thrilled to be sharing the back seat with bags.

We got into the car and waited for the queues of vehicles to start moving forward. Like a series of illuminated dominoes, the tail-lights in front lit up the ferry's sides. They were soon followed by the sound of engine ignitions chugging into life.

'Mum? Dad?' Suzanne piped up from the back. 'Wouldn't it be funny if the car didn't start and we were stuck on the boat?'

'Suzanne, don't be silly,' said Jane.

'It would be funny, wouldn't it, Dad?'

I made sure that both girls were securely in their seats before turning on the ignition. There was a click as the key turned, followed by silence.

'Oh, all rather predictable, funny man,' said Jane, giving me a sly glance. A cheer erupted from the back. The vehicles in front departed allowing daylight to illuminate the hold.

I turned round to Suzanne in the back. 'Jinx.'

'Come on, Mike,' said Jane. 'That's enough. Everyone's gone.'

'I'm serious,' I said as I made a second, third and fourth attempt at turning the ignition. 'The battery must be flat or the starter motor's packed in.'

Within ten minutes we were being towed off the ferry by a forklift truck and parked in the loading area. Three dock workers came over. 'We'll give you a bump off,' said one. They pushed the car and at the first turn of the key it coughed into life. Within minutes we were driving through the deserted streets of Dublin.

Halfway to Cork, we were parked up in a supermarket car park. It was another unplanned stop, thanks to numerous warning lights flashing on and off on the dashboard.

After ninety minutes of being assured by the breakdown insurers that the mechanics were on their way, a tow truck arrived. A faulty alternator was diagnosed. The mechanic advised that he could only put the battery on a fast charge for an hour as the garage was closing 'but that'll be sufficient to get to Cork'.

The weather was foul for the rest of the journey and the car was losing so much power that I had to continually extend the choke to keep the revs up. Like chucking sand from a hot-air balloon, anything that needed the battery was switched off – headlights, radio, heating and, last of all, the windscreen wipers. Arriving at the cottage, the car died with not even enough power left to turn the clock.

After tucking the girls into bed, Jane and I sat together in the lounge downstairs, sipping two whiskies and watching the rain pour outside.

'That bloody car,' sighed Jane, letting out a laugh.

'Oh well, it got us here, just. Maybe Dad's right, we need a younger car. There's barely a month goes by without something going wrong.'

'It was quite spectacular today, though.' Jane leant back and stretched her legs across me. 'Just sit up a bit, Mike, you're making me uncomfortable.' I sat, careful not to spill any whisky. 'At least without the car you won't feel the need to see the whole of Ireland and we can just relax. Ow, bony legs.' Jane laughed, digging her heels in harder. 'I was really pleased with the girls today and how well they behaved when the car broke down.'

'Yeah,' I agreed. 'I know they've said we can't have any more kids, but we couldn't get two better ones.'

'We've been lucky,' said Jane. 'I could have ended up never having children. But, not being able to have any more doesn't mean I don't want more.'

'I know,' I took a sip of Paddy's. 'Fancy another? Whisky, that is.'

'Both. Whisky for now. You can get it, though.'

JANE

As the ache in my left arm increased and its mobility decreased, I found myself, yet again, under investigation. But when the results came back saying that the problems were not related to any spread of my cancer, I was referred to the pain clinic to help me to find a way to cope on a daily basis.

Dr Thaw was a tall man, sandy haired, with a North American twang to his voice. He sat relaxed, ready to listen. On my first appointment, he made me stretch my arms up and out to the side. Rotating my shoulder, he manoeuvred me so I held my hands out with my palms facing upwards and asked me to push up against his hands, which were trying to force mine down. Afterwards, he sat back at his desk and scribbled some notes.

'I think physiotherapy will help,' he said. 'But for immediate relief I suggest steroid injections into the joint.'

I nodded, just glad that there was something he could do to help.

'Right, well it will only take a couple of minutes to set that up.'

'Will it hurt?' I asked.

'It may sting initially. I'll use local anaesthetic but you will have a few aches and pains today. After that you should notice some improvement.'

The nurse was busy setting up the needle and surgical wipes on a trolley and, while I removed my top, Dr Thaw drew up the solution into the syringe.

'Don't be alarmed by the long needle,' he said. 'I need to be able to get into the joint space for this to work.'

He wiped my shoulder with a cold swab, then prodded and poked. I gasped as he pushed the needle in. It prickled uncomfortably and then stung like hell. It was over in seconds and I gulped in air in an effort to breathe normally.

Dr Thaw was right. Within hours I experienced deep cramping aches but, as they diminished, I had relief from the shooting pain in my arm for the first time in weeks.

Over the next few weeks I had more steroid injections and attended physiotherapy regularly. As I practised daily the movements I had been taught to do, and followed the stretching exercises, I began to experience some longer lasting relief from the pain. I resumed swimming regularly and gradually felt as though I was making a return to the fitness I'd had before the operation. More like the Jane of old.

I was becoming increasingly familiar with the X-ray department and, although I had much to learn, I was feeling more confident dealing with patients. I was pleased to be able to take responsibility for the films I produced, discussing them with the doctors where I felt necessary.

It was a very physical job. The equipment was heavy and all day I would be stretching my arms high above my head as I moved it from side to side. Not only that, I also had to push wheelchairs and trolleys into the X-ray room and assist patients to stand or sit where necessary.

It wasn't surprising that, at the end of each day, I was weary. But the physical demands of the job couldn't explain why, every month, I would be brought down by excruciating stomach pains for three or four days. Some months, the pain would be so bad that I ended up in casualty. But even after several gynaecological examinations, ultrasounds and X-rays, the doctors could not find an explanation.

Following another admission to casualty, my gynaecologist decided that he would admit me for some investigations. I was taken to theatre for a laparoscopy. A small opening was made by my belly button and a camera inserted so the surgeons could look round my ovaries and uterus. Again, they could find nothing, but the episodes continued. The aches in my belly and the dull pain in my back preceded each heavy period.

Since they had only started when I had begun to take Tamoxifen, I asked if this might be the cause.

Discussions between my gynaecologist and oncologist continued. They were concerned that my endometrium – the lining of the womb – was slightly thickened. There was a known risk of endometrial cancer associated with Tamoxifen and so eventually I decided to stop taking it.

It was a hard decision to come to, and was made after lengthy discussions with my oncologist and my gynaecologist. The drug gave me the best chance of not having a recurrence of breast cancer. On the other hand, I was a young woman who was regularly spending a lot of time in hospitals, perhaps due to the very drug that was supposed to keep me safe.

Gradually, when I stopped the drug, the problems subsided and I could concentrate on my studies.

MIKE

Jane sat reading, as she had been doing for the last two hours, turning the pages of her book with the regularity of a metronome.

Both girls were in bed asleep and we had a couple of hours to ourselves. Throughout the summer the importance of Jane's final year had become increasingly obvious. Our savings had dwindled, Rebecca's nursery fees had rocketed and Jane's grant would no longer cover them. At the end of the summer, as a result of a changing bank policy, a property management company had taken over our Peterborough house and we were guaranteed only £42,000. We faced a mortgage we couldn't really afford.

Jane also had demons, a fear that upon passing her cancer would return: the ultimate sick joke. She was also worried that there were more newly qualified staff than jobs, and that she would need someone sympathetic to an ex-cancer patient to even get a start. This had destroyed her motivation. I could envisage her years of effort being wasted. I'd thought for a while how to broach the subject – this seemed an opportune moment.

'You really need to pass this year,' I said. 'If you think you're going to fail it would be better to drop out now, as we can't afford for you to fail later.'

Jane looked up, a pained expression on her face. 'What?'

'It's costing us a lot of money, especially savings. I don't think you've been working particularly hard especially seeing as it's your final year.'

She gave me an intense glare, but didn't say a word so I continued. 'We've invested a lot in the last two years, too much for you to blow it now. Apart from losing two years' wages, the kids have missed you being at home.'

It was at that moment that I realized my well-intentioned pep talk had gone awry.

'I can't believe you're saying this,' she said, tears welling in her eyes. 'I work as hard as I can. I can't do any more and all you think about is bloody money. How dare you put all the pressure on me? How would you feel if I started saying you'd better not get made redundant?'

'It's not the—'

'You're so selfish, Mike. And rude. I can't believe you sometimes.'

She got up, throwing her book down on the sofa, and stormed off to the kitchen. I went upstairs to bed, wondering how I could undo some of the damage. As I prepared for bed I thought, on reflection, perhaps my timing was a little off. She had, after all, just finished an eight-hour shift, made dinner for us, done some studying and ironing, while I hadn't done a lot to help. Plus, she'd already mentioned how tired she felt after the journey home from work – yes, I could have handled it better.

On my lunchtime walk through Leeds, I was still feeling guilty as hell. I spotted the aqua colours of the new Pink Floyd boxed CD set, *Shine On*, in a shop window. They were her favourites and although I didn't have the money to spare, I bought it anyway.

As I walked in from work, Jane hugged me tightly. 'I'm sorry,' she whispered.

'Me too,' I said and produced the present from my bag.

'What's this for?' she asked.

'Just because,' I said.

But, in all honesty, I considered it an investment for our future. Something had to stimulate Jane into studying. These CDs would encourage her to get her head down to the books in our uncomfortable compact bedroom. Because there was no way she was putting the damn things on downstairs.

JANE

I checked the mirror and indicated, easing the car kerbside, and gently put more pressure on the brake pedal until the car came to a halt. Pulling on the handbrake, I relaxed slightly, having parked successfully.

'Damn!' The car lurched forward and stalled as I took my foot off the clutch.

'Don't be doing that in the next hour, Jane,' my instructor Dave warned. 'Don't worry, you'll be fine. Remember, no jokes and be polite. Your driving is okay.'

Afterwards I walked back into the test centre. Dave greeted me.

'Well?' he asked.

I nodded and smiled. I had a full driving licence. Mike would be horrified. The last time I'd driven with him had been on our holiday in Scotland, where the car had nearly ended up in someone's front room. He hadn't dared take me out since.

As well as driving lessons, I had been continuing with my studies, which, in my final year, were proving to be intense. As I prepared for my exams, the weekends were spent surrounded by ever-growing piles of books on the bed. I would be tucked under the quilt unable to stretch out my legs for fear of knocking one of the larger piles on to the floor. Occasionally, there would be a soft knock at the door as Mike would bring me a cup of tea.

'How's it going?'

'There's no way I'm going to remember all this,' I'd say. There was so much to take in and I had never even seen half of the equipment I was supposed to describe in detail. The current exam system was archaic and was in the process of being replaced, but we still had to cover areas that were now obsolete, apart from at the most underfunded hospitals. But I was determined to pass. I had to. I could not be a radiographer without my diploma.

More difficult still was finding a job in a highly competitive market. I sent out CVs and visited several local hospitals where they all seemed encouraging, but had no jobs to offer. With so much time and effort invested, and knowing that our financial situation was not improving, I felt pressurized to find work.

I rang X-ray departments around the region on a regular basis and, even if there was only a sniff of a job, I would be on the phone asking for an application form. I filled in countless forms and was called for several interviews, but all to no avail.

I became the recipient of that most depressing of calls – the post-interview apology.

'You were a very good candidate, but we decided to fill the post with a more experienced person,' they would say in the politest of put-downs. No one seemed to want a recently qualified radiographer, when they could have their pick of people with two or three years' experience.

I was finally offered a post by Chris Rhodes at the Leeds General Infirmary, one of only four posts going in the radiography department I was training in. I was overjoyed. This was perfect, just a bus ride away from home, and a department I enjoyed working in and was pleased to be associated with. Now I just needed to know I'd passed the exams.

On results day, I arrived at the hospital to find individual brown envelopes laid out on a table with the students' names written on them. I was so nervous. If I had failed I would have to resit and that was something we could ill-afford. I tore open the envelope and read the first piece of paper. It was an application form for the Society of Radiographers; that could only mean one thing. I took the official results slip out which confirmed I had passed. I was now officially Mrs Jane Tomlinson DCR(R) – holder of a diploma of radiography in diagnostic radiography.

I found a phone and called Mike. I could hear the pride in his voice.

'I knew you would pass. Well done, you deserve it.'

But it wasn't all good news. Although I had passed, I still didn't have the security of a full-time job. I had only been given a six-month contract and knew I would have to work my socks off if it was to turn into something more permanent. Only then would I feel that my three years' hard graft which had taken me away from my family for so long would really have been worthwhile.

MIKE

The revolving door spun me out into the warm June air. Parked cars littered the roads, their drivers ignoring the double yellow lines so they could pick up their passengers and be on their way.

After a hundred yards, Phil and I reached the dual carriageway and found ourselves playing chicken with the speeding cars coming out of Leeds. Nimble-footed, we managed to weave through the traffic, escaping through a small gap in the wall opposite into a small secluded park. It was an oasis of calm, broken only by a group of ten lads half-heartedly playing football. The drone of traffic behind us was silenced temporarily.

'I can't give you a lift home tomorrow,' I said. 'I'll be at hospital with Jane.' Phil's granite face showed no emotion. A big powerful man with a gentle nature, he had worked with me during the dark days in Peterborough, where we were two Yorkshiremen desperate to return home. Our paths had crossed again in the last eighteen months working in the debt recovery department. During that time he'd been an unwilling but unbiased backseat referee as Jane and I had our daily playful bickering in the car.

'Sure,' he said. 'Everything all right?'

'Yes. It's just the three-month check up. I'll be okay to give you a lift in though.'

'Thanks.'

We carried on walking a few paces.

'You'll be quids in now with two wages,' he said.

'Yeah, not that I'll see any of it.'

Once the children were tucked up, though maybe not settled, the night belonged to me and Jane. That evening, after a game of tennis outside, we settled into the living room. Jane read while I watched the news. Turning a page, she looked across to me.

'Is there anything you want to ask tomorrow?'

The days preceding a hospital checkup were always tense. We'd skirt around the subject, especially through the weekend, so as not to spoil it. But there was always an edge to most conversations. After a moment's reflection, I said, 'No.'

'What about the lumps?'

'What do you think?' I moved the *Radio Times* on to the pine table. Outside, I saw Keith's head momentarily appear above the hedge as he pushed his mower. Jane, noticing my loss of concentration, grabbed the remote control.

'Maybe I can have your full attention, Mike?'

Within a second the TV sparked into life again, the result of an existing fault.

'Apparently not.'

'Bloody thing.' Jane's face scowled.

'Look,' I said. 'We always said we'd get them removed when you qualified.' I'd regularly examined Jane's breast and two lumps we had noticed beside her implant had become so familiar, they almost passed unnoticed. 'Let's see what Mr Brennan suggests.'

Next morning at the clinic, although we weren't waiting for scan results, I still felt that sense of anxiety you get when entering the unknown. The waiting was always the worst part and this time – two hours – left my mind as well as my backside numb.

Mr Brennan was his usual self. After some opening pleasantries, he cut to the chase, and asked us about the two lumps. Had they grown? Changed shape or position? After an examination he asked for our opinion. We concurred that although they had not changed in shape or size, they had, nevertheless, been there for nine months and we asked whether, as a precaution, he thought they should be removed.

Mr Brennan agreed. There was an operations list on Friday. Jane's name would be on it.

Silenced by how quickly he had decided to operate, we were soon in the car driving to work. Both of us had assumed she would be placed on the waiting list. Immediately a whole new set of tensions came to the fore, but at least the lumps would be removed and those doubts as to whether it could be cancer would be quashed.

JANE

On the Thursday evening Mike dropped me off at the hospital. With surgery the following day, it meant I only had to be away from work for one day and with the weekend to recover, I could be back in the X-ray department by Monday.

Next morning, I had been awake a few hours when Mr Brennan's senior registrar came round to check the patients on the theatre list. He expressed his surprise at my age and the fact I'd had breast cancer, but I was used to that by now.

He examined the two lumps and nodded sagely.

'I don't think you have anything to worry about,' he said. 'Almost certainly fibro adenomas.'

They were not the words I wanted to hear. My stomach flipped as I recalled the last time I had been told it was only a 'fibro adenoma'. But worse was to come when he said I would have the lumps removed under local, not general, anaesthetic.

'What?' But before I could protest further, he had moved on to the next patient.

Fighting back tears, I tried to quell the rising panic in my body. I knew that a 'local' was the safest and most sensible method of operating, but I was terrified of being awake during theatre. What if they didn't use enough? What would I be able to see? To hear? Would it hurt? The biggest lump was only the size of a pea, so I knew nothing major was going to happen. A part of me was still petrified that I would make a fool of myself.

One of the nurses approached the bed, noticing I was upset. I tried to explain my nervousness, but my sobs stopped me from making any sense and as hot tears ran down my cheeks, I brushed them away, angry with myself that I was behaving like a small child. As a compromise, the nurse suggested I be given some sedatives a couple of hours before the operation. By the time I would be wheeled into theatre, I would be feeling more relaxed.

After the dinginess of the hospital corridors, the sterile white light of the theatre was something of a shock. I screwed up my eyes.

'Don't look so worried,' said one of the nurses. The anaesthetist jabbed the needle into the back of my hand. I felt a slight scratch and the nurse attached a drip to the tube.

'Hello, Jane,' I heard a voice say from the foot of the bed. It was Mr Lansdown, Mr Brennan's registrar. 'Let's see what we're doing today.'

He prodded my breast, feeling for the lumps.

'We'll get you cleaned up and ready,' he said. 'It looks straightforward enough, so it won't take too long. It shouldn't hurt and you must let us know if it does.'

There was no way out. A nurse moved my right arm above my head and put a board under my left shoulder. I focused on the shiny chrome of the theatre lights in a bid to stop the tears rolling down my cheeks. Someone was talking to me. Were they trying to distract me? I couldn't concentrate on what they were saying, so let their words drift through my head without comprehension.

Green surgical sheets were draped over me so that just my breast was exposed. I was unable to see what was going on. A nurse gripped my hand tightly to reassure me.

'Hey, Jane, keep talking to me,' she said. 'We're nearly ready.'

A few seconds later I felt the needle sear into my breast. My toes curled up in pain.

'This might sting a bit,' said the surgeon as my body arched and tensed. He withdrew it slowly and I began to relax, only to stiffen again when I felt another needle go into a different part of my breast. More stinging, more pain.

'You won't feel much more after this,' said the surgeon. 'Just some prodding . . . Keep breathing, you're holding your breath.'

I tried to remember to relax and flashed the nurse a smile. I could see very little, but the weird tugging sensation was disconcerting. I knew they were cutting into my breast and I could smell burning flesh, so I was aware they were using a diathermy, which cauterizes the flesh to stop too much bleeding. The smell was acrid, like when hair is singed, but heavier and more persistent.

When the surgeon placed two bloody bits of gristle into two specimen pots I watched with revulsion. I couldn't get my head around the fact that they had been extracted from my body.

'Nearly finished,' said a voice. 'We're just going to stitch you up.'

I was relieved, pleased I had not shown myself up. When he had finished, I saw a red line on my white breast, two small beads at either end fixing the invisible stitching. The whole experience felt remote from me. I hardly dared to move, fearing I would split my breast apart. The beads seemed too small to stop the wound opening.

I was fit enough to go back to work the following Monday. I avoided lifting heavy equipment all week. I was sent to work in the paediatric unit where the patients were lighter and less lifting was required.

By Friday I was looking forward to the weekend as I was still feeling tender. But when the opportunity to do a Saturday shift came up, I was under no illusions. If I turned it down, the chances of my temporary contract becoming permanent were slim.

When I returned home that evening I was surprised to find a note from the district nurse, who had called round to remove my stitches. When I rang her the next day, she was surprised I'd been working but agreed that the stitches could be taken out at a later date. As the conversation ended, she asked, 'And how are you in yourself, Jane?'

I felt as if I had been struck across the face. What did she know? Had they found something in the lumps and not told me? Although I tried to dismiss the thoughts, fear of what might be kept playing round and round in my head.

Mike didn't help when I relayed the conversation to him that evening. The frown and furrowing of his brows, his insistent questioning all added to my growing apprehension.

He tried to be his usual upbeat self as we sat in the clinic waiting room a few days later. As ever, he failed miserably. His corny jokes and puns were as crass and unnecessary as ever. I didn't need them, but they seemed to keep him happy.

'Well?' he said as I took my seat next to him.

'What?' I replied.

'How far down the pile are you today?'

'How do I know?' I replied. I scanned the tottering pile and thought I could see my notes in the second waiting pile. 'It's going to be a long morning.'

MIKE

My eyes scanned the page, although its contents didn't register. After a half-hearted attempt at reading, I closed my book. Looking enviously at Jane steadily turning the pages of her book, I wondered how she could seem so absorbed as we sat awaiting the pathology results.

'Jane, do you want to come through?' said an auxiliary nurse, clutching a buff folder containing Jane's notes. This was a pleasant surprise. I had envisaged at least an hour's wait, not ten minutes. Taking us into a consulting room, she motioned to two seats and then quickly departed. Within seconds Mr Brennan appeared, followed by what seemed like a junior doctor and some students. Avril, a senior nurse, also arrived. She would be staying, Mr Brennan informed us.

My heart sank as if it were dropping through a crevasse to the bottom of my stomach. I felt a wave of nausea and the desperate need to cry. I looked at Jane, who looked as if her world had collapsed. Her hands were gripping the chair as if seeking some stability in a room that had just tipped on its side. She glanced across at me, forcing a weak smile.

'I'm sorry to tell you that the two lumps were cancerous,' said

Mr Brennan. Jane dissolved into a flood of tears. I got up. I had to get out. I left the room, went out of the hospital and sobbed uncontrollably until my chest heaved, gasping for oxygen. Jane didn't need to see me like this.

Within days, the familiar cycle of scans had commenced. Eager to retain a sense of normality, we continued to work full time. When we explained to Rebecca and Suzanne what had happened, their reaction was to help more than usual and pray.

When we arrived at the hospital just after nine for the scan report, there were few seats left. It was half an hour before Jane and I could sit next to each other. Jane reached across, putting her arm around my neck, kissed my cheek and whispered 'I love you.' My hands were clammy. I could feel the irritability bubbling away inside slowly turn to frustration. Waiting, waiting and waiting. Uncomfortable seats, no leg room, too hot, too cold.

'Mike, sit still,' said Jane. 'Are you all right?'

'Just scared.'

'Me too.'

Forty-five minutes later, Jane's name was called.

'Here.' Jane rose slowly.

Mr Brennan was waiting for us.

'Good news, Jane, everything is clear,' he said. I managed a smile while Jane sat showing no emotion.

'Thank you.' She took a deep breath. I shut my eyes and let my head drop.

As a precaution, however, we were told Jane should have some chemotherapy and radiotherapy.

'You need to be seen by Professor Joslin in Oncology about the chemotherapy,' Mr Brennan informed us. 'He'll liaise with Dr Roberts about the radiotherapy. You'll be in good hands. Make yourself an appointment to see me in three months.'

Leaving the room, I felt washed out and relieved. But I felt no obvious sense of joy; there was no cheering, just quiet acknowledgement that, for today at least, there was no death sentence. Every ounce of nervous energy had been spent and I think we were both conscious that any joy might be temporary. There was also a sense of abandonment; I felt like we were being cast adrift from a ship and now we were waiting for another vessel to come along and assist. Mr Brennan had taken us as far as he could.

Within a week, we'd seen both Professor Joslin and Dr Roberts. Jane would have three sessions of chemotherapy at three weekly intervals, two weeks rest, followed by four weeks of radiotherapy, then a final three chemotherapy sessions. In the two weeks' rest, they both felt a holiday might be a good thing.

At work, only my close colleagues were aware of our situation. Phil and Mike were fantastically supportive, ensuring my first responsibility was at home. It was a surprise, therefore, to be summoned into a meeting with them early one Monday morning. Having no time to prepare meant I had no time to be anxious, although as soon as I stepped into the room, I had serious misgivings.

Phil started. 'Mike and I have been thinking hard about how best to manage your needs to be at home with Jane, while she has chemotherapy, against our needs in the department.'

Where was this going, I wondered.

'You've clearly got a talent for IT, a good knowledge of recovery work and we thought we could marry the two. There's a new laptop coming. You could have six months away from normal duties to build us a recoveries database.'

I sat, silently, staring at them.

'It's a real opportunity,' said Mike. 'A chance to prove yourself. I can't promise you an upgrade, but if you do a good job there is a possibility.'

'I don't know anything about IT,' I said.

'You know more than the rest of us,' Phil said.

'Is that meant to make me feel better?' I smiled.

'You converted the provision spreadsheet from Lotus 123 to Excel,' Phil pointed out.

'That was an accident.'

'Yes, but no one else knew what to do. You have a flair for it. We'll give you every assistance, a course, books, the job lot.'

I have a flair for resting in bed, I thought. How about a sabbatical?

At home, Jane was as pragmatic as ever. Would I enjoy the challenge? It was another skill. I'd be at home with her when she needed me and my bosses would be happy. It soon became clear that I didn't have much of a choice.

JANE

My appointment for the first lot of chemotherapy was set for Monday. I tried to feel positive about it, but it was strange to think that, although I felt well now, the thing that was going to make me better in the long term was going to make me feel ill. It had been a hard decision to make. Although I could have refused treatment, I knew I was being offered the best chance of living a life without the cancer hanging over me. But I was very scared as to how I would cope.

The following Monday, Mike and I drove to Cookridge. I'd worked there during my training so I was familiar with the hospital, but still needed directions to the outpatients chemotherapy department.

'Can I help you?' asked the woman behind the reception desk.

'I'm here for my chemotherapy,' I said, passing her my letter.

'Have you had your bloods taken?'

'No, not yet.'

As my blood was analysed, I sat pressing the small round of sticking plaster over the tiny puncture. Mike sat in silence next to me in the small haematology waiting area. His glances at his watch became more frequent, but before he could voice any complaint the nurse returned with my results.

'Right,' he said. 'We'll be seeing you in three weeks, Jane. Take it easy.'

Mike and I returned slowly to the outpatients clinic. It was only a short walk but as we approached the grey building, I began to shake, my knees feeling like they could give way with every step. I heard Mike saying something, but his voice was distant. I was imagining the sickness and tiredness I might feel just hours from now.

In hospitals, time seems to take on a different quality; life seems to play out at a much slower pace. Although there is a diversity of waiting areas, they all seem to be themed around the delay of the patient's time. I looked around this new holding space, noticing the carefully chosen colour scheme, the way the light caught the notice board. Even as my mind wandered, I listened, leaning forward ready to move once I heard my name, aware of my eagerness to be called even as my thoughts drifted haphazardly.

Finally it was my turn. I took my seat near the window. At my side was a metal trolley loaded with several syringes, some small, some large. They were full of liquids, a couple clear, one yellow, another red.

'Hi, I'm Mary,' said the nurse. I drew my eyes away from the trolley, trying not to worry about its contents. 'I'm going to give you your chemotherapy. I'll tell you what I'm doing and what the drugs are as we go along. Okay?'

My stomach clenched, my mouth was dry. I nodded.

'You might feel sick but that will only last a day or so. We'll give you some anti-sickness stuff now and some to take home.'

I was desperate to take on board what she was telling me, to store it in my memory in case it was important. But all I could think about was how ill I was going to be. Still shaking, I put out my arm and Mary gently took my hand and held it.

'It won't be too bad,' she smiled, a practised smile, a smile that makes you think it might just be all okay. She tightened a rubber tourniquet around my arm and felt for veins on the top of my hand. I could feel her wipe a surgical swab across my skin and then felt a tiny stab as the needle went in. I watched her as she drew the needle partly back, leaving the tube in my hand. A small droplet of blood appeared on my hand as she screwed a cap into place.

'That's in now,' she said. 'I'll just secure it into place.'

A drip was attached to the end.

'Relax,' she said. 'Take a few deep breaths.'

I had been holding my breath, my chest was tense and still with fear. I imagined myself diving into a cool blue pool of water, swimming along with smooth, clean strokes. With each stroke my lungs expanded more fully, my breathing gained its natural rhythm, calmer and less laboured.

'That's better.' Mary was holding another small syringe. 'Now, this will make your bottom prickle.'

It did. And my head too, scratchy, my scalp pinpricked with minute concentrations of tightness, the crown smarting with pain. It lasted only a minute or so and after I'd finished squirming, Mary was ready with the next syringe.

Some drugs went in easily. I felt a grey white metallic astringency, deep down my throat, the same smell, bitter, in my nose. I could almost chew the strangeness, an experience so strong I could almost feel it as part of my face. When she came to a large red syringe, my fingers straightened and the muscles contracted as the liquid entered my veins. The sensation spread slowly, hardening my arm up to the elbow. My muscles carried on contracting. The spasm in my arm made me flinch away from the hands administering the toxicant.

'Ouch, that hurts.' The words seemed a feeble explanation of the harsh thrill of pain.

Mary nodded. 'I'll just ease off for a bit.' She opened the drip gauge fully to let a saline solution through, which eased the pain and stilled the cramps. After a few seconds, I was ready for her to continue. She pushed some more liquid out of the syringe. Again my arm contracted with exquisite cramps and she had to flush more saline through the drip.

'We'll take it really slowly,' she said.

By the time all the drugs were administered the clock had moved on nearly an hour and I felt vague, woolly-headed and my limbs were heavy with the turpitude of treatment. I was scared of swallowing, fearing I would gag and choke on my saliva. I tried sucking on a clear mint, the hard sweetness bringing relief from the nausea that was waiting edgily each time I drew a breath. My sense of smell was so heightened I could smell the dressing on the back of my hand. I thrust it into my pocket, trying to avoid the faint odour of the hospital as we stepped outside.

At home, Mike offered me a drink, but the thought of anything in my mouth made the bile rise in my throat.

'No, I . . .' I hesitated. I couldn't think of any words to describe how I was feeling. 'I'm fine, thanks.'

I slumped on the bed and lay down, my shoes still on. Pulling the covers loosely over me, the dip in the bed held me in sheeted familiar comfort. My body was heavy, listless and the colours in my bedroom seemed muted, almost grey. I shut my eyes.

I slept heavily that night, but woke early, desperate for a wee. As I lay in the darkness, I wondered what effect getting out of bed would have on me. Several minutes passed, but my bladder wouldn't allow me to wait and I slowly eased myself up and traipsed through to the bathroom. When I returned, Mike was awake.

'How are you feeling?' he asked as I climbed back into bed. Suddenly, my stomach rolled, I dashed out of the bedroom and retched violently, reaching the toilet just in time. I was sick, my body convulsing in waves to rid itself of the unwanted toxins. Each time I relaxed and breathed without panting, another wave of sickness rose up deep from my belly until I was retching noisily and emptily.

After several minutes, I returned to bed but no sooner had I sat down on the mattress than I was making a second dash to the bathroom. Again and again, the spasms overtook me and I sat clutching my aching stomach as I crouched by the toilet. This time the retching wouldn't stop and tears pricked my eyes. My face was wet with perspiration, my nose was running. Distressed, I felt panicked as waves of nausea rolled over and over and bitter acid rose in my throat again and again.

MIKE

Sitting at the dining table, the laptop had been staring at me, taunting me all morning. I was not going to admit defeat. I pressed the green button, powering up a familiar whir. I gazed, hypnotized by the display for so long that my glare was only broken when the computer switched into screensaver mode.

I tapped the keyboard, letting the blue screen flash up again and wondered how durable a laptop was. I put my head in my hands. I'd go into work tomorrow and admit there was a problem.

I got up and went to the living room, where I hunted for the *Radio Times*, but there was no way my conscience would permit me to watch television. I returned to the dining room and fired up the laptop again. Thumbing through the pages of the two database manuals that came with the software, the feel and smell of the pristine books was satisfying. Each contained over four hundred pages of long, complicated instructions and jargon. Opening the first, I turned to the contents page. Feeling daunted, I closed my eyes, then the book.

As I waited for the machine to load up, I heard a floorboard creak upstairs. It was followed by a painful-sounding retch into the echoes of the toilet bowl.

Sprinting up the stairs three at a time, I reached the top just in time to see Jane, who was crouching over the toilet, flick the bathroom door shut with her left heel. I stood motionless for a second, unwilling to move away.

'Are you okay?' I asked eventually. 'Have you taken your anti-sickness stuff?'

'No.' I waited. 'Of course I've taken it, although it's just reappeared.'

'Can you take another?'

Jane continued to vomit. I'd been so careful after the chemotherapy, aware that every smell, noise or distraction could make her sick. It was obvious she needed some space so I crept back downstairs. I listened for any movement upstairs but heard nothing, so after thirty minutes or so returned to the landing.

'Jane, are you okay?'

'I feel desperately unwell. I can't move without feeling sick. It shouldn't be like this.'

'Should we ring the hospital?'

'No, leave it a while.'

'Can I get anything? Rub your back?'

'No. Just leave me alone, can you?'

I went to our bedroom and picked up a glass of water. The hospital had said Jane might be a little sick – 'some patients were'. I wondered how long someone could be sick without suffering from dehydration. I thought about phoning Jane's mum or her sister Anne – both of whom were trained nurses – but decided it would be better to wait.

'Mike! Mike!'

I sprinted upstairs using the banister as leverage for extra momentum.

'Jane?'

'What should we do? I'm beginning to feel faint.'

'I'll phone Cookridge. Do you have the number?'

'On my bedside table.'

I fumbled around on the table until I found it. The connection seemed to take an inordinate amount of time.

'Hi, er, Jane Tomlinson had her first chemotherapy yesterday and she's still being very sick.'

'How long has she been sick for?'

'Since yesterday, but it's worse today. She's feeling faint now.'

'You really need to bring her here straightaway. Can you drive or would you like me to send an ambulance?'

'I'll drive. Thank you.'

I knew I could be a fair way to the hospital before the ambulance had even arrived. I'd also be in control. Trying not to alarm Jane, I suggested we made a move. She was unsteady on her feet, hair dishevelled, her T-shirt covered in water splashes. I moved forwards to help her.

'Don't touch me, Mike,' she said quietly.

At Cookridge, we were told that, although it was rare, some patients could be affected like this. Because of the expense, a more powerful anti-sickness tablet was not prescribed until the patient had suffered a bout of nausea like Jane's. Jane was given a prescription immediately.

Back home, in the early afternoon, Jane disappeared to bed. As well as destroying the cancerous cells, the chemotherapy was also destroying her good cells which, naturally, made her extremely tired.

After three days of doing little other than sleep and eat, however, she was back at work, forced into a premature return thanks to her contract. She was barely able to function at a basic level and, by the time I met her at the car park at five fifteen that afternoon, she looked like a ghost. She went straight to bed for a rest. As I put the kids to bed, we popped our heads around the door to say goodnight. There had been no sound, no indication of life, for over two hours and, as our eyes were unadjusted to the darkness, we could see no trace of her.

'She's not here. Where's Mum?' Suzanne shouted, tightening her grip on my right hand.

A feeble 'Here' came from the bed.

Barely discernible from an extra fold in the quilt, Jane lay in a small bundle, curled up in the foetal position. Reluctant to disturb her, the girls edged quietly to the side of the bed.

'Are you all right, Mum?' asked Suzanne softly.

'Yes, I'm fine. Have you had tea?'

Rebecca piped up. 'It was rubbish, Mum. The fish fingers were burnt on the outside and frozen on the inside.'

'We told Dad, but he wouldn't believe us,' added Suzanne. 'He was going to make us eat them. He said we were being stupid.'

'Is that right, Mike?'

'Don't believe everything, they're exaggerating,' I said, my hands on their shoulders trying to manoeuvre them out of the room.

Suzanne was indignant. 'No, we weren't. Becca tried to cut hers and the knife went off her plate. They were ice.'

'And burnt,' said Rebecca.

'He could have killed us by food poisoning, Mum,' said Suzanne.

'Disgusting. They were, Mum.' Rebecca again.

From the bed, Jane inched towards them, giving each a kiss

and a hug. 'I'll get up and get some tea. Is the kitchen tidy?' she asked.

'He made us do all the washing-up,' said Rebecca. 'It's not fair when you're ill. We do everything.'

'Is that right?'

I delayed a couple of seconds before answering. 'Well, there may be some elements that are close to the truth but, as you know, it is never that simple.'

Suzanne butted in. 'All he's been doing is sitting down with his laptop, typing.'

'Dad's got a lot of work to do. Suzanne, you do need to help out, you are eight,' said Jane.

I flashed a smug smile and Suzanne looked away in disgust. We headed into their bedroom where Rebecca dived on to the bottom bunk.

'When can I have the top one?'

'Never!' As Suzanne climbed the ladder to her bed she flicked her left foot out to kick Rebecca.

'Get lost, Suzanne!'

The light in the room was in the shape of a hot air balloon, the basket holding a small teddy bear peering over the side. I swung it like a pendulum while we recited prayers.

JANE

The sickness physically exhausted me, but having been taken on by work under a temporary contract, I knew I needed to get back as soon as possible. By Thursday, the nausea had subsided sufficiently to allow me to drag myself into work. Tiredness drove me to bed as soon as I had eaten, leaving Mike to supervise the children.

By the weekend I was beginning to feel like the bedroom walls were pressing in. I was weak and weary, but desperate to get out of the house so I decided to pack up a picnic and head out for the day. The girls had new lunch boxes for school and jumped up and down with excitement when I suggested they could try them out. I packed sandwiches, crisps and orange juice and we drove to the other side of Leeds to Kirkstall Abbey.

The children ran ahead towards the sandstone ruin, losing themselves in the towering weeds that grew abundantly around the stones. I shuffled along behind, holding Mike's hand, feeling like some geriatric relative being escorted on a day out.

I watched as Suzanne and Rebecca screamed and laughed, chasing each other through the grass. We'd only been there a few minutes but already I was tired. Mike and I sat for a while, admiring the views of lavender and rosemary in the knot garden.

'Thanks for bringing us,' I said. 'It's good to be out of the house.'

'We ought to get out more often,' said Mike.

'I know, I feel as if I'm resting to make sure I'm fit for work. The people who miss out are the people who matter most.'

'We'll just have to make more of an effort.' He reached for my hand. 'I need to do more round the house to help. Give you a chance to rest and spend time with the kids.'

On the journey home, I slumped into the passenger seat. I was shaking with fatigue. I let my head fall back against the head-rest, shutting my eyes, then jerking awake as we pulled into the drive. Mike glanced at me.

'Go and have a lie down for an hour.'

'The washing needs bringing in,' I said.

'Don't worry about it. I said I needed to do more round the house, and I meant it.'

'Thanks.'

I headed for the stairs to rest for a couple of hours.

The weekend passed quickly. Setting off for work on Monday, I wondered how I would get through the whole week. Mike and the children helped out at home: Rebecca, standing on a kitchen chair, her tongue caught between her teeth, concentrating, as she wiped the pots clean in the sink, Suzanne dancing around the kitchen, humming as she dried the plates and cups, Mike in the role he played best, sitting supervising them.

One evening he even pulled out the ironing board and, following his mum's instructions, managed to work his way through most of the pile of ironing.

Dragging myself through the next couple of weeks, I gradually began to feel less tired. The three weeks passed quickly and it was time for my second chemotherapy appointment. It followed the same routine – travelling to the hospital feeling relatively fit and healthy and leaving three hours later feeling sick, grey faced, arm sore from the injections.

The doctor prescribed stronger anti-emetic drugs which meant I didn't vomit, but I still couldn't rid myself of the horrid metallic taste which made eating hard to contemplate. Sucking ice cubes satisfied my thirst and stopped me feeling sick, although the sound as I crunched them drove Mike to distraction. My lips were often chapped and sore, the chemotherapy made my mouth uncomfortable, and my eyes felt gritty all the time.

After three sessions of chemotherapy, I was given a break before I was due to start radiotherapy in November. We booked our first trip abroad – a last minute holiday to Crete. Although it was the end of the season we arrived during a heatwave. Suzanne and Rebecca delighted in playing on the narrow strip of white sand, running in and out of the crashing waves.

CHAPTER 5

JANE

Back in England, driving through my third set of red lights, I pulled into the side of the road and stopped the car. I took deep, long breaths to calm my nerves and stop myself from shaking. I wished someone had offered to drive me, but miles from home and still three miles from the hospital I had no option but to try to compose myself for the rest of the journey. 'Radiotherapy can't be any worse than chemo,' I chided myself, as I refastened my seat belt and turned the key in the ignition.

At the hospital, when my name was called, I was led through to see a doctor who told me what the treatment entailed and what the possible side effects were. She told me I would have twenty sessions, over the next four weeks.

'It will cause some reddening and soreness on the skin,' she said. 'But we'll give you some cream for that. You won't be able to wash while you're undergoing treatment because this can increase the redness, and can cause you to peel. We'll keep an eye on you, but hopefully the worst it will be will be like bad sunburn.'

I nodded my understanding. My knowledge of radiotherapy was scant, but I recalled the words 'damp desquamation' from past lectures and shuddered at the descriptive term.

'Be careful not to use deodorant as well,' she said. 'The metal ingredients could intensify the effect of the X-rays and make the burns worse. Do you understand?'

'Yes,' I said and she handed me a consent form to sign.

The radiographer led me down a corridor into a large room. There was an X-ray table in the middle, and I could see other members of staff through the long window on one wall. Another radiographer joined us in the room, she checked a few details, then asked me to take off my top and lie down on the table, describing what she was doing and telling me what was going on at every stage.

Placing my arm above my head, she adjusted the shutters of the machine until it covered the area of my breast to be irradiated. With a permanent marker pen she began to draw on my skin. I could hear her calling out figures; her colleague wrote them down on the chart.

'Be careful not to wash this off,' she said, having drawn purple marks on my breast crisscrossing the corners, delineating the area to be treated. 'Has Dr Roberts explained you can't wash or wear deodorant for four weeks?'

'Yes, she's gone through all of that with me. I think that's what is worrying me most. The idea of not being able to clean under my arm for a month is repulsive.'

'There's not a lot you can do. Some people find that dusting themselves with baby powder helps them to feel less stale. Make sure you've got some soft tops to wear just in case you do get a bit sore, they'll be more comfortable.'

When they had finished marking out the areas, I was free to go. I would return a few days later for the X-ray treatment itself.

On my drive home I passed a discount clothing store, and stopped to buy several large cotton T-shirts. I parked at Rothwell and called in at the chemist to find a soft powder brush and some talc to keep me dry.

The sessions continued every work day for four weeks. During some treatments I found I could compose myself by visualizing walking down steep stone steps, set into a cave wall. One step, two steps, three steps. I imagined running my fingers across the rough sides of the cavern towards a pool of water that glistened below. If I listened carefully I could even hear droplets of water running down the walls into the green water below. Sometimes I could make my way down the ten hewn steps, feeling the rough stone, cool beneath me feet. Immersing myself in the experience I found I could take time to look around me. It was relaxing and would take my mind off what was going on above me.

I would open my eyes, my concentration broken, when the noise of the machine stopped. In stupefied torpor I would climb from the table with the help of the radiographers, feeling as if I'd slept heavily.

I'd gone in to work for the first week of sessions but when my oncologist found out she instructed me to take some sick leave. As the treatments passed I found myself tiring, and was glad of the time away from work to rest.

After twenty sessions, I was expecting to be free of my daily drive to Cookridge. But my joy was short-lived – another five sessions on a different machine were prescribed to mop up any rogue cells from the skin of my breast, as the tumours had involved some of my epidermal tissue.

Eventually my radiotherapy was over. Once the reddening had faded I was able to wash again. The bliss of sitting in a bath able to soap the whole of my body for the first time in over six weeks was an occasion worth celebrating. Christmas festivities were upon us and I wanted to make the most of a final chance to feel well before my last chemotherapy sessions. They would fall just after Christmas which meant I would be able to enjoy some time with Mike and the girls without feeling too ill.

As soon as New Year arrived I was straight back to the hospital for my last three treatments of chemotherapy. I found it incredibly hard to drag myself to Cookridge for my final session. Although it meant I would soon be able to plan my life without having to think about the three-week cycle, I sat in the queue for bloods with a feeling of dread.

'You again, Jane!' Rob the phlebotamist seated me and drew my blood. I waited impatiently for the results to take back to outpatients.

'Your white cells are a bit low,' he said.

'What does that mean?'

'You might not get your chemo.'

Damn. Bugger. Bugger. I turned my head away from him, petulant at the possible delay. I should have been feeling relief at the thought of a week's respite but I wanted it over. I waited again to see the doctor.

'We can do this treatment today or we can wait until next week.'

'It's my thirtieth birthday next week.' I could hear the childish whine in my voice. 'I don't want to feel sick on my birthday.'

'How are you feeling?' she asked, beginning to examine me, feeling my neck, listening to my chest.

'I'm fine. Tired but looking forward to this all being over.'

'I think you're well enough to have the chemo, the white cell count is a little bit low, but as it is your last treatment you should be okay.'

She signed my prescription and I returned to the waiting room until my drugs came from the pharmacy.

Mary finished pushing the last lot of toxins into my veins.

'Don't take this the wrong way,' I said, 'but I hope we don't meet again.'

'Me too,' she smiled. 'But you know where we are if you need anything.'

Later in the afternoon, I was resting at home when there was a knock at the door. I opened it to find a woman holding a small basket of freesias. The yellow buds were just beginning to open and the fragrance carried sweetly to my nose as I brought them through to the living room.

I read the card. They were from Mike.

'Thank you,' I beamed, kissing him on the cheek. 'That must be the first time you've bought me flowers on Valentine's Day.'

'Don't go expecting them every year,' he said.

It seemed to take months for the weariness caused by the chemotherapy to subside but gradually I began to feel more like my old self. As my energy slowly returned, I was able to focus more on my work at the hospital, while at home I finally felt able to be more of a mum again to Suzanne and Rebecca.

After months of short-term temporary contracts I got a permanent paediatric job at the hospital. I had never considered working with children but I wanted the job so much I studied hard for the interview. It took several days for them to decide, and when they told me I'd been appointed I was overjoyed. At last, all the years of studying and training had paid off and someone was willing to give me a chance.

My first few weeks on the job were terribly nerve-racking, the children seeming to sense my inexperience. The more nervous I felt, the more the children struggled and the more effort it took to get everything just right. However, I was a keen observer, everyone had their own methods to ensure the cooperation of the children and I soon developed mine.

Suzanne and Rebecca were now nine and six; they seemed to have grown up so quickly during the last year. Rebecca had finished her first year at primary school and Suzanne was settling into her junior school.

One night, after tucking them into bed, I returned upstairs to watch them, their small blonde heads barely visible above their quilts. My body felt empty. I knew after everything we'd been through I had so much to be thankful for, yet I longed for another child. I'd never considered that Rebecca would be the youngest of two, until my surgery.

I had occasionally broached the subject with Mr Brennan but his response had always been negative. He had been forthright with me, he was fearful that the huge boost in my oestrogen levels could have a catastrophic effect on my body. I could end up with an aggressive tumour that could not be treated successfully.

At the end of another checkup when Mr Brennan had no specific concerns about my health, I asked about further children. His reply was unexpected and quite different from the response I usually received. The latest research showed that a pregnancy would make no difference to the outcome of my disease. There were still very few young women with breast cancer, so very few cases of women going through pregnancy.

Mike was reluctant to be drawn into talk about further family. There were few avenues of advice and this left me feeling very isolated. It wasn't that he didn't want more children, more that he was frightened of the risk I would be taking. As Mike slept at peace beside me I could feel the sense of loss building tangibly inside me.

Unable to sleep, I crept downstairs, turned on a lamp and sat silently on the sofa, tucking my legs underneath my chin. This wasn't fair. My cancer had put me and my family through so much pain and yet still it continued to hurt us. Tears prickled my eyes. How dare it affect my future? I could cope with the surgery, the treatments, but I ached to hold another child of ours in my arms.

I sat in the gloom of the living room, tears of anger and self-pity rolling down my face. I moaned out, allowing myself to sob, letting the frustration and anger I had been bottling up for months pour out. Mike stood at the door to the room, and seeing my distress held me. My tears finally made him understand how much this mattered to me.

Mike was always saying that our house would be too small for further family but even this obstacle was removed. We had advertised the house in the local paper on a Friday night. By Saturday it looked like we had a sale.

As the furniture was cleared, it was strange how the acoustics altered around the house. The voices and heavy footsteps of the three removal men seemed to bounce off the walls.

'Excuse me, love, the phone's ringing,' one of the removal men called upstairs, where I was on my hands and knees scrubbing a grimy skirting board. Dashing downstairs, I picked up the receiver and answered breathlessly.

'Hello?'

'Everyone keeps asking me why I'm not at home to help you— What?' I could hear someone calling to him. 'Ha ha. Phil says he knows why I'm here, he reckons I'd be about as much use as a chocolate teapot to you.' I laughed and could hear other people laughing at Mike from down the phone.

'I'll have to go, there's still loads to do,' I said as I ran my hand through my unruly hair.

'I'll ring again later,' he said before putting the phone down.

Unwinding the cord of the Hoover, I noticed the scuff marks and the scribbled heights on the door jamb – no dates, just initials – where the girls had been measured. I could see Rebecca as she wriggled.

'Keep still just for a moment,' I said, weighing her head down with a heavy book, and sketching a line.

'Have I grown?' Pink cheeked like a fine china doll, her blue eyes looked up at me.

'Yes, loads. Hey you're cheating.' She was standing on tip toes trying to make herself taller. We laughed as I pressed down on her head and she shrank an inch as her heels slid to meet the floor.

My priority, once we were in the new house, was to get the bedding out so the girls would be able to sleep that evening. They had separate bedrooms, their own spaces, I wondered who would sleep where. I made a decision; making up their beds to stop any arguments, I chose their rooms.

The living room seemed oppressively blue, blue carpet, blue curtains, blue everything. The dining room with its peach and green decor was not to my taste either but we had stretched our budget over its limit and decorating would have to wait a while.

I noticed headlights flash up the drive: it was mum with the girls. As they raced through the door they were unusually quiet, a little dazed by their new surroundings.

'I won't stop long,' said Mum, handing me an envelope. I opened the card and placed it on the windowsill in the kitchen. I showed Mum round our new house. 'It's certainly big enough,' she said. 'I hope it will be a happy home.'

The girls went upstairs to compare rooms. I could hear them

deciding whose was biggest. Mike arrived just as Mum was leaving.

'Do you need any help?' he asked and I raised my eyebrows.

'What, now?' I said.

'So, what's for tea?'

He ducked quickly, avoiding my punch and laughed.

'Joke! Joke! I'll go to Peggoty's for fish and chips.'

That night we ate fish and chips from the paper at the dining room table, surrounded by boxes. When the girls finally went to bed, I left Mike to unravel the wires for the television and video, while I ran myself a hot bath.

Soaking in the warm water, I stretched my aching limbs. It had been a long, tiring day but I was pleased with the progress and was relieved we were finally here. I noticed the bathroom tiles. Yet more blue, Ah well, they would have to do. I could hear Mike, he was swearing at the television. I knew it had been a wise decision to let him go to work.

MIKE

Since moving in November, there had been nothing further to stop Jane and I from proceeding with the decision to have another child. I had evaded the subject successfully for five months. Throughout the winter I'd been increasingly unhappy with the new house. There was nothing intrinsically wrong with it, it was just an irrational dislike.

Jane was happy to drift through to spring without discussing it, but by March she started pushing for a decision. We sat down to talk about when to start trying. Because of the financial implications, it was fundamental that the baby was due as close to 31 August as possible – but not after it. With only one school intake per year for children who will be five during that academic year, a child born on or before 31 August would start a full year before one born on 1 September. This could mean an extra year in pre-school childcare which could cost us up to £5,000. So we agreed to start trying in June.

Although Jane was not fully convinced, it brought me a further three-month delay in making a decision. But by June, I'd backed myself into a corner. Jane wanted to start trying for a family now while I was struggling for a reason for further postponement.

We knew Jane's cancer could be triggered by hormonal changes, indeed some of her treatments controlled those very fluctuations and, previously, had temporarily put her through the menopause. We knew if Jane got pregnant there would be a number of hormonal changes. Would these changes prove a catalyst for the cancer to return?

No one could give us a definitive answer. Mr Brennan knew of only one woman who had given birth after a mastectomy but she had already been pregnant when she was diagnosed. Jane's situation was entirely different. Research from the United States, Mr Brennan advised, showed that it had made no difference. I was concerned about the level of research, though, as there couldn't have been an extensive amount of cases. Jane however, was reassured.

I suppose my underlying question was: who wanted this baby? Was it just Jane? Did I want another child? Was my conviction strong enough? Was Jane just being complicit with my wishes? Did I have the right to refuse if that's what she so desperately wanted? Or did Jane have the right to go against my wishes? It was an impossibly difficult dilemma and, to her credit, Jane understood when I asked for another three weeks at the start of June.

Summer arrived and so did Euro '96. I had tickets for each round. But when I should have been enjoying some of the best football matches in the world, my thoughts were preoccupied with sex: how to avoid it.

It all came to a head one evening.

'I can't imagine anything but the four of us,' I said, climbing into bed next to her. It was an off-the-cuff remark after a very pleasant family evening. I'd not meant anything by it.

'Not something we'll have to worry about is it?' she replied tersely.

'What's that supposed to mean?'

'Nothing.'

'No,' I said, turning to face her. 'Say what you mean.'

She lay on her back, staring at the ceiling but didn't say a word. Knowing that she couldn't leave it alone I waited a couple of minutes before she said in clipped tones, 'If you don't want to have any more children say so. You've shown absolutely no inclination towards having another baby. In fact, Mike, I'd say you've made every excuse possible to delay. Is it me? Us?' she asked. I let out a large sigh.

'No,' I said. 'Nothing like that.'

'Well, what? Because I'm puzzled. You always said you wanted more family.'

I turned on to my side so my back was next to her. 'You wouldn't understand,' I said.

'Try me.'

I wished for darkness, an extra blanket of protection.

'Michael, I think I deserve an explanation.'

I didn't know where to begin. What was there to say? That I didn't fancy playing Russian roulette with my sperm?

'Well . . .' She seemed on the verge of tears.

'What?'

'Please, Michael, we need to talk.'

I moved to the wall and switched off the light.

'Oh well that's big,' she snapped.

'Look, I can't do this with the light on,' I said.

'Nothing new there then.'

'I'm finding this whole situation extremely difficult,' I began. 'I feel like I've got a loaded gun and that I'm going to be the one responsible for killing the person I love the most. Do you understand? I can't go through with it.'

'Don't you want a baby?'

'You're not listening,' I said. 'I don't want a baby if that means losing you. Rebecca and Suzanne would lose their mum. I can't ask you to do this, the risks are too great.'

'You're not asking me. If I didn't want more family I wouldn't have any. You heard what Mr Brennan said about the research – it won't make any difference.'

'You don't know that. They've already changed their mind once and there are no published cases in this country. So no one really knows.'

'Michael. I want a child more than anything in the world. It's the only thing I want. The risk is mine, I want to take it. If I thought I'd die and that Suzanne and Rebecca would lose me I wouldn't even think about it. But this is so important to me.'

'I understand. Really, I do. But it's not easy. I don't want to be complicit in you dying. I couldn't live with myself or face the children if I forced you in to having a child and you died.'

Jane reached across and hugged me. I could feel that her face was damp with tears. I had never seen her so passionate about anything. I knew she was desperate for another baby but I had to be certain that it was what *she* wanted, not something she was doing because she thought it would make me happy. For five minutes we lay in the bed, our arms and legs entwined, silent apart from the rustling of bedclothes. It was Jane who broke the silence.

'I love you, Mike,' she said. 'Please let's have a baby.' As if reading my thoughts she said: 'It's not for you. It's for both of us. It's my choice. Surely I have got the right to decide for myself. I wouldn't be complete otherwise.'

I acquiesced, never enthusiastic but went through the motions nevertheless. By doing so I fulfilled my obligations to Jane, while being able to live with myself. Ultimately the decision to have a child wasn't mine. I thought I wanted more children, but I couldn't face losing Jane in the process.

JANE

As the days started to shorten and the children settled back into school, I began to feel a familiar sickness, nausea that persisted day and night. The smell of my shampoo would make me retch as I washed my hair, the bitter taste of coffee wouldn't leave my mouth and even the smallest amount of tea was enough to make me nauseous. I began to feel incredibly tired, worn out after only a few hours at work and strangely, despite the sickness, I was ravenous for food. I was delighted. I knew what it meant – I was pregnant.

After the first two months, we decided to tell the girls.

'We've got some news for you,' said Mike. 'Mum's pregnant. You're going to have a little brother or sister.'

They looked at each other, shocked and silent, before the colour drained from Rebecca's cheeks and she started to cry.

'What's wrong?' I asked.

'You won't die, will you?' she sobbed and I pulled her on to my knee, shaking my head.

'No,' I said, stroking her arm to comfort her. 'The doctors say it's okay. The baby's fine and I'm okay. It's why I've not been feeling very well. This little one has been making me tired, just like you two did.'

Suzanne sat silently, studying her sister's reaction to the news.

'When is it due? Where is it going to sleep?' She had lots of questions and I answered them one by one.

'I'll need lots of help from both of you,' I explained. 'We've got a date for the beginning of May and we'll put a cot in our room to begin with.'

'That means we'll have birthdays in February, March, April, May and June. Can I help you bath it?' said Rebecca excited.

'Of course you can,' I replied.

'Are you having twins?' was the next question. I laughed at the thought.

'No, definitely not.'

'That would be great.'

'Maybe for you lot.' I smiled.

The nausea washed over me every day. Because I could barely face drinking, my lips became dry and bled when they cracked. But gradually, as I got larger, the sickness lessened until it only overwhelmed me when I was very weary. Work drained me, my protuding bump made it impossible to slip into the space between the mobile X-ray unit and the cots of the premature babies I was X-raying, and I would have to lumber round the room to check the position of the baby before I stepped back to make the exposure.

Mike, Suzanne and Rebecca helped out at the weekend, letting me rest after the long week. As my bump grew, my breasts swelled – or rather my breast.

'I've got a little bit of a problem,' I explained to the woman in Mothercare who was about to measure me for a maternity bra. We both looked down at my chest, one milky white breast more than filling my A cup bra, while the other remained the same, rounded dome.

'I'll just measure you as though you are the same size on both breasts,' she said, reaching round my back and bringing the tape to the front. After reading the result she disappeared for a few seconds, returning with several hammock-sized contraptions.

'I'd say you need at least a C maybe a D cup,' she said, passing me the bras.

The D-cup bra was perfect for my fuller breast but the other side looked like a deflated balloon. I would have to speak to my friendly breast-care superwoman nurse Belinda to see if she had any ideas about how to pad out the other side.

When I told her my predicament I could hear her snorting with laughter down the other end of the phone and pictured her face. But it was a kindly laugh, not cruel, and I started to giggle as well. She booked me for an appointment to get a fitted prosthesis – a sort of chicken fillet which helped fill out the bra cup.

As my pregnancy grew to comedy proportions, a cartoon likeness appeared on the staffroom noticeboard. Stick thin legs poked out from underneath an enormous belly.

On my last week at work, I was relieved to be starting my maternity leave. Laden with armfuls of gifts and flowers I was looking forward to having some time to put my feet up and take it easy for a while. No more dashing to work in the morning or crawling home exhausted in the evening.

My delivery date, 9 May, arrived. I arranged the pillows around me in the bed, grunting as I reached down and plumped up a cushion to support my back. Bottom on the edge, I rolled laboriously on to the bed, and brought my legs up feeling for the cushion to push into the small of my back. I turned to adjust my position when suddenly there was a pop and I felt liquid on my legs.

'Bugger.' I was too tired for labour tonight. I eased myself out of bed and went to the loo where another torrent of liquid escaped as my waters broke.

'Mike!' I clicked on the living-room light. 'My waters have broken.'

'Are you sure?

I gave him a don't-ask-such-a-bloody-stupid-question look. I phoned the hospital and was told they would be expecting me shortly on the labour ward.

This new person wasn't keen to show themselves, and my contractions waxed and waned for over eighteen hours before my labour began in earnest.

In a bare room at the hospital I rested my forehead against the cool glass of the window. A thunderstorm was making its way towards us and we watched as the flashes of lightning crept nearer and nearer from the horizon, the storm banging its way over the hospital, the rain lashing at the windows.

'Breathe deeply,' the midwife said, handing me an oxygen mask. I drifted in and out of sleep as the pain kept waking me. Mike left the room as I sat up with my legs apart and the midwife studied me.

'It's time, Jane, come on, push, push, push.'

I grunted, holding my breath, pushing and pushing, jaw rigid and teeth clenched close with the immense effort. I felt the hardness of my baby's head and the midwife eased it out.

'One more push, then this one's nearly here.'

I felt the tide of pain and the fingers pulling, the pressure was unbearable, but as the contraction subsided so did the pain.

'That's it!'

I looked down to see the purple scrunched-up face and mass of black hair of my new baby. Just one more push and he slipped out, the midwife blew on his face, his eyes were shut. The nurse gently blew on him again, I could hear the suction catheter being used to clear his mouth and nose, but still no cries. The nurse placed a tiny mask over his nose, my body filled with fear as I listened but could only hear the small hiss of gas escaping from the mask.

'Come on, little man,' I heard her whisper as she bent over the tiny body. Then the quietness was broken as my little boy screamed with indignation, his face screwed up. I began to weep, tears of relief and joy.

The nurse went to fetch Mike and he walked into the room and approached the bed, our heads touching as we gazed down on our little miracle.

Mike rang the girls to tell them they had a baby brother. They were thrilled. Over the next few days, visitors streamed in and out of the room. I tried breast-feeding but, with only one breast, I was too sore. Each time his soft little lips clasped round for more, I would wince in pain but I wanted to persevere. Lack of sleep and soreness made me give up on the attempt and I sent Mike out for baby milk and bottles soon after arriving home. The guilt and disappointment lessened when Steven's angry cries subsided into a full bubbling snore, a dribble of milk beaded at the corner of his mouth.

Being at home with Steven was like being a first-time mum. With Suzanne and Rebecca at school I had time to spend with him. Best of all there was none of that fear of first-time parenting. I enjoyed bathing, dressing and feeding him. Settling him to sleep, resting myself.

Filling the small white bath with water, Rebecca watched as I dipped my elbow into it.

'What are you doing?' she asked.

'Checking that it's not too hot or too cold,' I answered.

'Can I help?'

She cooed over her little brother. Steven's eyes followed her as she bent her head to kiss his nose. Easing small plump arms and legs out of the babygro, stretching the vest over Steven's round chubby head, I marvelled at the sturdiness of his neck, a masculine thickness defining him as a boy, so different to the delicate white stretch that had looked too fragile to hold Rebecca's head.

Steven smelt of milk. I stroked his face feeling the softness of his cheeks. I gazed at him in wonder. His arms flailed, and his legs pulled up. His face closed up and a frown crossed his smooth features as he opened his mouth to let out a cry. Scooping him up, I wrapped him in a fluffy white towel, washing his face gently with snowy white cotton wool. Then, just as his cries became more indignant, I offered him over to Rebecca.

'Here,' I said, as I eased the towel away. 'Make sure you're supporting his head and have got a firm grip on him.'

She picked him up. 'Is this right?' she said, looking across at me and then back at her little brother, concentrating on the small white body.

I nodded. 'Now lower him gently into the water.'

She shuffled her knees slightly and balanced herself as she lowered Steven into the bath. His arms and legs flew apart making him look like a small star. Then his feet started moving, his eyes wide with delight, his tiny toes curling tightly. The frown furrowed his brow, this time with concentration, taking in this new experience. Gurgling in a happy way he waved his foot and brought it down with a splash. Again and another splash. Rebecca held him, swaying him gently through the water, her eyes opened wide with wonder, her voice soft as she sang quietly.

I trickled water on to his back and gently over his rounded belly. It contracted and rolled involuntarily. His eyes screwed shut, and he squirmed in Rebecca's hands.

'Here,' I said as she started to panic. I lifted him dripping from the water before he could begin to cry. I swaddled him with the warm towel patting him dry. Head close to take in the familiar smell, I dressed him and even as I covered his innocent nakedness, his eyes started to droop, heavy with sleep. His arms and legs flopped to the sides as I lifted him and placed him on his back in his carrycot. I sat crouched, Rebecca by my side, as we watched his small red lips parting with each breath. I put my arm round Rebecca and wondered at how lucky I was.

I stayed at home with Steven all through the summer holidays. The girls helped me to look after him. There was no rush, no pressures of work and although the night feeds were tiring, with no need to be at work the next day it was manageable. A promise is a promise, though, and I knew I would have to return to work. We could probably have managed if I'd gone back part time but we were both aware of the financial constraints placed on Mike if something should happen to me.

I kept my side of the bargain and resumed my full-time job.

CHAPTER 6

JANE

My breast implant had ruptured and started to leak. Over the years, its shape had morphed from something resembling a breast to a flattened mass. There had also been a number of health scares regarding silicone implants so for my health and self-confidence I decided to have it reconstructed. The operation was straightforward and I had four weeks to recover fully in our new house at Rothwell, where we had moved after Steven was born. It was early summer, the children were still at school and, although I was still sore, I felt really well in myself, using the time off to study for my gardening course.

I had undertaken a correspondence course for the Royal Horticultural Society a couple of years earlier and I was steadily plodding through it in my own time. I loved learning about plants and the practical aspects of gardening; I even enjoyed botany, a subject I'd struggled with at school. Walking home from Rebecca's school one day, I made my way through a rolling meadow past an old stone house. I stopped to admire the long narrow kitchen garden – the slightly haphazard rows of blue-green rounded cabbages and small softer leaved butter-head lettuces. The rows were broken up by dahlias and lilies, their heavy blooms supported by canes and twine. A big, blousy lavender protruded through the fence separating the vegetables and fruit, raspberry canes were tied rigidly upright, fresh green leaves hiding the starred white flowers, strawberry plants were heavy with fruit. As I continued towards home I thought about my next assignment for my course – designing a herbaceous border.

Our own garden was barren, its hidden fruits were bricks left by the builders and twine and other scraps were baked hard into the clay. I sat on the bench with my gardening encyclopaedia open on my lap, poring over border choices for my essay. The building site was due to be turfed as soon as the landscapers could fit us in. I glanced up from my scribblings and looked at the thirty-foot space before me. Would it be another football pitch for Mike and the children or should I make the most of the blank canvas and have someone help me with something more ambitious?

We'd had several flyers through the letter box from landscape gardeners and I'd kept the last one. Reading through it, I thought 'Why not?' and rang the number, leaving my name. I had a good knowledge of plants and gardens but not the vision or the courage to create one that would be more than just three straight borders round a square of grass. If someone could come up with a design I felt sure I could create it myself.

When the landscaper returned my call, I made an appointment for when Mike would be home and we went through a list of things we wanted. No to a barbecue, yes to a greenhouse, a seated area, fruit trees and arches. I also wanted some sort of water feature.

The man measured out the space and he returned three weeks later with three designs. I chose a soft, curved design and was surprised at how little lawn was left. Only about a quarter of the garden would be grass – enough to lounge on but definitely not enough room for goalposts.

MIKE

I'd always loved New Year's Eve, an excuse to party and look forward, but this had changed with Jane's first diagnosis over nine years before. This year, though, it was Millennium Eve and there was a real sense of optimism. We invited our friends, Stephen and Melissa Ridgeway and their boys Christopher and Daniel. Mick West would also come down from Settle.

Stephen Ridgeway opened our front door with his sons Christopher and Daniel. Steven ran to them.

'Hiya, you two,' called Steven. Christopher was a couple of years older than him but Daniel was only three months older. They all scurried through to the living room while Stephen walked into the kitchen.

'Hi, Jane, where do you want these?' he said, holding a carrier bag in each arm, both crammed with beer.

'I'll put one in the garage,' I said. As I entered the hall Melissa was struggling to fit through the front door, loaded with quilts, overnight bags and the lads' toys.

'Where is he?' she asked.

'Steve, you're wanted,' I relayed to the kitchen. He looked round the door frame.

'That's it,' said Melissa. 'You just look after yourself. Here, do something useful if you can.'

Suzanne hurried down the stairs. 'Pass some to me, Melissa'

'Oh thanks, Suzanne, you're a lot more use than that lump.'

'You sound like my mum.'

'We have a lot to put up with.'

After we'd emptied the car Melissa, Jane and Suzanne sat in the kitchen while Steve and I proved our worth by multi-tasking in the living room, supervising the kids and generating garage space by sinking a few beers. By nine o'clock when Mick arrived all the young boys were, notionally at least, attempting to go to sleep in Steven's bedroom. Mick dropped his overnight bag in the dining room.

'All right, Steve,' he said.

'Fancy a beer, Mick?'

'I'll get it,' Suzanne said. 'What do you want? Beer, lager, wine, whisky. Can I get another, Mum, please?'

'Okay,' said Jane.

'Beer, please,' said Mick.

Suzanne returned handing Mick a can of Boddingtons. She flitted back to the kitchen holding a bottle of lager like a professional drinker. How different this was to last New Year's Eve. When Jane had had to work the late shift from 6 p.m. to 2 a.m., it was left to Suzanne, Rebecca and I to stay up to let the New Year in. At midnight, while Steven slept soundly upstairs, we'd poured a toast, thrown streamers and pulled the strings on poppers.

We'd thrown ourselves into the evening though the celebration seemed hollow as we all knew this could be a dress rehearsal for a future New Year's Eve. It may have been my fault – I just didn't have the required *joie de vivre* for that particular night – but I suspected it was mainly down to the underlying sense that Mum wasn't there.

Fortunately, a year later on Millennium Eve Jane's shifts were more sociable and, conveniently, we found ourselves working the same hours which meant we were both free to celebrate midnight.

Steven, Christopher and Daniel were too young to stay up for midnight but, now that they were fourteen and eleven, Suzanne and Rebecca took it for granted that they would be up. Indeed, Suzanne had already advised us of her liquid requirements; anything alcoholic.

She'd grown up such a lot in a year. In March I'd taken her to her first concert – Kula Shaker – and before setting off I'd ridiculed her bright orange jacket.

'They'll never let you in in that,' I'd said. She'd stood out a mile as being younger than the other fans. The doorman outside the Town and Country club had looked at her suspiciously, querying whether she should be allowed in and it had taken some persuasion on my part to let her through. By the time we took her to see the Stereophonics a week before Christmas, she looked more grown-up wearing jeans, black T-shirt and jacket. No questions were asked.

Rebecca, too, had matured. She had started secondary school in September. Jane and I had fretted about the journey which involved a 7.30 a.m. start from Rothwell and a change in

Wakefield to another bus to Sandal. Our worries had been need-less. Rebecca may have looked seven years old but she was fearless. Small in stature but made up of strong muscle and sinew, she had not an ounce of fat on her. What she lacked in height she made up for in aggression. As a child, Suzanne had always been timid, afraid to have a go at anything too chal-lenging, whereas Rebecca had no fear. She was popular, too. Even at nursery when we dropped her off, the kids would shout, 'Becca', like the cast of *Cheers* greeted Norm. But Rebecca would ignore them all. She was incredibly kind with her time but was always her own person.

Rebecca had been more excited than the rest of us about Millennium Eve and had watched the celebrations from cities such as Wellington and Sydney, which had already celebrated the new year. She tidied round, collecting glasses and empty beer cans and clearing food plates.

'Can I have a beer, Mum, please?'

'Only one.'

'But—'

'No buts.'

Steven too was growing up quickly. For a terrible two-year-old, his sunny nature and disposition were a joy. When Jane had been pregnant I had wanted it to be another girl, mainly because I knew that, if it came to it, I could bring up a girl by myself. But I loved having a son. Somehow, being a parent again after a nine-year gap allowed me to enjoy each moment with him more and I cherished each stage of his development. The urgency to see him walk and talk before he was ready wasn't important like it had been with the girls. For the first two years, we had kept him in a cot by our bed, not out of any overtly protective feelings, simply because we loved seeing him bounce up in the morning, standing looking over the cot rail. He didn't cry, just grinned.

'Mum it's nearly midnight, are you coming through?' Rebecca asked. Jane had fussed over preparing the food all night, barely stopping.

'Coming. Becca, will you get some wine glasses? Suzanne, will you get the champagne?'

'Do you need a hand with anything, Jane?' Melissa asked.

'No I've got it under control.' Rebecca came through clanking the glasses. Suzanne followed ripping the foil off the top of the bottle. Jane walked in, sleeves rolled up, beaming a huge smile. Big Ben appeared on the television and as it struck I opened the champagne and poppers flew from every direction.

I went round the living room hugging and kissing my family and closest friends. Just after the clock struck twelve, Rebecca opened the patio doors and we went outside to watch the night sky flooded with fireworks. The light from them illuminated strange dark markings, like crop circles all over the garden. Much to mine and Steven's disappointment, our football pitch was being altered, *Ground Force* style, into Jane's equivalent of Kew Gardens. I didn't mind, her excitement over the project had sustained her over some difficult months of extra shifts.

I stood inside two tramlines watching as Jane walked towards me, red-faced and wide-eyed from the champagne, her shoulder length hair flowing down over her thick black jumper. Saying nothing, her arms enveloped me and her warm breath on my cheek sent a ripple down my spine. She was more than I deserved as a life's partner.

Rebecca bounded up. 'Can I have a photo?' she beamed.

We smiled at the camera, our joy stored for prosperity. As the fireworks burst in the sky above Rebecca's shoulder, it was hard to imagine how life could really get any better.

JANE

A couple of ludicrously high quotes for the gardening work had left me with only one option – to do it myself. My brother Luke was encouraging and promised to get me started, while Mick vowed to help with the tougher bits of landscaping; the paths, edgings and greenhouse base.

I was excited at the prospect of scaling up the garden design to see how it would look. With a large tape measure, a can of yellow road-marking spray, long pieces of string and tent pegs,

Luke and I laid the plan out on the garden table and placed a brick at each corner to stop it rolling back on itself. Unable to wear gloves, our hands were soon frozen in the biting January morning.

By mid-afternoon, there were bright yellow lines marking all the paths and borders. I wandered round, picturing the finished garden, arches cascading with fragrant blooms, trees heavy with fruit, borders a patchwork of colour.

Over the next few weeks I started digging, shovelling mounds of grass and depositing them in the skip at the building works further up the estate. Mike helped out but would become exasperated if I offered any words of advice, often throwing his spade down in frustration. Storming off into the house like a petulant child, he'd mutter inaudibly under his breath, peeved that I wasn't appreciating his assistance as much as he'd like. I was a hard taskmaster but knew I had to remove all the couch grass and other perennial weeds from the borders or else they would be overrun in no time at all.

I rang round several builders' yards to price up the paving materials. Some would have to order the slabs and path edging in. At last I found someone who could deliver the order in a couple of weeks. I was beginning to think that this project would take years. I wanted to have the garden finished and at least half the borders planted up by the summer.

MIKE

Sitting with my back to the door, I had a full view of the kitchen. The blind was open but it was dark outside and rain battered the window so hard that the drops sounded like a tyre over gravel. Steven was eating a ham sandwich and the girls were making a racket upstairs.

'Tell them to be quiet,' said Jane as she leant over to get the oven gloves.

'Your mum says be quiet,' I said.

'Thanks, Mike,' she said sarcastically. 'I could have done that.'

She slammed the grill door a little too forcefully. The oven timer beeped and she turned off the hob. I noticed the time on the oven door, it was six-thirty already. There always seemed to be road works on the way home so what used to be a twenty minute journey was now taking fifty minutes, especially in these dark, wet wintry months. Still wearing her jacket and shoes from work, Jane looked weary, her movements were laboured and it seemed that every one was taking her last energy reserve.

'Can I work a late shift next Thursday?' she asked.

'It shouldn't be a problem,' I replied.

'Are you sure?'

'Yes.'

'Because I wouldn't like to get in the way of your work.' There was a slightly acidic tone to her voice. 'By the way, I got the photographs back from New Year, they're on the top.'

I scanned the worktop but it wasn't immediately obvious where they were. The top was cluttered with two weeks' worth of post, circulars, magazines, letters from numerous credit card companies, Steven's paintings, small bags from the shops. Infuriated by my cack-handed search, Jane came over and, with her bony elbows, nudged me out of the way.

'Here!' she said. Glancing through the snaps, I stopped at a fantastic picture of Jane under the night sky. She looked radiant. But who was the fat bastard she was next to? I looked as though I'd been filled with helium. Disappearing to the toilet, I studied myself in the mirror as though I were looking at myself for the first time. There was definitely no shortage of chins. Thinking back to Christmas, I recalled my dad mercilessly ribbing me about my weight and my receding hair. I returned to the kitchen.

'I think I'll join that gym at work,' I announced. Jane sniggered.

'Marshalls will be here at eight in the morning,' she said.

'Who?'

'The builders. Will you start moving the sand and gravel to the back? The paving stones will need to go in the garage or at the side of the house.'

'Where are you going to be?'
'At work.'

The early commute the following Monday was dreadful, a soggy January morning with everyone driving at a snail's pace. The low lying mist looked liked it was in for the day.

'I'm in Sheffield tomorrow,' said Jane as I drove. 'Can you give me a lift to the station and pick me up afterwards?' Although Jane's days at university were only supposed to be occasional, they did lengthen the day. With us setting off at seven-thirty every morning and arriving home at six on a normal day there was no need for an extension. Our free time each day seemed squeezed into an ever smaller space. It would inevitably tire Steven.

What kind of life was this? This wasn't living. It was existing. A constant treadmill of juggling work, two older girls and a toddler. Jane and I had lost the plot. Gone were the days of sitting peacefully for an hour doing the *Guardian* crossword, playing cards, weekend walks, lazy Sunday mornings with the paper or seeing friends.

The sky was grey and foreboding, the rain more of a nuisance than heavy. The outlook for me this week looked just as gloomy. Each day and night seemed crammed with duties and obligations and even the weekend would be spent labouring as Mick was starting on the garden. In the boot of my car, my running kit constantly reminded me that my stomach was overhanging my trousers and that my belt would only tighten to the second notch.

At work I had a report to write that I'd been putting off for two weeks but now the deadline was pressing. How I hated writing; if only I could just sit down with some code in front of me, solving some queries. Was there anything worse than spending your day cooped up in an office typing into a laptop? The only daylight I'd experience today would be a cold damp lunchtime run.

JANE

The hours of back-breaking work were paying off, my garden was taking shape. Most days I would come home from the hospital, put the tea on and dash straight outside to make the most of the limited daylight. Life seemed to be frantic.

My passion for paediatric radiography had led me to look for courses to study at postgraduate level. I loved working with children, helping them in their journey through the hospital experience: greeting a young person and explaining what their X-ray examinations would entail in a language they could understand, drawing them out of themselves to help them relax, trying to treat them with all the respect they deserved. I gained immense satisfaction from seeing a pensive look turn into a positive smile. I wanted to show people the experience and expertise I had developed within the department – and I felt the best way to do this was to back up my practical skills with an academic qualification.

Today I'd had my first day of lectures at Sheffield Hallam University. The journey to Sheffield meant I found myself sitting on a metal bench at Woodlesford station waiting for the train. Through my thick coat, the icy seat was numbing my buttocks and the cold was creeping down my thighs and cramping my calves. The station lights were on, but the sun was just beginning to creep over the bare trees that surrounded the platform. I was startled out of my chilly reverie by the metallic voice on the loudspeaker announcing my train.

Arriving at the campus I was sodden and squelching from the torrential rain. The corridors were stifling with the smell of old, hot radiator paint. I made my way towards the dining room. There, half a dozen equally drenched people sat self-consciously so I joined the queue for a coffee.

It was an inauspicious start to a long, hard day in which I realized just how many new skills I would have to master: computer skills, literature searches, indexing systems. My mind felt numb as I packed away my newly filled folders and prepared for my journey back to Leeds.

I felt despondent on the way back home, the eagerness of the morning dulled by my inadequacies, unsure whether I really wanted to spend so much time learning new skills that I might not be able to use in the job. By the time the train had pulled into Woodlesford, I was almost certain I would not be returning the next day. I didn't feel I was motivated enough to see the course through.

I arrived home still cold and my shoulders ached with carrying my book-heavy rucksack.

'How was it?' asked Mike.

'Horrible,' I replied. 'I'm not sure I can face it again tomorrow. How was your day?'

'Pretty shit,' he said, tying his laces ready to go to fetch supper. 'I've got to go to Glasgow again next week.'

Since the New Year, Mike's job remit had expanded and he was required to travel to London, Scotland or Ireland at a moment's notice, leaving me to look after the children by myself. On top of everything, the constant travelling and hotel life had given him a greater sense of his own importance and he had become more abrupt and blunt, picking fights with me when he could sense I was too tired to argue back.

I knew that some of his agitation was due to his fear of flying, and the thought that he would miss his plane, but at other times I could find no reason as to why he seemed distant and aloof. He acted as though he were superior to me, which annoyed me. He no longer seemed to want to be a part of the Tomlinson family team.

The following week I was at home without the car. Mike needed it to drive to the airport. The bus would do for me. I shouted at Suzanne and Rebecca again to hurry, knowing that I was ranting unreasonably. Finally we were all ready. Suzanne marched up the road surly and uncooperative, Rebecca dragging her heels behind. Tired, I marched pushing Steven in his buggy, cajoling Rebecca to keep up.

Suzanne's lips brushed my cheek as we said goodbye.

'Have a good day.' I smiled.

'Yeah, right,' she said and turned her back on me to talk to her friend at the bus stop.

I hurried on, panting up the hill to the childminder's, where I deposited Steven, and Rebecca and I dashed off to catch the bus round the corner. It was full, standing room only, so I shuffled down the aisle and gripped the back of the seat next to me. We lurched forward, pulling to a screeching halt, and my bag hit the woman passenger in front of me.

'Sorry,' I mouthed and she just looked at me. For forty minutes we stopped and started, shoehorning more and more people on to the bus until we arrived in Leeds for another day at work.

In the evening, the process was reversed, although I ran down to the bus stop and queued early, so I managed to get a seat. Pulling a book out of my bag I started to read but was too tired and the same sentence fumbled repeatedly through my weary brain. On the way back from the childminder's, at least the walk was downhill. I pushed Steven back home, his little head drooping forward heavy with sleep. I lifted him out gently, carrying him inside and putting him down on the settee, easing his floppy limbs out of his coat. He grumbled at me briefly and then drifted back off to sleep.

I was peeling potatoes ready for tea when Mike rang.

'Hi, what sort of day have you had?' he said.

'Tiring,' I said. 'I'm just making tea.'

'Oh,' he said and fell silent. I could tell I'd irritated him by not being cheerful and chatty. 'I thought I'd phone now,' he continued. 'I'll be busy later.'

Yeah, I thought. Busy having a beer with your mates. 'Are you okay?' I asked.

'Yeah, but there are a few Leeds lads here. I'm just going to get a bath before I go and meet them.'

'Oh. That's nice. I will have to go, the kids are waiting for their tea. Any chance you could ring later, it would be nice to have a chat.'

'Not really, I won't have time.'

'Enjoy your night, then.' I hung up abruptly, before I could make some caustic remark about how some of us would be spending the evening making tea and looking after the children, while he was out enjoying a meal and beer with his mates.

MIKE

'When are you going to see your dad?' Jane asked.

'Friday night, after the op,' I said. 'I was going to leave it until Saturday but I can't bear not being able to see him the same day. I'd only worry if I didn't.'

'What about Suzanne and Rebecca, are you taking them?'

'No, if that's all right? I'll take them Saturday if he's okay. I'll take Steven as well. Presumably you won't be doing any work in the garden this weekend?'

'No, I can't. It's a bit frustrating but I won't be well enough.'

Jane was due in hospital on Thursday morning for a minor gynaecological operation but she would be home on Friday. When Jane was an in-patient it was always a rush. After work I needed to collect Steven and make tea before going to the hospital to visit. On Friday I would collect Jane before going to work in the morning; then after work I'd collect Steven, dropping him at home with Jane before going to Airedale to visit Dad. Although only twenty-five miles, I'd struggle to get there inside an hour especially during Friday-night rush hour. Visiting finished at eight but I gambled that the staff would allow me some flexibility due to circumstances.

Suzanne and Rebecca were a great help and would ensure Steven was looked after without Jane taking the burden.

Dad had been overjoyed at getting his hip replacement. Whether he actually required the operation was open to conjecture but he was happy and that's all that mattered. He'd wittered on for years about his poorly leg, although he was far from infirm. I think he had visions of outsprinting both girls.

Fortunately, I arrived at Airedale before visiting time finished, just missing Mum who had departed for home minutes earlier. Dad was sitting up in bed and wearing blue pyjamas.

He proceeded to describe his hip operation in graphic detail and I sat listening to him, unable to believe just quite how well he looked. I had been expecting him to be at least tired from the anaesthetic. He'd come into the hospital full of bravado but I suspected he was frightened. There's a risk at any age with a general anaesthetic, but at seventy-two it was a relief to see him chirpy. We chatted about Burnley's chances tomorrow and, before I knew it, visiting time was over. I was exhausted when I reached the car – two days of visiting different hospitals – now I just wanted to get back home to be with Jane. There would be more journeys to Airedale at the weekend.

Walking through the hospital car park with the children the next day I thought I could have planned this better. If we'd come an hour earlier, I could have visited my dad and nipped on to Burnley to see the game. Dad was sitting in the identical position as yesterday, same blue pyjamas, a bedpan in the same place, but the smile had been replaced by a scowl, which was so unlike him.

'About time someone came,' he said. By the tone it was clear he was serious.

'It's only one-fifteen,' I said. 'Mum said she would be here at half past.'

'I've been here four days and no one's been to see me.'

'Dad, I was here last night.'

'Last night? You've never been here.'

'I came after your operation – you've only been here since Thursday.'

He paused for a second. 'Rubbish. You've not been and neither has your mum. I went into Keighley for a pint with some of the blokes from across there last night,' he said, pointing to the two beds opposite.

The girls looked bewildered, Rebecca was particularly distressed and I spirited them off the ward, telling my dad I was going to get them a drink after the journey. A quick word with the ward staff elicited no useful information; they thought he'd been fine, although I'd noticed some lack of attention on the ward. Things became no clearer after Mum arrived. If anything, his anger was more intense. The children and I disappeared to the canteen and I asked Rebecca and Suzanne to keep an eye on Steven while I tried to figure out what was going on.

Dad eventually calmed down, soothed by comforting words

from my mum, his sister Joyce and her husband Robert. We sat and chatted out of my dad's earshot to discuss the developments. The consensus was that it was a delayed reaction to the operation and the anaesthetic. It would no doubt wear off after twenty-four hours.

Being so far away from him, I felt impotent and unable to help as much as I would have liked. And with Jane being ill, it all added to my sense of uselessness.

I visited each day, though there was little change in my dad's condition The doctors had been slow to respond, not fully appreciating the differences in my dad's demeanour. A stranger hearing his tales about some friends visiting him on the ward would have thought Dad perfectly coherent and normal. To everyone who knew him, it was a worrying development as those friends had all been dead for years. Jane was able to understand the medical jargon better than the rest of us, she would also probe with more insight the doctors' thoughts. Scans and tests were proving inconclusive.

As the days continued to pass there was a slight improvement, with his periods of confusion reducing. When he was discharged after ten days, while still being a long way from his normal self, he was safe to go home. His demeanour was more subdued, probably due to a lack of confidence in his memory, but there was little we could do but wait to see if he improved further; the doctors had been unable to diagnose a problem.

JANE

Work and the children took up so much of our daily lives that Mike and I looked forward to a day to ourselves. On those rare occasions, we would usually go walking in the Dales, followed by lunch at a traditional country pub.

March came and we indulged ourselves in a day together. Instead of driving into work we took the train up the Dales. The gentle rocking of the railway carriage made us feel light, like two teenagers playing truant. The tracks were higher up than the road and gave a different perspective of the villages and towns. The rolling green hills stretched before us and just being on the train journey felt like the beginning of our day, having time to sit and talk together.

I peered out of the window. We seemed to be leaving the blue sky over Leeds; up ahead the dark clouds massed over clefted hills. Typical, I thought, as I unfolded the map.

'Where do you fancy going?' I asked. We both looked at the map, tracing our fingers over possible routes, but even as the train slowed into the station at Settle, we still hadn't come to a decision.

'Settle to Malham it is, then,' announced Mike as he rose from his seat, folding up the map and putting it in his coat pocket. I gathered up my scattered belongings and we both rushed off the train. That route would be quite a challenge – seven miles over the tops and back again without the time to stop for tea and buns.

We made our way through the market square and up Constitution Hill, which soon leads out of Settle. Houses began to give way to high drystone walls, grasses and wildflowers straggling tall against the wind-gnarled limestone. As we rose higher, our cheerful banter stopped as we picked our way up the potholed lane.

The first big droplets of rain began to fall. Within minutes, we were walking through a Dales deluge, the water bouncing off the rocks.

We carried onwards and upwards, the rain lashing our faces.

I felt a sharp, taut pain in my right side. I gasped and drew a ragged breath in, hoping the stitch would ease, and tried to keep up with Mike who was now several steps ahead of me, striding across the rocky tops. Each breath seemed to make the pain worse and through my coat I pressed hard against my side over the area, hoping it might soothe the spasm.

We began to descend into Malham, the drops of rain thinning out until the sun appeared again, its warm rays drying out our hair and clothes. But the pain still hadn't passed. With each new breath, the tightness seemed to worsen, tearing at my side and eventually bringing tears to my eyes.

Mike was a good thirty feet ahead of me and, noticing I was falling behind, he stopped and waited. At that moment I missed my footing and stumbled, landing with a thud on my bottom.

'Ha,' laughed Mike, stepping over to come to my aid. I could tell he was about to say something at my expense when he noticed the tears in my eyes.

'Are you okay?' he said, concern etched on his face.

I nodded but couldn't speak, a little scared by the amount of pain. Catching my breath, I paused for a few seconds before holding out my hand so he could help me stand.

'Come on.' He hoisted me up. 'We won't have time for a pub lunch. Will a sandwich do?'

I held my side and we continued down the hill to the road.

'Are there any buses?' I asked, noticing the bus stop ahead. I was fearful that I would not be able to make the return journey.

'Not unless you want to wait until Friday,' joked Mike as we approached the shelter. The timetable was up to date and as Mike checked the times, I rested on the plastic bench, rubbing my side.

'I don't think I can make it back,' I said.

Mike looked at me, his eyes weighing up the situation.

'I could ring Mum and Dad,' he said. 'But you'll never live it down.'

'I think we'd better. I just don't think I can make it back.'

'That bad, eh?'

I nodded and stood up, the pain having eased slightly from resting. Slowly, we walked into the village, stopping at the first pub we came to by the river.

'I won't be a second,' said Mike, leaving me to sit on one of the outdoor picnic tables overlooking the water. I sat watching the ducks gliding up and down the river. I found that if I kept my breaths short and shallow, the pain was bearable. It was when I attempted to expand my lungs with a deeper breath that the pain ripped through my side.

Mike returned holding two pints of beer. Sitting opposite me, he placed my glass in front of me and smiled.

'They're on their way,' he said. 'You're in for some ribbing you know?'

I took a sip of the cold beer. I could handle Jack's banter. What I couldn't face was being airlifted to hospital from the hillside – now that I would never live down.

The cavalry arrived in their black Polo, with Jack barely out of the car before he was making jibes about my lack of stamina. Alice on the other hand was more concerned.

'Do you want to see a doctor?' she asked.

'No, I'll be all right, Alice,' I said. 'I'll see my GP tomorrow. If it gets any worse I'll go to casualty when we get home.'

The next day I visited my doctor. The pain had eased but hadn't subsided altogether. She examined me and listened to my chest.

'I can't find anything,' she said. 'And your chest sounds clear. It's probably just a pulled muscle. If it doesn't get better in a few days, come back. You may have got pleurisy, but I think it's unlikely.'

The pain didn't get better. I started coughing which made it much worse and I began to feel tired and listless. I returned to a different GP the following week.

'Could this be related to my breast cancer?' I asked.

'Very unlikely,' he said. 'It's a very acute onset so it's more likely to be pleurisy, which will clear up with some antibiotics.'

Reassured, I took my prescription home and read the instructions, confident the tablets would clear up the problem.

MIKE

The three-bunked cell smelled like a stairwell in a grotty tower block, musty and damp. It looked like the set from a TV prison drama but was, in fact, our family room at Castleton Youth Hostel. Cuddly toys on the waterproof blue mattress were the only reminder of home comforts.

We'd been sucked into Youth Hostelling after a couple of cracking experiences in the Lakes. We'd arrived in the mid-afternoon and, after checking in, we had found solace over a few pints in the local. But now, faced with the dimly lit room, any cheer had evaporated.

Steven wasn't bothered. He was quickly asleep. But I still had the indignity of getting changed in front of my teenage daughters, who made it perfectly clear that my training regimes weren't working.

'Leave your dad alone. He can't help being very big-boned,' was Jane's predictable comment.

'Thanks, Jane,' I replied.

She switched the lights off. The room was so dark that even when my eyes should have been accustomed to it, shapes could not be discerned. Drifting towards sleep my mind began to wander. I was glad my dad was better, still a little confused but better. I hope the car's all right. Did I lock it?

'Jane, are you asleep?' I whispered.

'Not with you snoring I'm not.'

'Did I lock the car, Jane?'

'Yes, and you went to check it twice.'

Walking down from Mam Tor next day towards the Speedwell caverns, Steven was flagging. A walking book I'd read had recommended one mile for each year plus one as a suitable distance for a child, so at five miles he had done well. Our cagouls had been off and on like the covers at Wimbledon, but it couldn't spoil our day. The grass looked lush, though it was the new lambs that held Steven's interest.

Jane was falling further behind, complaining again of tiredness and pain. She coughed sharply, shocking two birds nearby into flight. I was sure she wouldn't be so maudlin if she was working in the garden.

Steven, chuckling on my shoulders was draping his comfort blanket, a terry nappy, over my face, obscuring my vision. Tugging at it with my right hand, he gripped it tighter. I buckled my knees pretending to fall with him on my shoulders and he screamed just as I lifted back up.

'Be careful with him, Mike,' Jane shouted. His green and blue hat, shaped like a First World War flying helmet, covered his hair, while small walking boots caked in mud now deposited the muck on to my grey fleece.

'He's okay,' I said.

Rebecca, frustrated by our slow pace, was about fifty yards ahead while Suzanne kept Jane company at the back.

She caught up. 'Mike, can we go straight back?'

I was slightly relieved as Steven would not have to walk any further.

'What's up, not fit enough?'

'No, I don't feel too well,'

'What's up?'

'My legs are tired. My back and shoulder are aching too. It's probably all that gardening.'

I shouted at Rebecca, who was frustrated at having to retrace her steps.

'Okay, we'll get straight back,' I said.

Normally at the end of a walk, it's a great relief to take off your boots, rucksacks and walking clothes but that day it held no cheer. Back in the hostel, Jane began emptying our rucksacks of bottles and wrappers with ruthless efficiency. Suzanne and Rebecca sat on the bottom bunk until Rebecca banished her sister with a 'Get lost, will you?' Steven sat sucking his fingers, watching us all while holding his nappy.

That evening, on the verge of sleep, I watched as Jane stood up, moving stiffly like a Thunderbird puppet and emitting a shrill cough. No one said it – they didn't have to – we'd be happy to get home tomorrow.

JANE

Over the next few months my health went up and down. Some days I would have boundless energy, other days just getting out of bed exhausted me. It seemed to follow a pattern; every three weeks I would have an inexplicable ache or pain which would leave me incapacitated for several days. When it got to the point where I thought I should see the doctor, the pain and the weariness would lift as quickly as they had appeared.

Mike was still making regular work trips away during the week, leaving me alone. The responsibility of working full time while looking after the house and the children wore me down. Some days I would be too tired to even make dinner and the kids and I would have to settle for fish and chips. I was still travelling to Sheffield on occasion for my few days of supervised study. It required a huge amount of self-motivation; with little time allocated for study, I spent many lunch hours in the medical library, snatching time for essential literature searches.

Only my gardening felt like proper time off and it was rewarding to see the area develop. Luke gave me a hand but my main source of help was Mick. He kept a close eye on the work in progress and gave up several weekends to help with the laborious landscaping, the putting down of paving slabs and the securing of edges.

'My shoulder hurts,' I said to Mike one evening as we were getting ready for bed. A dull ache in my left shoulder had made driving difficult and I noticed it more when I tried to move the equipment round at work.

'I'm not surprised, what do you expect after all the work on the garden at the weekend?'

'No, it really hurts. It's not just an ache, it's more like a deep, dull pain. It won't go away.'

'Go to the doctor if it's that bad.'

I shrugged away from him, a little upset at his unsympathetic reaction. I didn't want to go to the doctor, convinced he'd think I was a hypochondriac. But the pain was beginning to worry me. The stitch I'd felt on our walk to Malham had never subsided completely and I'd been feeling weary and listless for weeks. But it was probably nothing. Besides, some days I felt completely fine.

Mike was working away again. He'd been distant with me at the weekend, abrupt and offhand and was critical about everything I did. I was tired; the week before he had spent three nights in Glasgow and the strain left on me was enormous. When he announced on Monday that a return trip was necessary, my heart sank.

He set off on the Tuesday. At least the bank had hired a car which meant I was able to drive into work instead of the dreaded bus journey. On Tuesday night I was tired and not feeling particularly chatty when Mike rang as I was preparing tea.

By the time I climbed into bed, my limbs felt heavy and aching. Next morning, my shoulder and the top of my back were still stiff. Stretching up to ease it, I then bent down to pull on socks and went to wake Steven. I sat on his bed and helped him get dressed.

'Keep still,' I snapped, as he wriggled about on the bed. 'You're hurting my back.'

Somehow I managed to get through the day at work, the pain increasing as the day wore on. I dreaded manoeuvring the car out of the multistorey car park in the evening. It was a heavy diesel without power steering and each tight, sloping bend pulled at my shoulder muscle.

Mike rang just as I was helping Steven out of his jacket. He had fallen asleep in the back of the car and I'd carried him in, placing him gently on the sofa.

'Just thought I'd ring now before I go out,' said Mike. 'I'm going for a run around Loch Lomond.'

'Right,' I said flatly. 'I've just got in, I'm a bit tired, can you call me back later?'

'How I'm supposed to do that?' he said, I could hear the short clipped tone of his indignation. 'I've got to eat sometime.'

The cold shoulder of the weekend, the shortness of his conversation, the feeling that I was inconveniencing him was too much. The tiredness that had been building up all day threatened to overwhelm me as I thudded heavily on to the stairs, crumpled with the phone in my hand. I thought about Mike swanning around in the lap of luxury at a four star hotel in Scotland, able to drive out of town for a run if he liked, living away from the unending grinding hassles of home. No doubt he would be going out for a curry and a drink this evening, while I made myself ill trying to ensure the house ran smoothly.

I knew I would not be able to face another day of driving, kids, work, shopping, tidying and cooking. The thought of ending the day in this much pain again was too much.

'I'm going to use some lieu time to book tomorrow off,' I told him and there was a silence at the other end. 'Is that all right with you?'

His response shocked me.

'No, not really. I thought you were going to save up the time to spend it with me.'

'I can't manage work tomorrow, Mike, I don't feel well and I can't face dragging myself in when I feel this way.'

'Whatever,' he said.

'What does that mean?'

'Do what you like,' he said.

I sighed, frustrated by his lack of understanding. I was about to explain how ill I felt when he spoke.

'Listen, I've got to go, I've arranged to meet someone down-stairs. I'll see you.'

And with that, he hung up.

I sat holding the receiver for a few seconds, anger causing my whole body to shake, my knuckles white with pent-up frustra-tion. I slammed the phone down.

I made the decision that night and took the next day off. After dropping Steven off at the childminder's, I returned to bed where I slept for several hours. Waking around midday, my body felt heavy, the pain had receded. I felt more refreshed and climbed into some clothes and started tidying the house.

I only just heard the knock at the door over the music I had blasting out. When I answered it, I was greeted by the sight of a large bouquet of flowers, blocking out the face of the man hold-ing them. They were from Mike. I couldn't understand it, he rarely sent me flowers, why was he doing this today?

When he got home, not only was everything clean and tidy but I had been to the travel agent and picked up some holiday brochures. Mike had been saying for months that we should have a holiday. If I found something suitable he wouldn't be able to put off booking it.

MIKE

Throughout the night I felt unsettled. Jane must be very poorly, nothing else made sense. She had been fobbed off at the doctors' for too long, the cough should have cleared but it seemed permanent. She was taking sick days from work – which was very unlike her – she suffered pain, listlessness, a lack of enthusiasm. Something was seriously wrong.

By the time I reached home, I was feeling a mixture of relief and trepidation. Morris and Prudence jumped down from the wall on to the bin before bounding up to me. The door was locked so there was some fumbling for house keys before I opened the door, only for the cats to shoot in in front of me. Their dirty paw marks on the door was a sign Jane had kept them out all day.

Jane was kneeling in the squat position, legs folded double.

'Oh, hello,' she said.

I looked at her as if seeing her for the first time. Her brown hair hung loosely over her white T-shirt and her thin arms were highly toned after days of gardening. A small tickly cough banished any notion that I'd been unnecessarily concerned over the last few hours.

'Don't sit down, we're going out,' she said.

'Why?'

'Do you have your Visa card with you?'

'Yeah, why?'

'We're going to book a holiday.'

'When? What for? What are you talking about?'

'We've been talking about spending some time together and so we're going to. In Brittany.'

'I can't drive in France.'

'You can't drive in Britain. It's only a short journey from Cherbourg. One week in August, that's all.' She thrust a brochure towards me and I dropped my bag, caught completely offguard. No discussions about alternatives; the fact I didn't want to drive was ignored.

'We need to talk' Jane said.

'I know,' I said. 'Let's just watch the closing part of the stage.'

Once the Tour de France programme ended, I turned off the TV. We sat on opposite couches. Jane placed her book on the rocking chair.

'I don't think you're well,' I opened.

'I don't think I am either.'

'I know it's a little more tiring for you when I'm away from home, but it's only two days a week and I don't have to go again.'

'Until the next time.'

'That's the job. You knew what it entailed in January.'

'I didn't marry someone who worked away. I didn't agree to it in January. It's too disruptive to the family, your job's not worth it.'

'I agree, but there are things you need to change as well.'

Jane swung her feet down from beneath her and sat more upright on the couch. 'You've always got to turn things around. This is about you working away.'

'But it's fine for you to spend your weekends in the garden, take a holiday and not spend it with the kids, or have a day off with me?'

'I'm tired, Mike. Up at five on Tuesday, ferrying Steven to and fro to Jo's, looking after the kids – you try it.'

'Okay.'

'If you have to work away, to compromise I'll drop a day, take Friday off. I can do the weekly clean, shopping and the other bits. I've spoken to Gill and she thinks it should be all right.'

I sighed.

'What?' she said.

'We agreed.'

'We can afford it, Michael. I'm too tired to live like this. It's no fun.' Her voice was showing real passion.

'It's not about the income, Jane. One day a week is twenty per cent of your wage, which will affect your death cover. We need that. Anyway you're not well.'

'I know. But we don't need to spoil the holiday. If it's serious, let's find out afterwards.'

I gave her a look of disbelief. She relented. 'But to please you, if this cough is still here after the holiday, I'll go back to the doctor again. If there's still no joy I'll make an appointment to see Mr Brennan. For God's sake, though, let me have a holiday in peace.'

'I'll keep working away to a minimum,' I said. 'I'll speak to Kev and let him know. It's not worth risking losing everything if that's the way you feel. When we get back we'll look to reduce your hours. You're right. There must be more to life than this. It's not just work, Jane. With you in the garden and me at the football, we seem to be spending more time apart. There needs to be a better balance. Would you come to the football with Steven and me after the holiday?'

She looked hurt. 'Of course. I need to feel there's more to life than work and home. Everything just seems to be one big grind.'

'I know. I love you.'

'I love you, too. We can make this work.'

We both stared at the television. We hadn't raised our voices. Maybe we both appreciated that the stakes were higher than normal and a more measured approach was required. Jane picked up her book, only to close it. 'Do you fancy a whisky, Mike?'

'Thanks.'

JANE

The Friday before we went away, I went swimming with my boss, Gill. As I swam through the water, doing alternate lengths of front crawl and breast stroke, I found myself panting for shallow breaths of air at the end of each length to try to alleviate the rasping feeling at the back of my throat. I couldn't ignore the sense that every time I tipped my head to the side to gulp in some air, it felt as though I was breathing through a straw and someone was placing their finger over the top of it. I was struggling to get enough air into my lungs.

'That was hard,' I said, as Gill and I pounded back up the hill to work an hour later.

She looked at me quizzically. 'You were doing better than me.'

'I'm a bit worried about my breathing. I've promised Mike I'll go to see someone when we get back from our hols.'

The thought of a week away with the family made me so annoyingly cheerful that Gill eventually succumbed to my good humoured smiles and let me leave early. Released from work, I bounded out of the hospital, thrilled that I wouldn't be returning for another fortnight.

On the Saturday, Mick and I built the greenhouse. Following the hieroglyphic instructions and the incomprehensible diagrams we pieced together the glass jigsaw which was piled outside on the patio. Putting the eight sides together we burst out in tired laughter, frustrated to find that the door was set the wrong way around. Turning the drawings around we discovered our error.

Mike arrived home with the children as we were sliding the last piece of safety glass into the frame. We stood back and admired the structure, hands enclosed in protective gloves. The green frame looked elegant and finished the garden.

Now the garden was complete I could concentrate on preparing for our holiday. I spent the next couple of days washing, tidying and packing for our camping trip in France. There was an air of excitement at going away, a week together in Brittany. I hoped the beaches at Benodet would be worth the long journey.

CHAPTER 7

MIKE

The grey skies over Brittany had provided rain of biblical proportions on the first day of our holiday. The torrent of water
battered the roof like peas on a drum, trapping us in our static
tin can. There was little chance of anyone being able to show off
a tan when we got home.

Suzanne on the other hand had something better to show
off – a chap, called Robert, who, rather conveniently, was
located in the next caravan. 'Bob the Boyfriend' provided the
rest of us with an endless pot of humour and the pair of them
spent the entire week together, holding hands as if they'd had an
unfortunate accident with superglue.

On the last evening of our trip, as Rebecca and I headed
down to Benodet beach, we spotted the Siamese twins desperately trying to make the most of their remaining time.

'Hello! Hello!' I chirped in Suzanne's left ear and Bob's right.
They jumped apart, startled.

'Is Mum coming?' Suzanne asked.

'No, Steven's tired. And Mum's back's sore.'

'Is she okay?'

'Yeah it's just the bed.' The holiday caravan was adequate but
Jane had found the hard mattress particularly uncomfortable.
For the whole week, she had been unable to travel very far or

even function for more than two hours at a time without needing to stop to rest. It had been somewhat limiting as far as day
trips or activities were concerned. Suzanne looked concerned.

'Don't worry, we're all a little stiff,' I said.

Rebecca's red, long-sleeved shirt with the word 'Millennium'
across the chest reminded me of the last firework display we'd
witnessed. Tonight pyrotechnic explosions lit the sky as the
orchestral accompaniment kept perfect time.

'I'm glad we didn't bring Steven,' I said, as one particularly
large rocket boomed overhead.

'He's a wuss,' Rebecca sneered.

'He's three!' I replied.

'Okay, he's three and a wuss.'

'Becca!' Suzanne was always quick to defend her little brother.

'Well, he is. A right daddy's boy.' She was developing the
habit of being unable to let a conversation end without making
the final comment. In one respect she was right, Steven *was*
sensitive – at the first bang he would have dissolved into tears,
screaming to go home. On the ferry to France after only twenty
minutes at sea he'd asked, 'Can we go home now?' It had been
the family catchphrase for the entire holiday.

When we arrived home from France – as part of our agreement
to try and spend more time together – Jane accompanied Steven,
Mick and me to the football.

'Daddy, is that Burnley stadium?' Steven gripped my right
hand tightly, even though with an hour until kick off, the
crowds were light.

'Yes,' I smiled. 'Welcome to the theatre of disappointment.'

For Steven, today was a rite of passage, his first football
match. Fittingly, it was at Turf Moor where both my dad and I
had witnessed our first games. For all the banter and despite
being a Chelsea fan, I'd watched Burnley play hundreds of times
since my first visit in 1967. From childhood matches with Dad,
through to university years with my mates, until now with
Steven. Mick turned around.

'Is Colman coming?'

'Who knows? He rang Thursday but didn't know whether he was playing golf or not.'

As we entered the stadium, Steven's eyes grew wide. The smell of fried onions, stale beer and cigarette smoke hung in the close summer air. Our tickets took us to ear-popping altitude at the rear of the upper tier, yet Steven found the energy to sprint up the last few steps to our seats. When Jane reached our row she was struggling to breathe. She straightened her back and, momentarily unbalanced, she looked as though she were about to topple back down the steps she'd just climbed.

'You okay?' I mouthed across Steven's head.

'Yeah, I'm absolutely fine,' she said.

Behind us, the shouting had already started.

During the second half, Steven's interest waned. On my knee, he grew tired, his head resting against me. I doubted whether Steven would remember this, his first match ever, in years to come.

I lifted him off my knee and he yawned and looked up at me.

'Can we come again, Dad?' he said.

JANE

The next day, after a heavy Sunday dinner, Mike and I drove back to Leeds. The children still had another two weeks of holiday, which they would spend with Jack and Alice, but sadly we had to return to work. On the drive home I had to fight to keep my eyes open. My chest was tight and my breathing uncomfortable. Feeling as though I was gasping for each breath, I tried in vain to keep it quiet and regular. The dull ache in my left shoulder hadn't eased either.

At home, I felt no improvement. Dragging my heavy bag upstairs I tipped out the contents and began to sort out the laundry. Stooping down to pick up a bundle of white shirts, I then stood up but before I could steady myself the floor tipped away from me. The room seemed to spin gently around me.

Mike was sitting in the living room watching the football

when I walked in, lowering myself carefully into the smaller settee. Misjudging the height, I thudded down into the cushions.

A little worried about the light-headedness, I put it down to tiredness after all the travelling and I wondered whether a bit of fresh air might do some good.

'Do you fancy a quick walk?' I asked Mike.

'Not really,' he said, turning his attention back to the TV.

'I think I'll go. I won't be long,' I said, pushing myself out of the settee.

I walked slowly down the street, concentrating hard on coordinating my feet. Every step I was aware that I was wobbling towards the wall or the kerb. Experimenting, I closed my eyes for a second and took a few short steps, opening them just in time to stop myself from falling into the road. It felt odd, as though I were looking through a goldfish bowl, distances hard to judge and movements dizzying. My changed perception gave everything a crystalline quality.

I took a deep breath in and could hear my chest rattling, making me cough. I was so frightened I wanted to cry. I steeled myself and continued down the street. I would walk to the next village of Carlton and back. If I still felt the same when I returned home I would not go into work the next day.

'Don't be so pathetic,' I thought to myself. 'There's bugger all wrong with you. You're just panicking, making it worse.'

I braced myself for the return journey home, hoping that if I concentrated on my footing and my breathing, it might lessen the tingly sensation in my body. It all seemed fine until about five hundred yards from home, when the whole world seemed to lurch madly away from me.

'Here, you've forgotten these.' I passed Mike his sandwiches and drank the dregs of my lukewarm coffee, throwing my own lunch and uniform into my bag. Just about to leave the house, the keys already in the door, I remembered and stooped to look under the dining-room table.

'Come on, you,' I ordered. Prudence the cat's pair of big green eyes, which had been watching me closely, looked away in disdain. 'It's time to go out.' Backing away, she finally took the hint and rushed out into the garden. I picked up my bag, and locked the door.

It was an easy journey into Leeds. With the schools on holiday, there was relatively little traffic and we were soon pulling off the ring road towards the multistorey car park.

'See you tonight,' I said, leaning over to give Mike a kiss.

'Don't forget to ring the doctor,' he said. 'And ring me if you're not well.'

I smiled at him, closing the door and waving him off from the pavement. I walked towards the hospital joining others for another day at work.

'How was your holiday?' asked Trevor, holding the door open for me.

'Great. It rained a couple of days but it wouldn't be a proper Tomlinson holiday without rain,' I said.

'Are you doing any extra shifts over Bank Holiday?' he asked.

'Supposed to be.' I coughed. As I struggled to keep up with his long stride, my breathing became more shallow and raspy. 'But I'm not feeling too well.'

Trevor slowed down and looked at me.

'You don't sound too well.'

'I know, I know.'

'Do you want a coffee?'

'No, I'm all right, thanks, some other time. I'm going to ring my doctor, see if he can do anything about this cough. I'll see you later.'

I left Trevor to go in the opposite direction and headed down the link corridor towards Clarendon wing, slowing my pace considerably in order to regulate my breathing; it was laboured and heavy and I was starting to feel dizzy. I arrived at the radiology department and checked the worksheets for the day; we didn't seem too busy apart from the skull X-rays clinic and a full screening list.

I continued through the corridor, almost bumping into Helen, the department nurse, who was wheeling through a trolley laden with supplies.

'Hi, Jane, how was your holiday?' She smiled.

I opened my mouth to respond but I was too breathless to speak. The room began to spin and my skin felt clammy.

'Are you okay, Jane?' said Helen as she came near me and held my arm. 'Come on, come with me and sit down.'

I followed her through to the prep room, with walls lined with boxes of syringes, gauze and tubes, and sat on the plastic chair by the door, putting my head down through my knees.

'I don't feel too good,' I said. My chest felt like I wanted to breathe in deeply but I couldn't, my heart thudded noisily, my throat was dry. Helen crouched down beside me looking concerned.

'Do you want a drink?' she asked,

'No thanks. I'll just get my breath back, and then I'll go and get changed.'

Slowly my breathing became less laboured and the light-headedness subsided.

'What time is it?' I asked.

'Eight-thirty,' said Helen. The GP's surgery would be open by now.

On my third attempt I could hear a ringing tone. I asked to see a doctor urgently, and I was surprised when the receptionist offered me an appointment for that morning.

'I don't think it's anything to worry about,' said the doctor, barely looking up from his notes after he had examined me. 'Possibly just an inflammation of the bronchials from a past chest infection. I'll prescribe an inhaler which should relax them and ease your breathing.'

He passed me a prescription form and as I rose out of my seat I turned to him. 'What if I don't get any better?'

'Come back and see us but you'll probably feel a difference within a couple of days,' he said. I picked up my prescription on the way home and phoned Mike.

'Are you going to phone your breast care nurse and tell her what's going on?' he asked.

'I don't think so, it's probably nothing.'

He paused. 'Well, I'm not happy,' he said. 'I'd be happier if you talked to Belinda.'

'Okay, okay,' I said, feeling myself tense up. I didn't feel comfortable troubling her with something that was so trivial. I expected to hear Belinda's answerphone message as I dialled the number and listened to the rings, so I was a little taken aback when she answered in person.

'Jane, how are you?' Her tone was upbeat and vibrant.

'I'm all right,' I said. 'I'm just ringing because Mike's a bit concerned about me.'

'Why? What's going on?'

I explained about the shortness of breath and the pains in my chest.

'How long has this been going on?' she asked.

'Since about March,' I said. 'My GP isn't too worried but I promised Mike I would see someone about it when I got back from our holiday.'

'Does your GP know your relevant medical details?' she asked.

'Yes, but he doesn't seem bothered. I don't think they're taking it particularly seriously that I feel this lousy.'

'Let me see what I can do. I'll try to get you an appointment. I'll ring you back shortly.'

I began to stack the dishwasher. The phone rang. 'Hi, Jane, it's Belinda,' she said, efficient as always. 'Can you make it to the hospital at two-thirty tomorrow afternoon?'

'Yeah, of course I can. I'm really sorry to trouble you with this, Belinda.'

'No problem, chuck, that's what I'm here for. Besides, it sounds like you've been putting up with this for far too long. The least we can do is put your mind at rest. See you tomorrow.'

'See you,' I said and immediately phoned Mike to tell him the news.

MIKE

Tuesday. For some reason, the traffic always seemed heavier. It was irrational, I know, but I despised the day. Maybe, subconsciously, it was because clinic days were always held on Tuesdays.

Walking from the lifts at work I followed a makeshift corridor of lurid green dividers, which separated individual departments in the open-plan building. My skull felt as though it was being crushed in a vice. I made a conscious decision that I was not going to engage with anyone in conversation if I could help it. I was going to keep my head down, get on with my work and hopefully be left alone. Unfortunately my desk was plastered with Post-it notes and before I had time to sit down, the phone went.

'Yes?'

'Tommo, no one can get in the database.' It was the recognizable voice of William, a former colleague from recoveries.

'Is there an error message?'

'I'm not sure. I'll ask.' I could hear the question being bellowed throughout his department. 'Yes, but it was complicated, too complicated to write down.'

'Okay, I'll get back to you.'

'How long will it all be off?'

I thought, how the fuck would I know, you dozy sod? No message, no details. What am I, a fucking clairvoyant?

'I'll get back to you,' I said.

I looked across at Darren, one of the most capable members of the team who could work unsupervised.

'Daz, the usual are off, will you do a repair?'

His sleeves were already rolled up, his eyes bloodshot. He looked like he'd not moved since I'd left him last night.

'Are you all right, Tommo?'

'Why?'

'You look like shit. I know you normally look like shit but today you're worse.'

'I'm fine,' I said, way too abruptly. I scrunched the Post-it notes up and chucked them in the bin before wandering out to get some water. Darren noticed.

'Are you getting a brew?'

'No.'

I walked off, desperate not to bump into anyone. I couldn't face anyone's banal questions or pointless small talk. I resolved to sit at my desk until nine-fifteen when everyone would be in the building and then I would get some fresh air.

The feeling of claustrophobia eased as soon as I left the building. It was impossible to be alone at work, meeting rooms were too few and never empty. Now I just craved twenty minutes of solitude, enough time to clear my head so I could get on with the morning. I was meeting Jane at one o'clock so there wasn't long to go. Just the morning to get through.

Glancing up, I noticed Carol Dunne, a family friend and occasional babysitter, some twenty yards away having just walked past me. I was relieved she'd not seen me. I'd forgotten she started work at the bank at nine-thirty and if I'd remembered I'd have come out later. I watched her disappear into work and my attention was drawn to a university van negotiating a ramp that dissected the steps. I let my head droop down again, and tried to empty my mind, listening to the footsteps on the pavement below. After a few minutes some footsteps stopped in front of me.

'Mike.' It was Carol. 'Are you okay?'

'Not really,' I said. There seemed little point in lying. She sat down beside me.

'I saw you as I walked in but thought you didn't look like you needed company. When I got inside I thought I'd better come back. I'd best not be long or I'll get into trouble, you know what it's like. What is it? Jane?'

'Yes, we're at the hospital today.'

'Checkup?'

'Yeah, but at our instigation. She's not well, the cancer's back.'

Carol's shoulders slumped a couple of inches. 'How do you know, has she had any tests?'

'No tests, it's her first appointment, but I know.'

'Mike, you've been this concerned before and it's always been all right, she'll be fine, she looked fantastic before you went away.' Carol forced a smile.

'This time it's different. There are a lot of things. Coughing, breathlessness, back pain, shoulder pain, dizziness and struggling to walk far.'

'She'll be fine, she'll be run down, we all get it occasionally. Has she been to the doctor?'

'Yes.'

'What did they say?'

'They've been useless. I think they've just been fobbing her off. I had to get Jane to ring St James's or we wouldn't have even been going today.'

'Don't worry,' she said. 'You know where we are.'

The conversation drifted – you can only discuss cancer for so long. Talking to her didn't alleviate any of my worries, but I did at least pretend to perk up and accompanied her back to the office.

By twelve fifty-five I was in the car waiting for Jane. I could see her appearing fifty yards away. She was wearing black jeans, a sleeveless round-necked black shirt and her rucksack was on her back. Despite hobbling a little, she looked well, her cheeks were flushed and, as she reached the car, she smiled and waved. The car bobbed slightly as she shut the boot, depositing her rucksack inside, and she opened the passenger door putting her handbag on the floor between her legs.

'Hi, had a good morning?' she asked.

'Yes,' I lied. 'You?'

'Not really.'

'Why?'

'I'm not sure we should be going to see Mr Brennan.'

'Why?'

She buckled the seat belt before moving her handbag strap which had wrapped around the gear stick. 'Because there's nothing wrong with me. I'll just be wasting his time. He'll think I'm a neurotic, paranoid woman like the GPs do. Anyway, I'm only doing this for you.'

'That's bollocks,' I said and was surprised by the tremble in my voice. 'You know that, as well as I do.'

'I'm not going.'

'You bloody well are. You promised.'

'It's my life not yours. You're always interfering. I don't even know why you come with me to the clinic. I don't want you there. I'm a grown-up, I decide about my health, not you.'

I chucked my book to the back seat, turning ninety degrees to face Jane. Her face was reddening, her hands were tucked under her legs. She looked tearful, like a little girl refusing to go to school.

'You're going today,' I said. 'After today you can go by yourself, it'll be a bloody relief for me not to go again. If you'd said that to me ten years ago you'd have saved me a load of trouble.'

'Who are you to tell me what to do?'

'You're poorly. If you don't go today, you'll have to go at some point soon. Mr Brennan will want to see you, Belinda said that to you yesterday. You're not wasting anyone's time and no one will think so. He won't mind you wasting his time, it'll mean you're well. At least it'll stop that bloody coughing.'

'Shut up, just fucking shut up.' Jane was sobbing uncontrollably. I reached across to hug her but she pushed me away. The second time I tried she said: 'Just leave me a minute.'

'We sat in silence. I concentrated on the squashed insects on the windscreen. Jane reached down to her bag for some tissues, snuffling. 'We need to go or we'll be late,' she said.

Mr Brennan looked concerned for Jane, who was still red-eyed. He probed for symptoms.

'It's probably nothing,' said Jane, and immediately I felt my jaw clench. As she described her 'slight cough' and the 'odd muscle ache' I began to tense.

'Is that right?' Mr Brennan was looking at me.

I raised my eyebrows and hunched up my shoulders before turning to Jane. The silence hung. Eventually, Jane opened up slightly, explaining the cough in greater detail although she was still far from candid. Mr Brennan listened, nodding occasionally, and asked questions. His immediate reaction after she'd finished was to ask for a chest X-ray. There followed another agonizing delay in the X-ray department.

After thirty minutes a female radiographer came up to Jane.

'Hi, Jane, has someone taken your card?'

'No, it's at reception.'

'You should have said. We'll get you done now, staff shouldn't have to queue. Let's face it, we don't have any other perks.'

Jane disappeared, leaving me in the waiting area. When she returned she smiled.

'We can go.'

'Well? Did they say anything?'

'No, how many times do we have to go through this. I don't ask. It's not fair to put someone on the spot. What happens if they tell me incorrectly and say it's okay, then a radiologist spots something when they're going through the films.'

'I just wondered. You're not just not telling me, then?'

She stopped walking, put her left hand across my chest and looked at me. 'Mike.'

'Well, the chest X-ray shows nothing,' said Mr Brennan, when we returned to the breast clinic about an hour and a half later. 'Can you just retrace the history over that time?'

Jane explained again her symptoms over the last few months, with a frankness missing from our previous conversation.

'How on earth did they think it could be pleurisy?' he said, shaking his head as Jane told him about the GP prescribing her an inhaler. He disappeared again, leaving the door slightly ajar. Although his tone was sharp his voice was barely audible over the background noise of a busy clinic.

He bustled back into the room, moving slower than he had in previous years.

'I would like you to have some tests and scans. We could get these done quicker if you were admitted.' By the tone of his voice, I sensed he wasn't really giving us a choice. Jane looked down, with a resigned expression.

'I'll come in and be admitted,' she said, closing the zip at the top of her bag.

'Someone will give you a ring. Leave Avril your contact details.'

We stood up to leave.

''Bye, Jane,' he said.

'Thanks,' we said in unison.

As we were walking back to the car, Jane turned to me. 'You're not still going to the football, are you?'

'Yes.'

'I'd like some company please, Mike. Let's go out for a drink maybe?'

'I'll be back before closing time.'

'I don't believe you.'

'How many times do I get to see Chelsea each season? Anyway, John Bird will be expecting me.'

'Oh, you decide what's important,' she said.

JANE

Sitting on the bench at the bottom of the garden, I noticed that the fresh golden green of the hops had begun to yellow; the end of summer was on its way. The vines were studded with small papery husks of hanging hops, the green canopy was lit from above, almost like stained glass, by the low evening sun. I rested my arm along the back of the bench, tugging at the entwined tendrils climbing through the trellises, vibrant green against the brown. Snatches of steam from my coffee mug rose into the air and I slipped my feet out of my shoes and buried my toes in the dark, cool bark beneath my feet.

Anointing the garden with the dregs of my coffee, I rose and walked slowly across the sun-warmed slate, being careful to distribute my weight carefully so the sharpness of the stone didn't hurt my feet. Below the kitchen window, the herb garden was lush with bronzed feathers of fennel, its umbrella-like seed heads scented with aniseed. Underneath, the bright green of lemon balm showed through. I pinched a soft green tip and released its fresh, tangy oil, with its light, citrus scent. The soft silky heads of the apple mint released their pungent odour as I eased a weed from its roots. I crushed some thyme beneath my foot and enjoyed its savoury smell as I edged round the herb patch.

Memorizing every small detail of my beautiful garden I hoped might alleviate some of the fear I'd felt all day. After all, I told myself, until anyone told me otherwise, there was nothing to be frightened of. The red ball in the sky sank behind the trees and the light dropped. I walked gingerly back up the path to retrieve my shoes. I could hear a warm murmur of chattering next door and a clinking of ice against glasses.

'Did you have a good holiday, Jane?' Terry's head appeared above the fence.

'Hello. Yes, we did. Thanks for watering the plants. Did you pick any beans?' I pointed at the dark green foliage with the curved purple pods hanging abundantly.

'I didn't like to,' said Terry.

'Oh, you should have. They won't get eaten otherwise.'

Cynthia appeared beside Terry.

'Where's Mike tonight?' she asked.

'Bradford. He's gone to watch the match.'

'Are you on your own?'

'Yeah, the kids are in Settle with Mike's parents.'

'Come and join us,' said Terry.

'No, you've got company,' I said, nodding towards the couple sitting in the garden enjoying their drinks.

'I insist.' He smiled warmly. 'Come and share a nip of whisky.'

I slipped on my shoes and took my mug indoors. I locked the door and made my way down the side of Terry and Cynthia's house to the back patio area where Terry was carrying out a dining chair for me. He passed me a whisky, its smooth warmness soothing my throat.

'You look lost in your own world tonight,' said Terry. I hadn't entered into much of the conversation, happy to be a quiet observer while I sipped my drink.

'I'm all right,' I said, suddenly aware that four pairs of eyes were on me. 'I'm just waiting to go into hospital for some tests.'

'And Mike's at the football?' asked Cynthia.

'He's had the tickets for weeks,' I tried to explain, sensing her surprise, but deep down I felt resentment as once again I'd come second to precious bloody Chelsea.

'You know where we are if you need anything,' she added.

'Thanks, Cynthia, but really I'm fine.' I took the last sip of my drink and stood to leave. Terry led me to the front door and squeezed my hand as he said goodbye.

'You going to be okay?' he asked.

'Yeah, really. I'd better get back.'

Just as I began to unlock the door, the headlights from Mike's car lit up the front of the house as he came up the drive. Winding down the window he shouted, 'Come on, we'll just make last orders if you hurry up.'

In the snug bar, Mike attempted to reassure me, buying me a pint to make amends for leaving me alone. I listened to him, nodding absent-mindedly and allowed the alcohol to numb the panic.

We tried to keep everything as normal as possible the following morning but it was hard. Mike bent down to kiss me before leaving for work and I sat in the garden in my pyjamas writing a letter to my friend Amanda. What could I say? I couldn't write anything about my family; I needed to wait and see what happened to me before I could send news of them. I ripped up my scribblings and threw them in the bin, going upstairs to run myself a bath.

The day passed slowly; waiting for a phone call was tiring. When the phone finally rang, it was a welcome relief. A bed would be ready at 8 p.m. that evening. Could I be there? I placed the phone back in its cradle, feeling a mixture of emotions. There was relief that I would finally have some sort of answer, agitation as to what the answer might be but also embarrassment that I might be wasting everybody's time.

I packed some pyjamas, underwear and toiletries into an

overnight bag, cramming some gardening books and coursework in on top to distract me on the ward. I heard the car pull into the drive.

'Jane, where are you?' Mike was home.

'I'm upstairs.' I heard his heavy footsteps thud up the steps.

'What are you doing?' he asked.

'They've got a bed ready for me at eight o'clock,' I said.

'Great. I'll just pack my football kit. We can go for a curry afterwards if you like.'

He reached down to open one of his drawers and took out his kit. 'We'll have to leave by seven-thirtyish in the morning, though.'

'No, Mike,' I said. 'It's eight o'clock tonight.'

I saw his eyes narrow, obviously thinking hard.

'That's okay,' he said. 'I'll have finished in time to drop you off at the hospital.'

I glared at him, hoping he could feel my rage burning into him as he rummaged oblivious through a pile of jumbled-up clothes next to his bedside. The selfish, selfish bastard, more concerned about letting down the five-a-side team than making sure I was at hospital on time.

'No, Mike,' I said, my tone surprisingly measured for the amount I was shaking inside. 'I need food before we go and there's nothing to eat in the house.'

He looked at me, almost despairingly, as though this wasn't part of his plan. 'But I've got to play,' he said. 'They're expecting me. I haven't got any of their phone numbers at home.'

'It's just not possible, Mike,' I said. I would refuse to capitulate, refuse to be abandoned for a second night running.

Mike's face flushed with anger and he threw the gym bag down on the floor, grabbing the keys from the chest of drawers and heading out of the bedroom.

'Where are you going?' I asked, suddenly alarmed.

'Off to Darren's to tell him I can't play,' he bristled. 'Is that okay with you?'

He stormed off like a child who had been told he couldn't play outside, no grace as the doors slammed behind him. I listened to the car engine start and willed myself to calm down. I would not be riled by his petulance. I studied the pile of books next to my bedside table and reached down to pick one out. I thumbed through it casually, dreading his return.

MIKE

Arriving at the new entrance to Lincoln wing, I walked through the usual array of smokers lining up getting a quick drag. It never failed to amuse me. Some were in pyjamas, some dressing gowns, many attached to drips or in wheelchairs. Some looked barely capable of drawing breath, let alone smoking. I opened the door for a man on a drip whose speed belied his condition.

'Ta,' he said as I followed him through.

The ward still looked new: its floor tiles gleamed, the reception area's wood was still untarnished and the beds had more privacy than older wards. I peeled to the right to find Jane propped up in bed and Belinda sitting next to her.

'Oh hiya, Mike.' Belinda motioned to the spare chair, which I gladly slumped into and stretched my aching legs under the bed, accidentally knocking the metal protection bar.

'Careful, Mike.' Jane looked in discomfort. 'Only here a minute and already I'm feeling worse.'

'Sorry, are you okay?'

'I was.' She smiled.

'That's told you. Did you enjoy the football Tuesday?' said Belinda.

'Not really.'

'Good,' she said. 'Jane's been telling me. Don't know how you had the nerve.'

I thought it best to move the conversation on. 'How were the CT scan and X-rays? Did they show anything?'

'No.' Jane shook her head. 'They wouldn't tell me, it's not professional and I'm not going to ask and put someone in an awkward position.'

'So you couldn't see anything, then?'

She widened her eyes and looked at Belinda.

'See what I have to put up with, Belinda? No, I didn't. Don't you listen, we had this conversation on Tuesday?'

'I just thought . . . you know.'

'No, I don't.'

Belinda and Jane both smirked conspiratorially.

'Did you get out for a run today?' asked Jane.

'Yes, a slow four mile.'

Belinda looked across; she couldn't contain her smirk. 'I didn't know you ran, Mike – is it just to keep fit?'

'We can't all be coal carrying champions.' Jane and I had been surprised a year ago when we saw Belinda running on the local news with a hundredweight of coal on her back in a race with an obvious nod to Yorkshire's mining past. From her slight frame it was difficult to believe she could run a mile carrying a hundredweight of coal on her back in an astonishingly quick time. I shook my head: 'I'm embarrassingly slow, Belinda. It's also not a pretty sight, me in lycra shorts.'

'Mike, please don't put that image in my mind,' she said.

'Do you do any other running?' Jane asked Belinda.

'I did the London Marathon last year. I haven't done much since.'

'I haven't the determination to do anything like that,' I said. 'I don't like pain.'

Jane interrupted. 'I've always fancied doing the London Marathon.'

I leant forward and shook my head in mock astonishment. 'What?'

'I have,' she said. 'It's something I've always fancied.'

'You fancy it for thirty minutes every April when we're watching it on telly.'

'What would you know?'

'I know you,' I said. I was finding it hard to contain my laughter, mimicking her voice: 'I can't run with my knees.'

Belinda looked across at her. 'It's quite a big commitment, Jane.'

'Belinda,' I said. 'She could just about run a bath, that's her limit. She's a martyr to her knees. We played badminton last month, she managed ten minutes before she was whingeing. She's been taking the piss out of me running for years.'

'If I get out of here and I'm okay, I'm going to do it,' Jane said, staring at me.

'You're taking the piss, wait till I tell the kids.'

Belinda turned to Jane. 'Anyway, before you start training, how about a pint?'

'Yes,' said Jane. 'Let me know when you're free.'

'I meant tonight. We're having a curry night later, we could nip across the road to the Florence Nightingale.'

I could tell Jane was sceptical about Belinda's seriousness. But this was Belinda.

'I'll go,' I said.

'Women only,' said Belinda.

Jane looked a little taken aback by Belinda's invitation. 'Are you serious?'

'Of course, you're not a prisoner. My treat.'

'No, I'm not really up to it. This contrast from the CT scan is sloshing about, I've been on the loo most of the afternoon.'

I studied her face. I knew she wasn't well but really thought that two hours out of the ward would do her some good.

'Why not go, Jane?' I said. 'The offers aren't exactly lining up tonight?'

But she was not for moving.

'No, I'm not up to it. I'm out tomorrow, plenty of time for beer then.'

JANE

I had a restless night snatching moments of shallow sleep as I lay, heavy-limbed and aching, on the hospital bed. When the light began to filter through the windows, I gave up any hope of rest and resigned myself to rising. My eyes felt gritty and sore, my mouth was dry, and a dull pain throbbed in my forehead. I sat up against the pillows and through half-closed eyes, observed the other patients as they shuffled about the ward. As the breakfast trolley was rattled off the ward a young nurse approached.

'Mike's on the phone,' she said quietly. 'Do you want to speak to him?' I nodded wearily and pulled back the covers to get out of bed. Putting my arms through the sleeves of my dressing gown seemed to require a complicated effort. The nurse led me to her station at the end of the ward and I picked up the phone.

'Hello?'

'Hi, how are you?'

'Fine,' I said. 'A bit tired.'

'You don't sound fine,' he said. 'Do you want me to come and sit with you?'

I could tell he was distracted. Even as he was asking the question I could hear the rustle of paper and the quiet clicking of the keyboard and knew he was studying his computer screen, not really paying attention. Hoping to stem the tears that were beginning to form in my eyes, I shut them tightly, immediately relieving them of their prickliness.

'No, I'm fine,' I said. 'I'll ring you after the ward round.' I passed the phone back to the nurse and returned to the ward, picked up some of my course notes and began studying the anatomy of the plant leaf. I took out some paper and began to sketch a diagram of its epidermal layers, carefully labelling each component.

Time dragged on. Every time a nurse entered the ward, I looked up, eagerly awaiting some news or even for someone to tell me what to do next. The monotony had become too much.

'Excuse me,' I said, approaching two nurses, interrupting their conversation. 'I thought I was due a bone scan today?' They looked at each other quizzically and the taller one reached down and looked at my notes. Flicking through the pages, she shook her head.

'It doesn't say anything here about that,' she said. 'But let me check with the doctors about it and I'll get back to you.'

Grateful someone was finally paying some attention I seized the moment.

'I don't know what's happening,' I said. 'Do you know when someone will be able to tell me my results and when I'll be allowed home?'

The other nurse raised her eyebrows and took my notes from the first nurse and turned to me.

'There's a ward round later,' she said. 'The doctors will be able to tell you more then. I'm sorry we don't know any more ourselves.'

I smiled my thanks and returned to my bed. My purse was on the top of my bedside cabinet and I checked it for change. I had hoped to be back at work by today.

'Hi,' I said, pushing the several 10p pieces into the slot. 'Is Gill there?' There was a short pause before Gill came on to the line. I could picture her standing over the radiographer's desk in the office.

'Gill, I'm still on the ward waiting for some test results so I'm none the wiser, I'm afraid,' I said.

'I've had Chris from casualty on the phone asking if you're still all right to work Monday, Tuesday next week.' Damn. I had forgotten I had put my name down for a couple of extra shifts.

'I'm not going to be able to do them,' I said. 'Can you ring her and apologize?'

'Sure. I'll need a sick note from you, Jane, you've been off work for more than a week. But no rush, I'll get it from you when you come back to work.'

'Oh.' I hadn't been expecting that and realized I would have to speak to someone at the hospital about arranging it. It was a trivial demand but it left me feeling slightly persecuted and I returned to my bed a little tearful. Half an hour later I was dressed and felt more composed. It made me feel less vulnerable.

The morning continued to drag on; each time the ward door opened all eyes looked up expectantly, waiting for the doctors on their ward round. It was after lunch before a nurse came over to my bed.

'The doctors won't be too long now, Jane,' she said. 'Miss Richards, the senior registrar, said she'll speak to you in a separate room after the ward round.'

I swallowed hard and nodded, fighting the increasing sense of panic welling up in my insides. My head buzzed with questions. Should I phone Mike? If I did, he'd never be here in time. Is everything going to be okay? Why shouldn't it be? I knew I needed to get out, away from the ward for just a few minutes, to be by myself and calm down before I saw the doctor.

'Is it okay if I go for a walk?' I asked the nurse.

'Sure, you've got at least twenty minutes,' she said, and I put on my shoes and left the ward, holding the doors just as the parade of doctors walked in.

Outside felt fresh and cool after the airless, stuffy ward. I made my way across the car park to the medical museum where there was a small knot garden with miniature box hedges surrounding the herbs. I noticed the skeletal remains of an artichoke plant, tall, silvery and spiky, and had a go at identifying some of the other plants, picking some French lavender. The smell, pungent and cleansing, cleared my head.

I glanced at my watch and turned to walk back to the ward, passing the red brick chapel on my left. It had been several years since I had attended a service there but I walked up the ramp and turned the heavy, ornate doorknob. The door was open and I pushed it just far enough for me to be able to squeeze into the church. It was full of brown, scarred pews. I approached the book of remembrance and traced my hands over the black copperplate writing of the most recent entry. Light through the stained-glass windows caught the dust motes, lighting them up like tiny angels. The smell of incense and candles pervaded as I walked quietly up the aisle, stopping to kneel and cross myself. Sitting on one of the hard wooden benches, I placed my elbows on my knees and cupped my head in my hands, looking hard at the altar.

I wasn't expecting a miracle, I knew I couldn't change anything about the news I was about to hear, but now seemed as good a time as any to pray.

'Dear God, help me to understand and hear the news the doctors have to tell me. Give me the strength to cope with whatever is going to happen next in my life and help me find calmness, a peace with which to live through whatever the future holds. Remember Mike, Suzanne, Rebecca and Steven and give us all the strength we may need after today.'

The tears that I'd managed to hold back all morning felt hot and heavy in my eyes and I let them slide silently down my cheeks. I let out a small sob, but then grew gradually calmer. I genuflected as I left the church, shutting the door with an echoing thud and made my way back to the ward.

I sat beside my bed, a book open but unread as my mind fluttered through the possibilities of what might be said. I glanced up when the doctors arrived at the bottom of my bed.

'I'll speak to you in a little while, Jane,' said Miss Richards, moving briskly on to the next bed. I scanned the page of my book and willed myself to refocus on the words but my eyes were misting over and the letters were all hazy. I looked down, pretending to read. After what seemed like an age, the nurse came over.

'Would you like to come this way, Jane?' she asked. 'The doctor is waiting for you.'

I followed her into a small room where another nurse and two doctors were waiting, seated, looking at my scans on a light box. I took a seat in the semicircle around my scans.

'I've had a talk with one of the radiologists,' said Miss Richards. 'Apparently the X-rays of your back and neck look normal but we have some concerns regarding the CT of your chest. There is definitely an abnormality on your lungs. It's obvious even to me, but we really aren't sure what it is.'

I sat stunned. What did that mean? I asked her to point out the enlarged nodes she was describing. With her biro she indicated an area, following it through successive images.

'We feel it's most likely to be related to your breast cancer,' she went on. 'The appearances aren't typical and I think we need to carry out some further tests to confirm exactly what the nature of these areas is. We'd like you to come back next week for a bronchoscopy so we can take some biopsies and find out exactly what is going on.'

It didn't feel like the news was getting any better. I understood. I had some abnormalities on my CT scan and although they were not 100 per cent sure that it was secondary breast cancer, they were telling me that it was the most likely explanation.

The people circling me seemed a long way off as I sat trying to focus on the explanation of the bronchoscopy. It was easier if I regarded it dispassionately, as I would if I was seated at a professional discussion of a patient, as so often happened at work. The doctors would need to pass a tube down my windpipe while I was sedated so they could take a closer look and try to confirm the diagnosis from the biopsies to decide what to do next. Tearful and shaking, I tried to make a sensible comment.

'Could it be anything else?'

'It might be,' said Miss Richards. 'But looking at your past history and taking into account your symptoms, it looks likely that we'll be making a diagnosis of metastatic breast cancer.'

As well as the bronchoscopy, they wanted to carry out bone scans the following week and booked me in for a head CT to check out any other reasons for my light-headedness and loss of balance. I had tried to prepare myself for terrible news and this was terrible. But there is no way that anyone can prepare for such news. The senior registrar shook my hand warmly and said she would see me next week.

'There's no reason for you to be in hospital,' she said. 'Go home and have a rest before the tests.' I was crying and asked if there was a phone as I needed to call Mike. Left alone in the room with the house officer, I sat sobbing.

'I'll wait with you, Jane, until your husband gets here,' he said. 'Then I'll go through it again with you both.'

'Thank you,' I said, trembling as I stabbed at the phone trying to pluck Mike's work number from my shocked brain.

'Mike, you should come here please,' I said. 'I've just had the CT results and it's not good news. There's some sort of tumour in my lungs, they're not sure but they think it's my cancer that has spread.'

MIKE

Replacing the receiver, I sat for a moment and looked around
the office. Daz was studying some lines of code, Alec was going
into the technical support area with a PC under his arm, and my
boss Kevin was walking down the corridor towards me, carrying a standard issue A4 red notebook, mobile phone to his right
ear.

'Daz,' I said. 'Will you pack my stuff away? I need to go.' I
reached underneath my desk and grabbed my gym bag and
stood up, heading out of the office just as Kevin was coming in.
He was still talking on his mobile phone as I mouthed 'I have to
go' and he pointed one finger in the air indicating for me to wait
a minute. I stood, impatiently, with my head down, comparing
his spotless shoes with my more scuffed black lace-ups as he
continued his conversation.

'Jane's called,' I said when he had finished. 'I'm needed at the
hospital, something's wrong.'

'No problem. Just get off, we'll sort everything. What did
she say?'

'They found a lump in her chest, they're certain it's cancer.
The doctor needs to see us now.'

'Shit, Mike. Don't worry about anything, you know where I
am any time. I'm not doing anything at the weekend that can't
be cancelled. If you need anything – help with the kids, anything – just give us a ring.'

I thought he was going to cry so I averted my eyes. I felt a
chill run down my spine forcing the hairs on my arms to stand
to attention. I needed to go before my own veneer cracked.

'Thanks, Kev.' I hurried out of the building, taking the stairs
rather than the lift. It was a lonely walk to the car. My mind
raced as I tried to weigh up all the potential options for Jane.
Without knowing the full details, it was frustrating.

The thought of being left on my own with the kids flashed
into my head. Could I cope? Steven was so young, the girls were
both at secondary school. It was too much to think about.

Arriving on the ward, I saw Jane sitting perched on the bed, dressed, ready to come home, bag resting on the floor. She stood, and we embraced. I'd anticipated her to be a wreck; she was so calm, considered. Unnerved, I held her tight, feeling her breath on my neck. I stroked her hair, desperately trying to make sense of things.

'The doctor's just gone away, he'll be back in a minute, he's hanging on to see us.'

'What did they say, Jane?'

'Just that there was a growth in my lung which was restricting my breathing. They can't definitely say it's cancerous at the moment.'

'So what else can it be?' I spluttered through the words, my mind working faster than my mouth.

'I don't know, Mike, although they're not one hundred per cent certain it's cancer. It could be TB or pneumonia. They are ninety-nine per cent sure it's cancer, though; they're just dotting the i's before saying for definite.'

'What will happen? Can they get rid of it? Operate?' I was aware of barking the questions, without wanting to.

'You're asking me questions I don't know the answer to.' Jane's voice sounded panicked.

I held her tighter. 'I love you, Jane.'

JANE

I drew the curtains around the bed to keep prying eyes away. Heads were turning, curious faces questioning my reddened eyes. Placing my bag on my bed, I started to empty the bedside cabinet, stuffing my clothes in any old how. I opened the drawer containing my toiletries, and behind them was the inhaler prescribed by my own GP. I picked it up and looked at it, holding the grey weight in my hand. Sweeping the curtain aside, I marched to the end of the ward, stepped on the pedal of the bin and threw in the useless object. It landed with a clang.

'Inflamed bronchials, my arse,' I thought angrily and stormed back to my bed. I finished packing, feeling better for the show of rancour. Checking with the young nurse at the station, I was asked to return to the ward the following Tuesday night. She smiled and, as my face fell, she stood up, stepped round the desk and put her arms round me reassuringly.

'Go home and enjoy some time with your family,' she whispered. 'You don't know how things will turn out yet.'

Mike shouldered my bag and, as we walked out of the exit into a beautiful summer's afternoon, he wrapped his free arm round my waist and squeezed me. When I looked into his face, his smile back to me was half-hearted and he looked as frightened of the future as I felt.

'We should call at Mum's,' I said. Mike nodded in agreement.

'Hi,' Mum greeted us, with a smile. 'Do you want a coffee?' She busied herself in the kitchen as Mike and I wandered slowly through. She looked at me.

'Are you all right?' she asked. 'You look a bit upset.'

'No,' I said. 'We've got something we need to talk to you about.'

Passing me a mug, we went through into the living room where Mum sat herself down on the edge of one of her high-backed ornate dining chairs looking at us apprehensively. I suddenly felt like a child again, unsure where to start.

'We had some test results today and it's not good news.' My voice began to falter and Mike jumped in.

'They think Jane's cancer may be back,' he said. 'It looks like it may have spread to her chest.'

Mum's face paled, her eyes widening as she tried to comprehend.

'Do the children know?' she asked.

'No.' 'We're going home and then we're off to Settle to tell them. I've got to go to hospital for some more tests next week.'

I told Mum about the bronchoscopy, bone scans and head CT as she sat listening, grave-faced, her jaw working as it clenched and unclenched, her head nodding slowly.

'You know where I am if you need anything, Jane,' she said, placing her mug on the table. 'Any help at all, just call me any time.' I stood up and hugged her.

'Thanks, Mum,' I said and at that moment felt my self-control fail and I began to tremble.

The journey back to Rothwell took for ever in the rush-hour traffic and Mike concentrated on the busy roads. I was too caught up in my own thoughts to talk, glancing up occasionally when Mike swore with malice at other road users. We headed south along the M1, stopping and starting in the snarl of traffic until finally we reached home.

In the driveway, he turned to speak to me; I shook my head in incomprehension, unable to concentrate on his words. Indoors, we went into the living room, Mike slumped on to the settee and I left him, crawling wearily up the stairs. I lay on the bed, brought the covers over my head and shut my eyes against the strong sunlight, hoping it might also block out some of the horror of the afternoon.

In my head, the doctor's words played over and over again: 'secondary cancer', 'spread to the chest'. I hiccupped down my tears, burying my face in the pillow to try to eradicate the last few hours from my memory.

Thoughts of the children caused a shuddering sob to roll through my body. The force of the sorrow relaxed the tension sharp across my shoulders, where fear had tightened muscles in my body. I sat up, blew my nose and looked at my bedroom with the make-up scattered across my dressing table, the mirror askew, the alarm clock blinking redly. It seemed so normal, so everyday, and nothing had changed. Except, suddenly I didn't seem to fit, my whole world seemed to have turned just off true. My future was in doubt and everything felt rotten.

I stood up, ignoring the dizziness, and stood by my bed. Feeling as though I was aboard a ship on a rough sea, I stumbled over to the door, missing the doorknob the first time I fumbled for it and banging my hip on the door jamb as I made my uncoordinated journey downstairs.

'Hi,' said Mike softly, standing up to hug me. Comforted in his arms, I stood motionless in the warmth of his body and thought about the children.

MIKE

At the brow of the hill, we could see the shape of the Craven Fault and views of Ingleborough over twenty miles ahead. Rathmell Bottoms was to our left beyond the Settle to Leeds line and we could see the edges of Giggleswick, including the magnificent chapel dome. The original copper shade of the dome had recently been restored from the oxidized green, but that was the colour I'd been accustomed to throughout my childhood; with the restoration came a loss of character.

On any other occasion, I'd have felt a sense of overwhelming pride approaching my home town, where I really still belonged. Today I only felt hollow, as if I'd left my spirit in Leeds. Jane was in the passenger seat, wearily gazing out of the window. She'd hardly moved, let alone spoken, since we set off more than an hour earlier. I felt the same. Nothing we could say to each other would help what was to happen next week; pointless conversations couldn't change anything.

'We should get it over with straightaway, Jane,' I said, as we drove through Meerbeck. 'We can't hide what's happened and you know what Suzanne's like, she'll notice.'

Jane kept staring out of the window ahead. 'I just need the loo first, Mike.'

'We are doing the right thing telling them, aren't we? We've never lied before, I don't feel like it now.'

'Yes, they need to know, both girls are old enough. Steven won't have a clue.'

'The only alternative is to wait until we know everything next week.'

'No, they need to be able to trust us.'

'At least Aunt Edith is visiting until Tuesday, it will take my mum and dad's mind off things.'

'I don't think it will but she's very sensible.'

'Michael!' Mum gasped, caught by surprise at our early arrival, having not expected us for another couple of hours. She was busy laying the kitchen table which had been extended so it filled most of the room. Six plates of lettuce and tomato salad were laid out and three eggs were bubbling away in a pan on the hob. 'You'll have to wait, I wasn't expecting you yet. Hello, Jane, the kids are in the front room with Jack.'

Edith appeared in the doorway of the kitchen, bronzed and looking well.

'Hello, Michael, Jane.' She moved to give us both a hug. As a child, our family had spent a week's holiday with her and her late husband Maurice each year. It had been over a year since Jane and I had seen her. 'You must have had a good journey,' she said.

'We got away a little earlier than anticipated,' I said. 'Any chance of a brew, Mum?'

'In a minute, have some patience.' She continued to methodically lay out the cutlery.

'Standards are slipping,' I said, 'it must be your age.'

'Michael!' Jane said, she always felt I took my mum for granted.

'You're not too big for a clout,' my mum said motioning with her hand.

'Mum we need to have a word, can we go through?'

'Won't it wait until after your dad's tea?'

'Not really, it's best now.'

My parents' house was centrally divided by a staircase, small hall and the front door. I left the dining room, checked myself in the mirror in the hall and hung my fleece on the coat peg before bursting into the living room with a snappy Hello. Dad, who had been sitting in his armchair, was startled to attention.

'What!? You daft beggar.' Steven shot up from the floor, knocking aside wooden bricks

'Daddy, Daddy, Daddy.' He ran to me with his arms outstretched. I crouched down and he ran so fast into my arms it knocked me slightly off balance. I kissed his cheek, holding him close. It was a comfort to hear his heart pounding. He looked to have changed in only five days, taller, older, hair shorter. I picked him up, held him tight. Suzanne, who was stretched out on a three-seater leather sofa, rose slowly to give us a hug. Rebecca shouted 'Hello', then turned the TV over, barely averting her eyes.

'Rebecca turn the telly off,' I said.

'Why?'

'Mum and I need to have a little chat with you.'

'What about?'

'Well, when you've turned the telly off and Grandma gets here we'll tell you. Where is she?' I looked up towards the door. 'It's like waiting for Christmas waiting for her. Go and chivvy her along, Suzanne.'

My dad interjected, 'She'll be coming.'

Rebecca flipped off the TV, chucking the remote to the floor as a protest. 'We know what it is, don't we, Suzanne? Grandma said you'd be wanting to talk to us.'

'Don't bring me into it,' Suzanne said. I held Jane's hand, giving her a quizzical look. Her forehead scrunched as if to say 'no idea'. My mum dawdled into the room.

'Waiting for me?'

'Do you want to sit down, Mum?' I asked her. A white plastic garden chair had become a permanent fixture in the living room thanks to my dad's hip problems.

'I'm okay,' she said, positioning herself so she was leaning on my dad's armchair. My dad looked up with a cheeky grin.

'You can sit here, Alice,' he said, tapping his thighs.

'Get lost, Jack,' she said.

Jane looked at me, prompting me to speak.

'You know how your mum's not been feeling too well over the last few weeks?' I started, moving my eyes to each of the children in turn. 'Well, we went to see Mr Brennan on Tuesday and he decided it would be good if Mum went into hospital for some tests. After those tests, they found a lump in Mum's chest which is causing her some of the problems she's having. The doctors aren't sure yet, but they're fairly certain that it's cancer.'

We had Rebecca's undivided attention and she quickly chipped in. 'But they're not certain, are they, Dad?'

'It's not one hundred per cent,' I said. 'But it doesn't look like it could be anything else. You need to get it into your heads that it's cancer and just deal with that.'

'When will they know, Dad?' Rebecca again.

'Mum's got to go back into hospital next week and we should find out by next Friday.'

There was a delayed shock before both girls started to sob gently. Mum steadied herself on the back of the chair and Dad leant back in his chair saying, 'Oh no.' Jane went over and hugged each girl in turn, my mum sniffled into a tissue, while my dad looked grey and breathed deeply. Edith came in with a tray of drinks rather like a secretary walking into a boardroom meeting.

'Oh sorry,' she said, realizing straightaway that her timing wasn't perfect.

A reverential silence filled the room; it felt like afternoon tea at a wake. Steven started to build a new tower before sending it crashing down. The noise reverberated throughout the room.

'Dad, will you play with me?'

'Come on, Mum, get the tea sorted or it'll be supper,' I said.

'Not much for me, Alice,' my dad said.

My dad picked up the *Craven Herald*, folded it and put it back in the paper rack. Jane stood up.

'I'm just going to the loo,' she said.

Suzanne slowly built Steven a tower. As it reached a foot tall each additional brick caused it to sway gently, prompting Steven to giggle. My mum got up and headed to the kitchen. As I sat with Steven, I nudged the bottom brick sending the tower crashing on to the hearth. My dad's eyes were shut. As the toilet was flushed, I left the room to meet Jane on the landing.

'Are you all right, love?' I asked.

Her face was damp. 'Yes, you?'

'Yes.'

'How's your dad? He always takes things worse.'

'He's quiet.'

'I'm going to have a lie-down.'

'Do you want me to stay with you?'

'No, if you can make sure the kids are all right that would be more useful.'

I kissed Jane on her cheek and she headed off to the bedroom that the kids had been sharing.

CHAPTER 8

JANE

On the Saturday morning we travelled back to Leeds. I still needed to buy school clothes for Suzanne and Rebecca and, unsure when I would next have the opportunity, I asked Mike to drop us off in town to buy some essentials.

'Are you sure you'll be okay?' he asked as I turned to shut the door.

'I'll be fine,' I said. 'We'll just go to the three shops. If we don't find what we need, it's tough.' I watched as he pulled out into the stream of traffic and I turned to the two girls. Suzanne had grown over the summer and, at fifteen, no longer seemed like such a child; she was always so mature.

We tackled the dreaded task of finding shoes first. While Rebecca had her feet measured, Suzanne wandered the store, pointing out a pair of black shoes. Utilitarian, flat, thick-soled, ugly, they fitted the bill perfectly.

'These look okay,' she said. I was amazed they fitted her. Even more surprisingly, Rebecca appeared to approve. I mentally ticked the task off my list and we headed to a department store in search of a grey skirt. There was always a fine balance to tread: we had to follow the uniform code but allow enough leeway for their personal taste to show through. Suzanne noticed my weariness.

'We don't need to do this today, Mum,' she said.

'I'm fine. We'll just get Rebecca's skirt and some more pyjamas for me. I'll be all right.'

Another week in hospital meant I needed something comfortable to wear. Rebecca found a straight, slim fitted skirt and I found some pyjamas with a vest top and a buttoned long-sleeved top, perfect for entertaining on the wards.

'Where do you need to go to get your coat?' I asked Suzanne.

'I saw a nice one in Top Shop,' she said. I pulled a face. I always felt about a hundred years old wandering through the slim-waisted, snake-hipped teenage throng in Top Shop. It made me feel fat and frumpy. We walked through the shop, me interrupting Rebecca and Suzanne's musing over the latest fashion.

'You couldn't possibly wear that!' I said, holding a flimsy, pink tube. It deflated as I placed it back on the shelf.

We pushed our way past more youthful bodies towards the rails of coats at the rear of the shop. I felt ready to fling myself in the corner; tired, the effort of concentrating on not bumping into people left me light-headed. Suzanne tried the coat on. It was long, it fitted well enough and would see her through the autumn and winter.

'That's nice. Are you sure it's the one you want?' I asked.

'Yeah, if that's all right?'

'Sure. Let's pay before I change my mind or fall over.' We stood in the long queue waiting to pay, Rebecca holding carrier bags in one hand and holding on to my arm with her other. Shuffling on her feet, she glanced round the shop singing tunelessly and hanging off my arm. I tapped at her gently.

'Try not to tug on my arm,' I said. 'It's a bit achy.'

'Sorry, I didn't realize, Mum,' she said, her face serious. 'I'm really sorry. I didn't hurt you, did I?'

'No, don't worry, I'm okay. I'm just a bit tired.'

We shuffled forwards till we reached the front of the queue and after paying for the clothes finally headed out into daylight again. As we neared the exit Rebecca turned to me, her face serious, her eyes hooded with uncertainty.

'Mum, you know you told us the cancer might be back?'

'Yeah,' I said, wondering where this would be leading.

'You're not going to die, are you?'

Rebecca's directness stopped me in my tracks. I paused.

'I don't know.' It was the honest answer. 'The doctors don't know. That's why I'm going back into hospital to have some more tests.'

She looked at me, her eyes watching my face, looking for hidden meanings. I continued, 'I do know that we need to make the most of our time together. Things might be a little different after next weekend.'

'But you won't die, will you?' she asked again.

'I don't know. I might. But until anyone tells us differently we just have to trust that things will be okay. Now's not the time to be sad.'

Rebecca's head dropped slightly and she fell silent, deep in thought. I bent down to hug her.

'Come on,' I said. 'Let's get the bus home. I've had enough now.' Suzanne linked arms with her little sister, who in turn linked up with me, and we made our way past the rails of youthful commercialism laid out in Top Shop, down the street towards the bus stop.

The weekend rushed past and it was not long before we were dropping the kids back in Settle. We had thought about letting Suzanne and Rebecca spend some of the week at home, but Mike felt happier knowing they were with his mum and dad. It meant he wouldn't have an extra worry as he dashed to and from the hospital.

I walked back into the ward on Tuesday night.

'Hello, Jane,' said the nurse. 'We've put you in the smaller ward, the other is quite full, you don't mind, do you?'

I shook my head, following her through the wide, double doors, with Mike behind me, to a ward with two beds lined up on one wall. In one, was a young woman wearing headphones, bobbing her head in time to her music. In the other, an elderly lady, wrapped in a bed shawl was trying to sleep. The nurse led me round the corner to a bed just out of view, it would be good to have some privacy, away from other patients.

'This is all right, Jane,' said Mike. 'Better than the other ward.'

I smiled, noncommittal. Try as a might, I couldn't lift myself out of my low mood; being back in hospital meant having to face up to the tests I had put out of my mind.

'Come on, cheer up,' said Mike, a false brightness in his voice. 'You won't be here for long.'

'I know,' I said. 'I'm just nervous, I guess.'

When Mike got up to leave, I followed him slowly to the exit. Resting my head against his chest, I felt his arms envelope me and his cheek rest softly on the crown of my head. My arms circled his waist. I didn't want to let go, warmed in the familiar secure feeling of his embrace.

Eventually we pulled apart and said our goodbyes, Mike left the hospital and I reluctantly made my way back to the ward. I broke the evening down into small chunks of time, hoping it would help the slow minutes to pass – unpacking my bag, sorting my clothes, putting my books in my bedside cabinet. Slowly, the night passed until I noticed the dark sky outside was now the light grey of dawn. I looked at my watch, it was six-thirty. I wouldn't be getting any more sleep, so sat up in bed and picked up my novel.

It was no good. I couldn't concentrate. I gave up and searched my bag for the cards I'd chosen for my family. I scribbled 'Love you' messages to Suzanne, Rebecca and Steven. I wrote a short message to Mike. I got out of bed, dressed and walked out to the front of the hospital to post them in the red mail box.

When I returned to the bed, my brother Luke was waiting for me. Dressed in his nurse's uniform he was all set for another busy day in casualty.

'I thought you might like some company,' he said. 'Did you sleep okay?'

'Not bad,' I said. 'Mrs Thomas over there had a bad night and I'm a bit nattered about this week, if I'm honest.'

'You just have to last this one out,' he said. 'It'll pass and then you'll know where to go from here.'

My throat was dry with nerves as I thought about the tests. My breathing was still laboured and raspy and I worried the bronchoscopy would make it even worse. My throat was sore from the dry, tickly cough and it was making it difficult for me to speak.

A nurse appeared with my notes.

'Are you okay to walk round for your scan?' she asked.

'Yes, of course,' I said. I gathered up my bound orange folder of notes, more than an inch in thickness now I'd been a patient for so many years, and headed up to the scanning unit.

The radiographer introduced herself as Pat and she escorted me to the scanning room. I was halfway through telling her all about my postgraduate course when the first image of my scan was projected on to the screen in front of me. I could see the outline of my pelvis, the bottom of my back, my hips and the upper part of my legs, represented as fuzzy grey black dots, like pointillism pictures. As I studied it, I could see darker areas, one in my lower back, several in my pelvis, one in my left hip. I couldn't believe what I was seeing.

The darker areas showed an increased uptake of the isotope. I knew it could mean a number of things but, with so many sites, the logical explanation was that I had secondary bone cancer. I was stunned, unable to take my eyes off the grainy image, and was still staring at it when the machine bleeped. The radiographer got up and repositioned me in front of the machine.

'Is that me?' I asked, pointing at the image I could see.

'Yes,' she said. Her chattiness had gone, replaced by a friendly professionalism.

'We've got a few more images to acquire, it won't take long,' she said. 'I'll review them quickly at the end.'

I felt remarkably calm. I didn't collapse in floods of tears. I finally had the answer to the aches and pains I'd been experiencing. As the images continued to flash up on the screen, I watched them feeling a sense of detachment. More areas with more disease; my left shoulder that had given me so much pain recently.

'Funny, I thought I would have more pain than that,' I reflected as the darker areas became more prevalent. I'd been managing the pain of bone cancer with paracetamol. I'd always thought I'd have been drugged up to the eyes with morphine if I'd been this ill.

Sufficiently composed to walk out of the room, I greeted my mum who had come to visit me. Together, we returned to the ward.

'Here they are,' I said, passing my mum a wallet of photographs. I thought you might like to see the pictures of my garden.'

Looking at the recently developed pictures, Mum was impressed by how far the garden had come on. By now, the arches had fingered leaves of clematis climbing up them and the flowerbed, which I had been unable to plant up, I'd made to look like a French parterre. There were wigwams of red-flowered green beans at the corners, dwarf black beans curling in the plants radiating diagonally from the centre. The sides of the square were made up of the feathery leaves of carrot and the four triangles were full of four different-coloured leaved vegetables. Mum looked through them and the holiday photos of us all smiling and happy on the French beach.

Sitting in companionable silence I must have fallen asleep because when I next looked up Mike was sitting with Mum and they were talking in whispers. I sat up slowly and tipped my head forward as he lightly brushed his lips against my cheek.

'I'll get off, then,' Mum said, jangling around in her pockets for her car keys. 'I'll pop in tomorrow if I may.'

When she had gone, Mike asked, 'Anything new?'

I nodded slowly, desperately thinking what words to use, and picked at the cuff of my pyjama jacket, unable to meet his gaze.

'There are lots of hot spots on the bone scan,' I said eventually. 'Oh Mike. It can't be anything else. It must be my cancer back.'

MIKE

Everything seemed to stop; sounds, smells, every sense seemed to be suspended so Jane had my complete attention. I was unable to take it in. Jane spoke softly: 'You know what it means, don't you?' Her self-control seemed to contradict her words. I stood up and moved across to her. If she was going to die, why was she so calm?

'Yes,' I replied, but in truth I was confused. I struggled to understand what she was telling me. Her face showed no emotion. I didn't want to ask for clarification but I must have appeared puzzled.

'I'm so sorry, Mike,' she said.

I moved to sit next to her on the bed and we held hands tightly.

'I don't want to die,' she said. I sat still in preparation for some huge outpouring of emotion. For years I'd lived in fear of this moment but I just sat there, dumb, unable to comprehend that my soul mate, her warm body currently making my hands sweat, was going to die.

In the past, I'd always imagined that if I heard this dreadful news, I'd break down in some extravagant show of despair. But sitting here now, I couldn't cry or even articulate any words which would bring Jane some comfort. I started to shake slightly. My heart raced, making my whole body tingle as if a small electric current was running through it, tensing my muscles.

'How sure are you?' I asked.

'Absolutely certain,' she said. 'The radiographer was as shocked as I was. It was an absolutely classic case of metastatic breast cancer.'

A vacuum, like a black hole, sucked me in, making my surroundings disappear. I felt like we were the only two people in the ward, marooned on an NHS bed. I was unable to shed a tear, my head feeling like it was overheating, my senses deprived, completely and utterly bereft, impotent to the point of being punch-drunk. I felt my body rocking on the bed, gently as if in the arms of my mum. I could feel Jane breathing heavily, gasping for breaths.

For a long, long time, we sat still like that until Belinda appeared. When she spoke, I heard her voice but the words' meanings were beyond me. I moved to the chair. The two women hugged and the dams burst. I left, determined not to fold. Outside, I dodged the internal hospital traffic and walked to the multidenominational chapel. I had nothing pleasant to say to God, so I sat on the lawn at the front and sadness overwhelmed me. Touching the grass was comforting, a physical reassurance that not everything had changed. I plucked a couple of blades, both snapping at a height just above soil level.

A late-middle-aged lady accompanied her daughter at the bus stop, her nightdress hanging underneath her coat. Hospital staff walked past, followed by a man only slightly younger than me, with a toddler by his side, clutching a bouquet of flowers heading for Lincoln Wing and the maternity unit. I smiled, remembering.

My thoughts drifted to Jane lying a stone's throw away. Quietly, I said some prayers, asking for strength for both of us, hoping we had not been completely forsaken. In a desire to be proactive, I decided to amble to the ward. Forty-five minutes on my own was enough.

At the entrance an ambulance pulled up and the tailgate was lowered, a wheelchair appeared. I waited until the space was cleared before going back into the hospital. I didn't want to crowd Jane but I wanted to be with her. Peering at her bedside unnoticed, I saw Belinda and Jane sharing a joke. It seemed irreverent to try to add a comment so I joined them silently, took a seat and observed them.

Belinda turned to me.

'How do you fancy a cup of tea in the office?' she said, nodding towards the bay's entrance. For the first time in hours I became aware that my throat was dry and I'd not drunk anything, but I didn't want to leave Jane.

'No thanks,' I said.

Jane looked across at me. 'Go on, Mike, please. I need a bit of time to myself.'

'Are you sure?'

'Yes, please go. I'm all right, honest'

Belinda made to go. 'Come on,' she said. 'I've even got milk, I think.'

We walked a hundred yards in silence to the breast clinic. It was locked and dark when we arrived, like a school corridor without any children. Two receptionist's chairs were empty, the computer screens were blank, the desks bereft of patients' notes.

Belinda spoke: 'If we didn't lock these areas there'd be nothing left by tomorrow.'

'You're joking,' I said.

'You ask Jane,' she said. 'We've had people come into the children's oncology unit and steal the PlayStations that the kids use. They're completely heartless.'

Belinda unlocked her office and I followed her inside. It was a room I'd been to before, but without the daytime bustle the atmosphere was different. Like a mad professor's tutor room, the chaos wasn't confined to her desk. The shelves, the floor, the chairs were all cluttered with papers and folders. She quickly threw some pamphlets off a chair and told me to sit down. A tray with mugs stood precariously on one shelf, fighting for space with a box of prosthetics.

'How's work?' she asked.

'It's just work, you know,' I replied.

'Are the kids at your mum's?'

'Yes,' I replied.

'What's Jane told you?'

'Everything.'

'Do you understand all the implications?' she asked.

'It's a little confusing.' The thoughts in my mind fluttered like the opening frames of a film reel.

'It's important you understand everything,' Belinda said calmly.

'Yes, I know,' I said.

'The most important thing for you to understand is that Jane is going to die.'

It was as though she'd administered a dose of smelling salts. My mind was suddenly alert. She continued: 'There's nothing anyone can do. No miracle cures. Nothing. The cancer is in her bones, there's no point contemplating any reversal. It would seem very likely that the growth in her lung is also cancer. The bone cancer won't kill her, but it may spread the disease to other areas. People can live for quite a while with bone metastases, though it will be very painful and debilitating. The growth in her lung will most likely be the cause of death or alternatively the disease will spread to other vital organs. She's going to die, Mike, and you need to be strong for her.'

I nodded and muttered, 'I know.'

Her manner of delivery was hard but professional. She showed little emotion, ensuring that her message was getting through. 'I'm sorry, Michael, it's better this way,' she said as though reading my thoughts. 'No false hopes. There is no hope.'

I was on the verge of breaking down but I was damned if I was going to. An eerie silence followed as I looked out of the window. It had become dusk outside.

'Mr Lansdown will speak to you tomorrow. He'll go through everything, give you a referral to an oncologist who'll discuss treatment options,' she continued. 'Jane may be entitled to an allowance. It will be about fifty pounds a week but the condition is that you're expected only to live for the next six months.'

Like cold steel ripping through my skin, those words tore me apart. February, six months is February, she won't even make her thirty-seventh birthday.

Belinda saw my reaction. 'I'm not saying that she will or won't die in six months, Mike,' she said. 'All I'm saying is that she may be entitled to that money. And I'm guessing you could use it. Weekends away, that kind of thing.'

'Every cloud, eh?' I said flatly.

'There's a leaflet here.' She turned and started rifling through pamphlets, throwing them over her shoulder like discarded rounds from a machine gun.

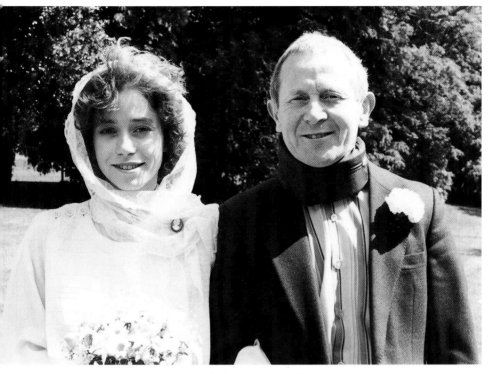

Jane and her dad on our wedding day.

Our daughters, Suzanne and Rebecca, in our first house.

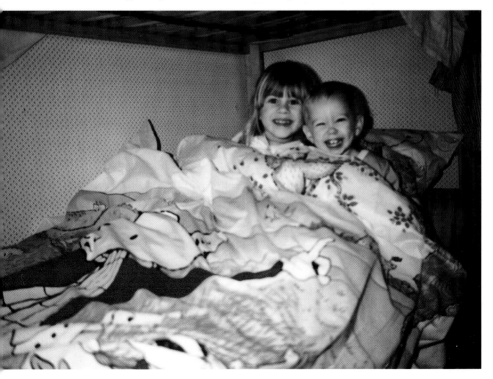

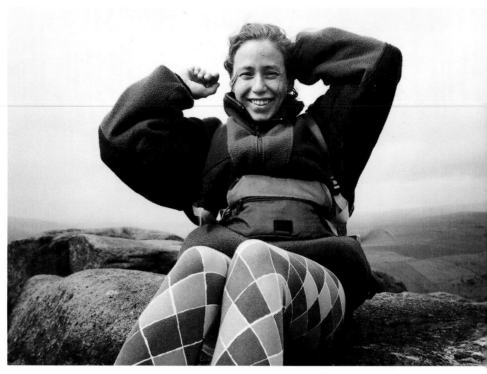

Jane's choice leggings.

Jane, Suzanne and Rebecca at Ingleton waterfalls in 1992.

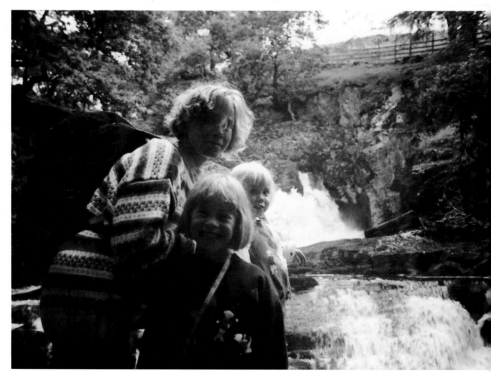

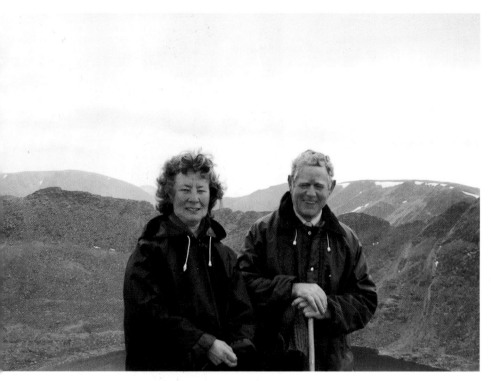

Mike's parents, Alice and Jack, on Helvellyn.

Jane and her mum at
the Yorkshire Women
of Achievement
Awards in 2002.

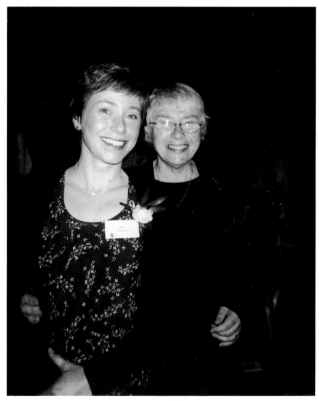

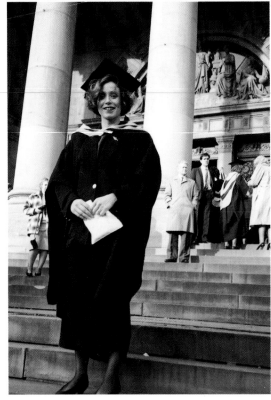

Jane collected her Diploma in Radiography at Leeds Town Hall in 1993.

Steven at one day old in 1997.

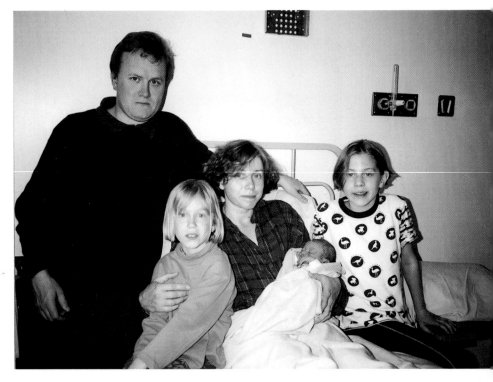

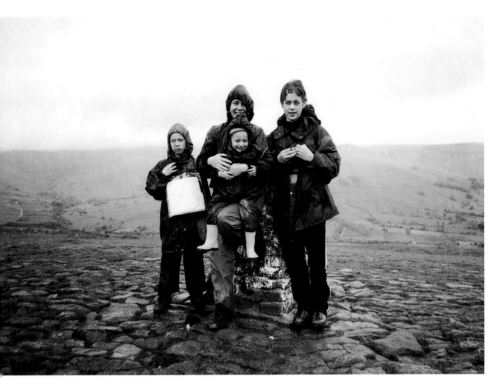

Another beautiful day in the Peak District: a family walk in April 2000.

Summer evening in the Lake District: a quiet moment without the children.

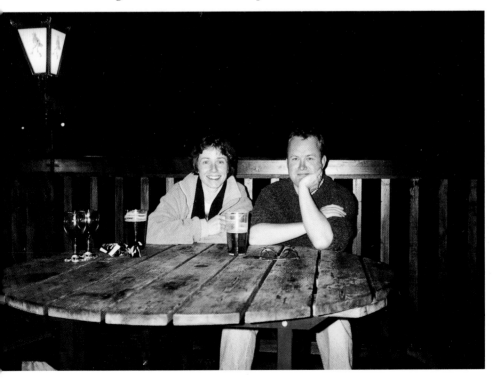

It's people not places that count.

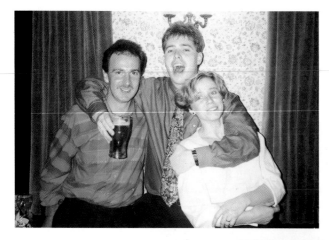

Mick West, Stephen Ridgeway and Jane at Stephen and Melissa's wedding day in 1991.

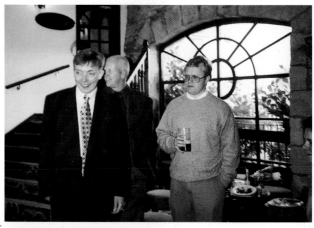

Stephen Whiteside, Jon Colman and Mike.

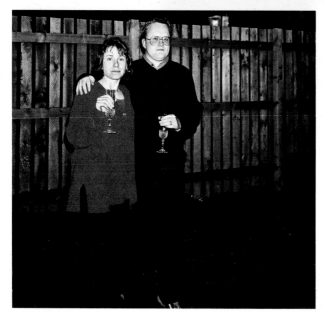

Millennium Eve: Helium Man puts his arm around Jane to stop himself floating away.

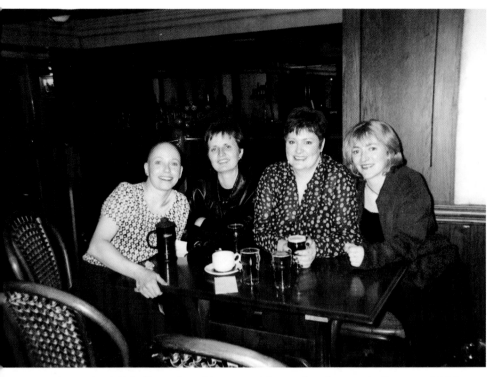

Jane, Amanda, Michelle and Jackie on a girly weekend away in January 2001.

Celebrating with Belinda on Jane's birthday.

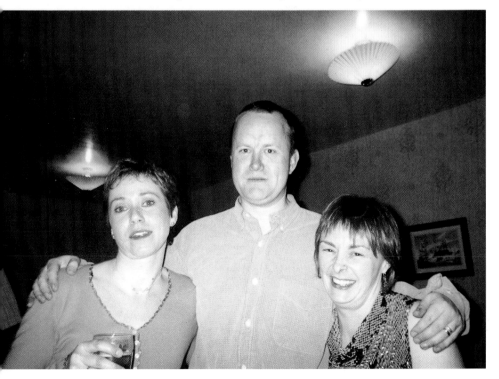

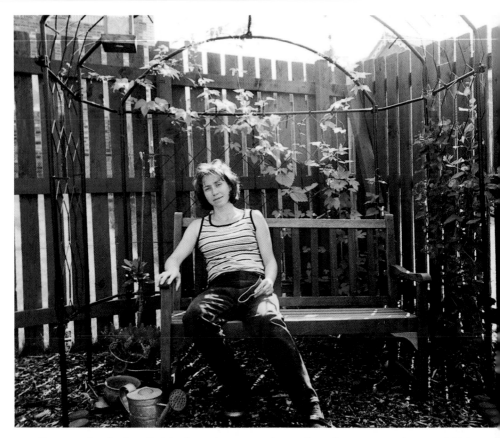

Jane resting in her finished garden just prior to her diagnosis in August 2000.

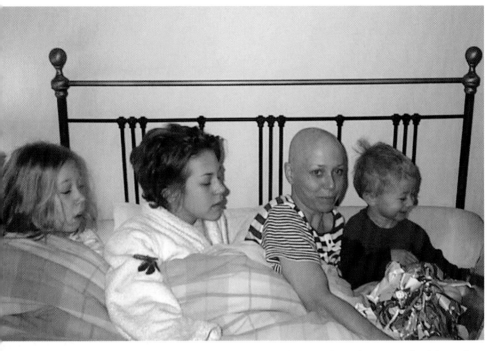

Christmas morning in bed, 2000: Jane worries needlessly about having a bad hair day.

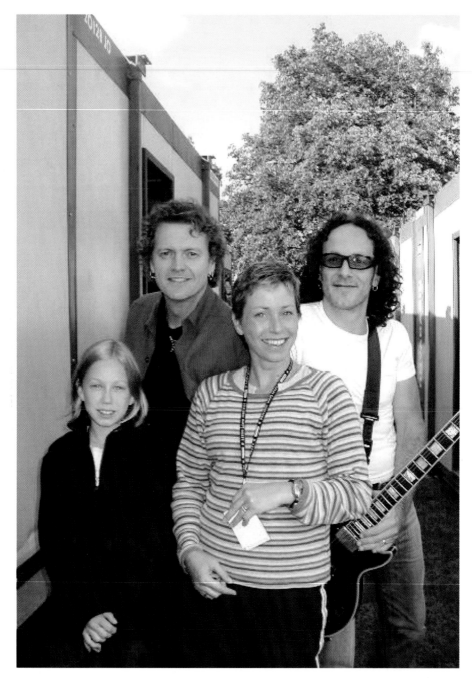

Posing with Def Leppard, from left to right: Rebecca, Rick Allen,
Jane and Vivian Campbell.

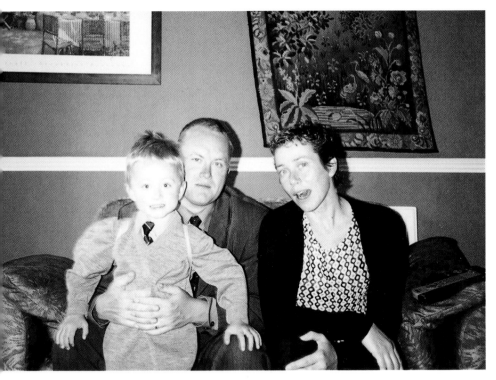

Seeing Steven's first day at school in 2001: another goal achieved.

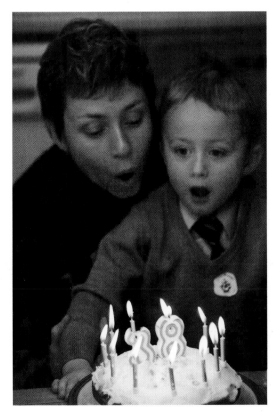

Jane's 38th birthday.

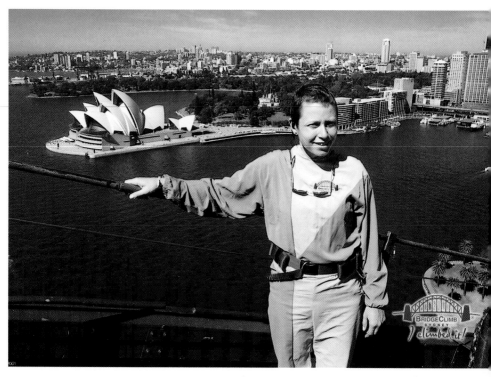

At the top of the Sydney Harbour Bridge, admiring the scenery after a strenuous climb

Holidaying in Australia, still recovering from chemotherapy.

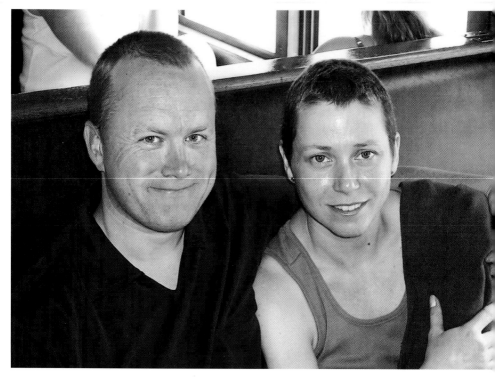

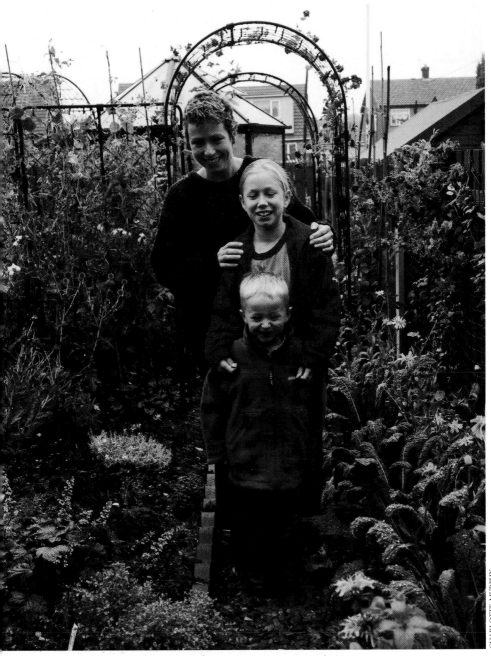

Jane, Rebecca and Steven in Jane's garden in autumn 2001.

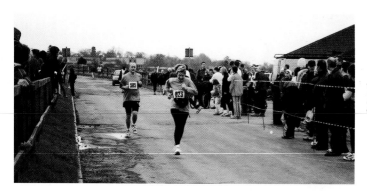

York half-marathon, 2002. We let Jane win!

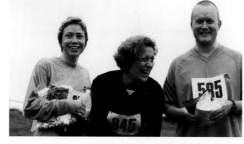

Jane, Delia and Mike after the run.

Mike and Steven crossing the finishing line of the London Marathon, 2002.

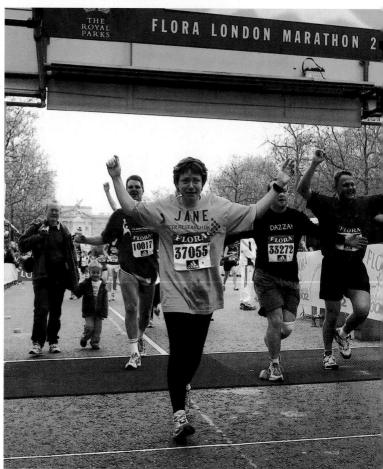

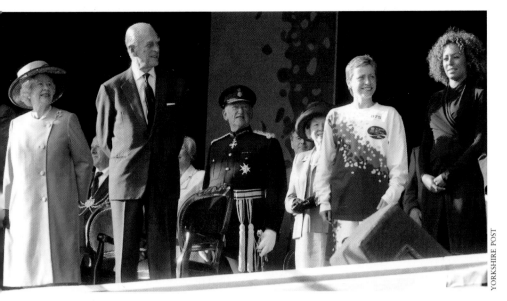

Jane after the commonwealth baton relay at Temple Newsam.

At the finish of the London Triathlon, 2002,
crossing the line in under three and a half hours.

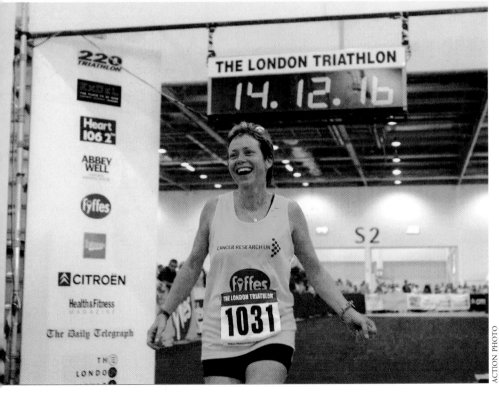

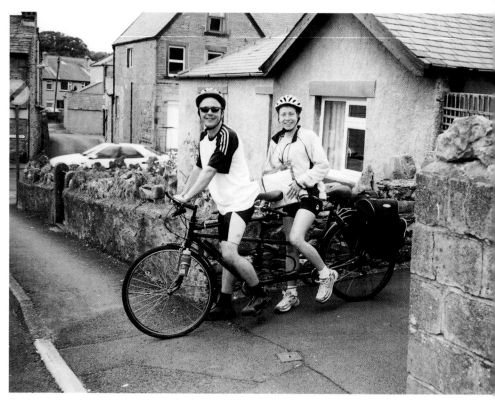
Luke and Jane set off on a tandem tour of the Dales in September 2002. Note their high spec tandem and optimistic clothing.

'Jane always said she'd make me rich,' I said.

'I'll need a consultant's signature,' said Belinda. 'That won't be a problem.'

'I'm not sure Jane will be too happy with it,' I said. 'Let me know if she's not and I'll use some sophisticated charm – or failing that, extreme violence.'

'She's also entitled to a disabled parking sticker and mobility allowance. She'd need to be assessed.'

'Jackpot,' I said. 'Money and we can park anywhere? Our luck's in tonight. She won't agree to that, though. There's no way she's going to agree to a disabled sticker, that's not going to happen.'

Belinda passed me a battered leaflet and then another.

'What's this?' I asked. 'Dying for dummies?'

She said, 'Listen, I'm here for you as well as Jane, if you need me.'

'I'll be fine. I won't let Jane down. I love her.'

Holding back the tears I needed to go. 'We'd best be getting back, she'll be thinking we've nipped out for a pint,' I said.

JANE

Belinda's pixie-like face appeared through the bedside curtains that I'd pulled around to give myself some privacy. She looked serious.

'Life's such a bastard,' she said and promptly burst into tears. Her loss of control was short-lived and she soon composed herself. 'Mike's gone for a walk, he just needs a few minutes on his own. I'm afraid I had to tell him some harsh home truths. He just needs some time to cope with them.'

I nodded at her.

'You know there's no cure, don't you?' she asked.

I nodded again, afraid that if I tried to speak tears would cascade down my face and I would not be able to stop.

'What about chemo?' I asked eventually.

'The oncology team will have some ideas,' she said. 'There are some new treatments but there's no guarantee they will be of any help at this stage.'

I watched her as she thought of something to say.

'There are some forms that need filling in,' she said. 'Are you okay for me to do those? You can get benefits if the doctors think you might die within six months. I'm not saying you will, I'm just saying it's money you're entitled to. Life's going to be tough and this might make it easier.'

'I don't feel that ill,' I said.

Belinda shook her head.

'Listen, just because the forms say you might die in six months doesn't mean you will. In fact, I expect you to be around for quite a long while yet. You're far too stubborn.'

She wagged her finger at me. 'So, you'll let me fill these out, then?' she asked.

'Of course,' I replied.

Mike returned, pale faced, and shoved a wad of tissues from my bedside table into his pocket. I could see him brave a smile but his red-rimmed eyes gave away his sorrow.

'Will you be okay?' I asked him.

'Don't worry about me,' he said. 'I'll be fine. I might call in and see Jon tonight. I can't face going home straightaway.'

After a few moments, we unlaced our fingers and I watched as he left the ward. The night stretched ahead and I lay there, wondering how I would get through it. One step at a time. I filled in the minutes, I showered, dressed and read a little. I made some more notes for my course. The evening drink trolley arrived and I sipped at the sweet, milky liquid. As I lay down, my cough started, dry and tickly. I hacked until my throat was sore.

'Are you all right?' A nurse appeared beside me.

I nodded, still coughing.

'I can get you some warm linctus,' she said. 'That might help.'

She went away and returned with some warm cough medicine, which felt soothing as it slid down my throat. I lay back, closed my eyes and thought of Mike and the children.

Holding Steven's woolly gloved hand as we walk up Watery Lane, he is laughing as he kicks his way through small snow drifts, watching the powdery snow scatter from the kick from his tiny yellow Wellington boot. Suzanne and Rebecca are running on ahead, Suzanne reaches up and pings on a branch and a white flurry descends. I walk with care, picking my way through frozen footprints, trying not to slide. Mike and his friend Steve Chapman bring up the rear. Steve, red cheeked and taller than Mike, wears a thin anorak. Mike is hidden in a brown duffle-coat. It's months since they've seen each other but it's as if they had never been apart, chatting easily with one another.

We carry on up the snowy lane, the cloudless sky heavy and full, pressing down on the white-capped peaks around us. We carry on across the road through a small stile into the field beyond and head for the wooded area. The stunted gnarled trees look like grotesque dwarves, the giant black trunks etched with white. Frosted spikes of grass crunch as we squash them with our boots, we cross the field in a diagonal, leaving a trail.

As we reach the other side, I hear a crack, like gun-shot. Suzanne and Rebecca are jumping on an ice-covered puddle, the small hole leaking muddy water. Their feet crash down again and cracks creep out to the outside edges, another whip-like crack as the ice separates. Small fluffy flakes catch in Steven's coat, he lifts his grey gloves, hoping to catch some of the larger ones, and brings them to his mouth, his pink tongue tasting the coldness. We carry on walking, dropping down on to the walled lane, the snow is falling heavily now and we are rushing to get home. My fingers are tingling with cold and Steven stamps his feet. Mike and I round the corner and I duck just in time to miss the compact snowball, turning to deflect it, it misses my head but hits my back. Cold snow cascades down the back of my jacket, making me shriek. I wriggle to try to get rid of the melting ice and look up just in time to see Mike hit full on in the face.

*'Right!' he shouts and bends down to scoop up a hand-
ful of fresh snow. Patting it into a ball he runs at the girls,
who in turn scream and run away as he lobs the snowball
at them. He turns his attention to his tall friend, throwing
two snowballs in quick succession, and turning his back to
avoid the retaliation.*

*Steven scoops a small handful of snow and throws it
towards the marauding group. He is laughing, his mouth
open, his eyes wide. Mike ducks and the snow intended for
him hits Steven in his face. His eyes shutting, his face
screwing up, he starts to cry. I bend down to hold him,
brushing the snow away from his face. A small pink mark
on his cheek shows where he has been hit. He quietens in
my arms, the hurt forgotten.*

I lay in my narrow hospital bed, unable to block out the harsh
white lights of the ward. I pictured my family last winter.
Suzanne and Rebecca shouting and laughing, their voices echoing in the cold air. Mike rushing at them, making them shriek in
horror. Steven, pink cheeked, his long lashes fringed with snow.
I wanted more memories to treasure, memories for *them* to
treasure. I didn't want to leave them, Steven was too young to
abandon. I wanted to be a mum and a wife for a little while
longer and I cried at the thought of my family without me.
Cried at the uncertainty of my future.

MIKE

The house was dark; the bowling club floodlights illuminated
the living room. Reflections from the front door window made
a pattern on the hall carpet from the street lights. Picking up the
telephone receiver I dialled the number.

'Hi, Carol,' I said. 'Is Jon there?'

'He's on a course, Mike, overnight at the resi',' she said.

Shit. I remembered now. Stuck for words, I released a stut-
tered 'okay'.

'Is everything all right, Mike?' she asked. 'Is it Jane?'

I didn't want to alarm her.

'No,' I said. 'Not perfect.'

'Do you want to come round?'

It was Jon I had wanted to see but the house was so damned depressing I couldn't face the thought of being on my own.

'Yes, I'll pop over.'

Within fifteen minutes I was parking outside their house. Carol answered the door and we made our way into the kitchen.

'Are Holly and Sophie in bed?' I asked.

'Yes,' said Carol. 'Do you fancy a drink – tea, coffee, or Jon's got some beer in the garage?'

'A tea's great,' I said.

'You don't look too good,' she said.

'Thanks.'

'No seriously, you don't. How's Jane?'

'Er . . . she's back in hospital,' I said, thinking about taking my fleece off but instead I just sat down at the kitchen table. 'We've had some bad news. The cancer's come back.'

'Oh no.' Carol put the kettle down and came over to the table, taking the seat next to me.

'There's nothing anyone can do.' I shrugged.

'What?' I could see by the quizzical look on her face that I needed to clarify. 'The cancer's in her bones. There's no cure. She's going to die.'

Carol winced, recoiling from the same bluntness I'd been on the receiving end of only hours earlier. Sensing she was about to dissolve into tears, I quickly added: 'Please don't cry. I need you to be stoical for me. If I start, I might not stop.'

'Are they sure?' she said.

'Yes. The breast care nurse said not to even dream that there might be a cure. Jane and I need to accept it and deal with it.'

'How do they know?'

'Because that's the way it is. We always knew that if the cancer ever got into her bones, that would be it.'

'I can't believe there's nothing anyone can do. What about the internet? America? There must be something in the world—'

'There's nothing, Carol,' I interrupted.

'But there must be—'

'No,' I said firmly. We sat in silence. After a couple of minutes I said, 'Anyway, what kind of caff is it here? The service is appalling.'

Carol got up, picked up the kettle and put it on. As she poured the tea she found her voice.

'How's Jane?' she asked.

'She seemed okay,' I said. 'Although there's bound to be a time when she crumbles. Neither of us wanted to break down in front of each other. We've been dreading this day for a long time. Ten years.'

'If you need anything, you know where we are,' she said.

'Thanks.' There was a pause. 'It's the kids. I just don't think I can face telling them and breaking their hearts. But I know we've got to do it.'

'Are you going to tell them everything?'

'Yes, they have to know. They have to be able to trust us.'

'Even Steven?'

'Yes.'

'Oh, Michael.' She looked at me sadly as I took another sip of my tea. 'Do you want to stay over? There's a spare bed. You shouldn't be on your own. I've got some wine.'

'Thanks but no thanks. I don't think the alcohol would be a good idea. I'd better be sober in case Jane rings and wants me to go back.' Jon and Carol's house felt too warm, too comforting. Something inside me needed to experience a sense of loss, pain and discomfort. Solitude had to be faced, after all there was a lifetime of it stretching in front of me. Better to get used to it now.

'Are you sure you'll be okay?'

'Yes, I've practised at being a grown-up. How's Holly doing at school?'

'Fine, fine,' she said and the phone rang. Carol spoke quietly although I guessed it was Jon. She called from the hall. 'Do you want to speak to Jon?'

'No,' I answered. 'I'll catch up with him later.'

I leant back on the chair and stretched out my arm on the

radiator. Cold, I craved that feeling where frozen hands redden and swell against a blistering hot pipe, causing any kind of tingling which would make me feel alive. I felt uncomfortable, as if I was wearing someone else's clothes. My flesh creeped from their touch. My thoughts wandered: how many times would I have to go through this conversation?

When she returned to the kitchen Carol had telltale red eyes. 'You soft sod,' I said.

At home, the loneliness took hold. Spying my breakfast dishes on the kitchen table, I realized I'd not eaten for over twelve hours, but I couldn't face food, I felt too nauseous. A full Talisker bottle on the kitchen worktop shone like a beacon. I went over to it and lifted it, reading the label. But common sense prevailed.

I brewed up and went into the living room. Turning on the amp I chose Led Zeppelin and programmed 'In My Time of Dying' and 'Kashmir' and pressed play. The mystical melody of the latter lifted my mood slightly after the bluesy first. I replaced the CD with Radiohead's 'OK Computer', its sombre, miserable tone fitting perfectly with my mood. As 'Karma Police' started, I felt the hairs on my neck stand up.

The neon lights of the CD player glowed in the darkened room, illuminating it with a blue tinge. The settee sagged in the middle so I moved to the left, out of the centre of the speakers. At least I was comfortable. I felt completely inadequate. How could I ever perform the roles that Jane performed?

I envisaged the garden being my albatross. There was only one way it could go – downhill. I had premonitions that it would turn into something resembling a rainforest. Everyone who visited would comment. The decorating? How would I manage? A friend always said, 'If you can piss you can paint.' I seemed to be the exception. I panicked.

The kids. How could I be mum to them? My thoughts wandered to Jane. How was she? I was tempted to ring the hospital to check but figured no one would thank me for that, so I decided to ring first thing in the morning.

I changed the CD again, unable to find music to suit the moment. Every time the thought that Jane was going to die overcame me, thousands of unanswered questions appeared. Tears welled up again but who was I going to cry for – myself? Or Jane? This had to stop, my emotions had to be controlled, I had to keep my strength, I couldn't wallow in self-pity. Depression would only be self-serving and I knew once I started it would never stop. Something Carol had said earlier in the evening resonated.

'You must be angry,' she'd said.

I felt a lot of things, too many to understand, but no angst, so no anger, no self-pity, no depression. I prayed quietly for Jane to be given enough strength for the following months.

Awake by four, up by five, I spent a couple of hours tidying the house and watching the news. It was a relief to get to seven o'clock and have the normal routine of the day to go through. It was puzzling that even though I'd been awake so long it was still a rush to get ready – wash, teeth, suit. I'd planned to go into work, arrange a few days off and go to the hospital.

Running downstairs, I grabbed my fleece and put it on, emptying the pockets of tissues, paper, Steven's toys. Sitting on the bottom stair I picked up the phone and called Jane's ward.

'Hi, it's Mike Tomlinson, Jane's husband. I'm just ringing to see how she is.'

'She's fine,' said the nurse. 'She's sitting up in bed reading.'

'Can you tell her I'll be there soon?'

As I spoke, the shadowy outline of the postman approached the front door. The letterbox opened and an envelope with what appeared to be a card fluttered through the door. I recognized the handwriting but couldn't figure out whose it was. Postmark Leeds, nine-thirty, yesterday morning. I ripped the seal open, it was a card of the Little Prince, an angelic infant boy sitting on clouds with the line, 'It is only with the heart that one can see rightly; what is essential is invisible to the eye.'

It could only be from Jane. I opened the card.

Dear Mike,

I saw this card and thought of you!!!
Thank you for all your support this
week. I love you more than I can
ever say and always have. I'm missing
you tonight. You're my best friend &
I'm sure we can get through this
together!

All my love for ever
Jane
xxx

My body jerked with uncontrollable sobs. Every ounce of control gave way and from my seated position on the stair I fell tearfully into a foetal position on the floor. I lay there, crying out, paralysed by the thought that I was losing the only person I'd ever loved. My world had dissolved. There was no future.

JANE

I spoke to the Mr Lansdown, the consultant, on his ward round, early next day. Mike made sure he was there to be with me.

'We want to see an oncologist as soon as possible,' I said. 'I know there was something on my bone scan and I want to know what my options are.'

Mr Lansdown hesitated. 'What did the bone scan show?' he asked.

I thought carefully as to how to phrase my reply, so I could convince him I wasn't panicking needlessly.

'Lots of active sites, there was increased uptake in several areas consistent with metastatic bone disease.'

He nodded and turned to one of the junior doctors beside him. 'Could you contact the oncology team?' He spoke with an authoritative tone. 'Arrange an appointment.'

Turning to face me again he said: 'You've an appointment for a bronchoscopy this afternoon. I still think it's very important that we carry it out. We need as much information as possible if we're going to decide which treatment is best for you.'

I nodded in agreement and watched as the party of medics moved on to the next bed. Later that morning, the young house officer returned.

'You've got an appointment at the outpatients clinic this afternoon,' he said.

'Thank you,' I said. He stood there looking lost for words so I added. 'I just want to find out what's going on so I can tell my kids at the weekend.'

Mike and I set off for my appointment after lunch. The oncology unit was on a grim, grey corridor lined with grey chairs.

A young man with thick-rimmed glasses called my name.

'Hello, Jane,' he said. 'I'm Dr Ward. If you'd like to come this way. One of the doctors from Mr Brennan's team has explained the situation to me,' he said once we were in his office. His voice was hushed and I found myself leaning in to catch the words. 'He told me you wanted to discuss the implications. It would appear that your disease has spread to your bones and that would be the likeliest cause of the abnormalities in your chest CT. The bronchoscopy this afternoon will verify this and might help us decide the best course of treatment at this stage.'

I nodded. 'Can you tell me what my prognosis is?'

There was a lengthy silence. He looked down at his desk before raising his head. He cleared his throat and looked over the rim of his glasses. His direct stare made me shift uncomfortably. I struggled to understand his words.

'You have months to a year to live, possibly two years,' he said. 'Your disease is advanced. There may be some chemotherapy options to consider but you will die of your disease.'

I sat motionless, stunned by the harsh knowledge. Tears fell from my eyes and I brushed them away. Tears had no use here, I needed to be composed to understand and contemplate the options open to me.

'Months to live.' The doctor's words echoed in a long corridor, dimly lit, with purple swirled carpet underfoot, hemmed in by dark maroon walls. I felt myself thrown against a brick wall. There was no way forward, this was how my life would end. My breath felt punched out of me by the shock. Where had my life gone? How would my family cope?

'That's not long.' The words fell from my lips. I focused my attention back into the room. Dr Ward leant forward in his chair, studying me, watching my reaction. 'You said something about treatment options?' My voice was hoarse, my throat dry.

'Yes,' he said. 'There's a trial you may be eligible for involving high dose chemotherapy but it would mean you would have to be nursed in isolation for up to six weeks. There's no promise that it would reverse your disease but it might stop it progressing for a while.'

He handed me a leaflet. 'This describes the treatment and the side effects you might experience,' he said. I took the piece of paper and glanced at the front page. 'You might want to think very carefully whether this would be the right option for you, though, Jane. You may find yourself spending time in hospital when you could be at home with your family. At this stage of your disease, I urge you to look to the present and not to the future.'

His words were delivered calmly and thoughtfully but with a quiet force. I felt the weight of a heavy decision fall on me.

'Read the information,' he said. 'There are many questions you might need answering. I'll try to explain things more fully when you've had chance to take everything in. This isn't the only option open to you. There are other combinations of drugs that may be worth trying.'

I could feel his dark brown eyes studying my face, making sure I understood.

Afterwards, Mike and I walked slowly back to the ward. We held hands, the small physical contact helping to ease the weighty silence. My head felt heavy with impossible decisions. The enormity of it all overwhelmed me. The void of no future exhausted me.

My life was going to end. I had nothing to hold on to, only certain death and, before that, the awful business of dying. The growing horror constricted my chest and I struggled for breath. Rigid with fear, I gripped Mike's hand as I imagined a gaunt, pale figure lying in bed, her eyes sunken, and her cheek bones prominent, her wrists painfully thin. It terrified me.

As we stepped into the ward, a nurse noticed us both and came over.

'I'll pull the curtains round,' she said softly. 'You don't need anyone looking in.'

'Oh Mike,' I said, looking up at his sad, stony face. 'What are we going to do?'

I didn't expect an answer and we sat in silence with our own thoughts. The only thing to stop me collapsing under the weight of the trauma was the prospect of treatment. It wouldn't cure me, wouldn't lighten the horizon, but might allow me to step back from the bricked-off future.

'Are you having some tea, love?' a woman's voice asked me. I sat myself up in bed.

'Yes,' I croaked, dry-mouthed. My throat was sore but I had not eaten since the morning so I took the tray of food and peeped underneath the metal lid. Liver casserole with mashed potato. I put the lid back on, while I summoned the energy to eat.

Just as I decided to give the meal a go, a voice said: 'You can't possibly be thinking of eating that.'

It was my sister Mary, who leant in to kiss me, with my boss Gill, who was scraping a chair towards my bed from the other side of the ward.

'I'm so hungry even this looks okay,' I smiled. 'You don't mind if I eat, do you?'

'Actually, I do if you're going to eat that,' said Gill. 'It looks revolting.'

'It'll be worse cold,' I said and started picking at the meal, separating the gristle from meat. I shovelled it down hastily, the warm gravy disguising the lumps in the potato.

'You need a medal for eating that,' laughed Gill. She reached into her bag, retrieving a pink envelope and a small parcel. They were from my friends at work – shower gel and other smellies.

'Thanks,' I said. My eyes were still puffy from all the tears shed that afternoon and I was touched by the warm wishes in the card. Another tear fell from my eye.

'Oh Jane,' said Gill gently, standing up to place her hand on my arm. Mary looked on.

'How's it going?' she asked.

'Pretty crap really,' I said, not knowing how to describe my day. 'I've seen the oncologist today and things couldn't be much worse,' I said, glancing at their faces in turn. 'They're talking about months, possibly a year.'

They looked horrified.

'What about treatments?' asked Mary.

'I've got a few options to go through, it looks quite positive and might give me a little more time. But it means I'll have to spend more time in hospital and that scares me.'

It was a conversation stopper and we sat there in silence until Gill spoke.

'Have you had your bronchoscopy?' she asked.

'Yes, couldn't get out of it. I had it this afternoon.'

'That makes you eating that mess even more impressive,' she said.

Mike was my last visitor of the night. We sat and talked about what to tell the children. We'd already decided that the kids would be told everything. No secrets. If we were honest with them from the start at least they would know we were not hiding anything from them. They were going to lose their mum. They had a right to know so they could ask if there was anything special they wanted us to do together. So they could have their own special memory in the future.

I didn't want to be alone and Mike stayed long after the bell chimed for the end of visiting time. Eventually he stood. 'I'll see you tomorrow. Ring me if you want to talk.'

We stood, clinging to each other, tears pouring down my face on to his shirt. I grabbed a tissue to wipe them away.

'I'm fine really,' I said, looking up at Mike's distraught face. 'You get off. I'm going to have a bath.'

He kissed me and left the ward, turning at the door to blow me another kiss.

The night drew out before me. I lay on my back, pulling the covers under my chin.

I had always hoped Mike and I would end up living in the Yorkshire Dales with the countryside on our doorstep. That dream was shattered now. There was no future. Only what I had. I ached for my family and knew right there that I wanted to have enough time to give Suzanne, Rebecca and Steven some happy memories. I wanted to enjoy some good times over the next few months, shying away from the important decisions I knew I'd have to face. I hoped for some help in making them.

'Please God,' I prayed. 'Give me the courage to guide me in my decisions, help me stay calm to deal with this. Comfort Mike and the children so we can all stay positive. Comfort my mum and help her deal with some of this sadness.' Although I was finding it hard to deal with, I knew it would be harder if it had been happening to one of my children.

I tried to think what it would be like for Mum. No parent should have to see their child die and I imagined her grieving.

Mum was my first visitor of the day, arriving before the ward round the next morning. I'd asked Luke the night before for advice as to what to say to her. He'd said 'Be honest.' Looking at her sitting next to me, her face furrowed with worry, I knew he was right but it was difficult.

Afterwards we sat holding hands in silence and Mr Lansdown walked in with his entourage of about a dozen nurses. I was to be discharged in the afternoon. After his rounds he came and sat with me for a few minutes and we talked about the trial.

'Think carefully about it, Jane,' he advised. 'It's been going on for some months now and there have been very mixed results. Not all the data have been gathered yet but the results are not as promising as they would have liked.'

I thanked him for his words and time and he left.

'Oh Mum, I don't know what to do now,' I said. I felt people were trying to dissuade me from taking that particular option but I didn't know which way to go. There were many small doubts and worries that I couldn't shake off. I didn't want to rush the decision and pushed the questions to the back of my mind.

At least I could leave the hospital. I began packing my things and clearing the bed.

MIKE

The silence at the other end of the phone made me wonder if the signal on the mobile had cut out.

'Did you hear me, Mick?' I said.

'Yes.' There followed another pause. 'Did they tell you how long?'

'A few months – March, April – maximum two years.'

'You'll need to be strong for her.'

'I know. I'll see you later.'

It was a completely unsatisfactory ending to a conversation between the closest of friends but there was nothing else to say. We both knew what we needed to do; that didn't include self-indulgent whingeing.

That night, I went out for a pint with a work colleague, Mick Parker who lived nearby. We rarely went out for drinks together but at least it got me out of the house, allowing the time to pass quicker and I knew he wouldn't overdramatize the conversation. His opening gambit of, 'I don't want you crying into your beer' set the tone.

We didn't talk about Jane or of cancer or of dying. We both realized the most appropriate approach was to be pragmatic and this couldn't be achieved by conducting a therapy session. But it hadn't dawned on me until then how impossible it is to conduct a normal conversation in these circumstances. Seemingly innocuous questions such as, 'Where are you going on holiday next summer?' or, 'Will you be spending Christmas at home?' can't be answered. Without wanting it, it was impossible to avoid the subject and the conversation went at a stuttering pace.

Telling the two Micks had been an exercise. They were my sounding boards, two chances to practise my lines before having to tell the kids. I had chosen them specifically, knowing their reactions would be deadpan, no matter how cut up about it they were.

Inflicting such misery on friends and family was going to be difficult. Constantly recounting the same bad news would be akin to reliving the death sentence again and again. It was impossible to know how folk would react. Experience told me that many would cry and I couldn't handle that.

On returning from the pub I decided to write a couple of e-mails. Steve and Karin Whiteside first. I rattled off the first few lines quickly, joking about football, asking how the kids were and, oh, by the way Jane's dying. Within five minutes I'd written a couple of hundred words and hit send. It was an easy and a soulless way of communicating the news as rapidly as possible. I appreciated it was an unfair way to deliver it but, however done, it wouldn't alter the situation. By sending the e-mails so late it ensured that no one would read them until tomorrow so at least it wouldn't prompt any phone calls.

'Bloody caravans,' I muttered as we trailed behind one on the road up to Settle. 'There should be a ban on the fucking things,' I said. 'Or they should only be allowed to travel between 3 a.m. and 5 a.m. each day.'

'Calm down,' said Jane from the passenger seat. 'There's no rush.' It was the same familiar car journey we'd made time and time again but today the Friday holiday-makers were out in force. Jane sat serenely, reflecting on what we were about to do – the heinous act of telling three children that their mum was going to die.

We needed to let them know the worst; it was a matter of trust and honesty, which would hopefully remove some uncertainty from their lives. Jane, even without having to impart the news, would have been tired from the rigours of the tests. She coughed every five minutes, was constantly dizzy and light-headed. Every day seemed to mark a further decline.

'We won't have to think about moving to Settle to retire,' she said.

'No,' I replied. My mind drifted as it had in the past to images of me and Jane as pensioners walking idly through Langcliffe together, looking across the Ribble Valley towards Stackhouse.

I looked at Jane. She looked peaceful. What a ten days it had been: you're fine . . . no, it's cancer . . . you're going to die . . . you've got months. The montage of all the conversations we'd had over that time replayed in my head like radio soundbites.

Before driving off to Settle we'd stopped at Luke and Karen's, seeking advice. Both were nurses and, as Karen worked for the Blood Service, Jane felt she would be in a good position to advise on the stem cell option.

Stem cell treatments would put Jane at risk of infection, which could lead to her premature death and would require a period of isolation. Research had not conclusively proved its use yet, although the feeling was that this treatment was the future, with potentially big gains.

Chemotherapy would be extremely aggressive, offering a cocktail of drugs to try to throw everything at the disease in one huge effort. Without being forceful, Mr Lansdown had steered us away from the stem cell option.

Arriving at my parents' house we were spirited into the lounge where all three children and my dad were sitting. My mother followed with unusual haste. Rebecca and Steven were sitting on the floor playing with Steven's train set. Rebecca jumped up to sit between Jane and me on the couch.

Steven called, 'Dad! Mum!' when he saw us. 'Dad, will you play with me?'

'Hello, Steven,' I said. 'Mum and I have just got to talk to Suzanne and Rebecca and then I will.'

'Hooray!'

Four faces, looking tired, anxiously stared at us in anticipation.

'Mum's had some more tests,' I began. 'We've had the results. The lump in the lungs is cancer but it's also spread to the bones.' Sensing my faltering voice, Jane stepped in.

'There's no easy way to say this,' she said. 'But there's nothing the doctors can do to cure me. I'm so sorry. I'm going to die.'

Rebecca howled deep, heartbreaking sobs that shattered me; she leant into her mum who cradled her to her stomach. Dad slumped back in his chair with the words 'Oh no', while Mum sobbed into a tissue she'd found in the pocket of her apron. Suzanne sat motionless, barely showing any emotion.

'Are you all right, love?' I asked her.

'Yes,' she said quietly. Jane, busy consoling Rebecca, looked over to her. Steven, distracted from his train track, watched us bemused. After a few minutes, Suzanne began sniffling into the sleeves of her jumper in a failed attempt to hide her tears. Jane beckoned her over to no avail, but after a few seconds she stepped over and the three of them huddled together, inconsolable, their bodies heaving in unison.

Steven, looking scared, came over to sit on my knee. The room was filled with sadness as the girls released their grief. Jane cajoled, offering the few words of comfort that she could.

'We'll have a fantastic few months,' she said. 'Memories to last a lifetime.'

Rebecca said, 'How do they know you'll die?'

'They just do, love,' Jane replied.

'But how?'

'Because there's nothing they can do about it.'

'Why?'

'Because they haven't found the right drugs to cure it.'

'Maybe they will.'

'Sorry, Becca, they won't. Not in time for me. Even if they make a breakthrough it would take years before they let people take it and I haven't got that long.'

'How long, Mum?'

Jane glanced in my direction and then back at Rebecca.

'Months,' she said. 'Maybe next spring. Two years maximum if everything goes well treatment-wise.' Rebecca broke down again.

'That's not fair,' she howled, sobbing into her mum's black jeans. Jane stroked her head, Suzanne turned to me and we hugged.

'Why you, Mum?' cried Rebecca. 'What have we ever done?'

'Nothing, Becca,' said Jane, calmly. 'It's just how life is.'

We sat there for a few seconds. Jane hugging Rebecca, me holding Suzanne.

It was Steven who spoke next.

'Mum? Will you play with me?'

Within a day, the sadness had been shared with most of those who were closest to us. After a tea that was barely touched by anyone, Jane and I set off to visit our friend Steve Chapman. He was unsure as to why we wanted him to accompany us on a walk; he came anyway, trusting us. He took the news badly.

I asked my mum to phone my sister Janet as I couldn't take any more.

Driving home with the children, it was Steven's cheerful demeanour which relieved the tension. But as soon as he slept, sadness hung over the car and we travelled until we were almost home in complete silence.

'Becca, me and your mum were a little puzzled this week.'

'Why?'

'Last week you said that you knew what Mum and me were going to talk about. What did you think we were going to say?'

'Nothing,' she responded.

'Go on, Becca, tell us,' Jane prompted. I noticed in the rear view mirror her head drop down as if she was embarrassed.

'It doesn't matter, it wasn't anything.'

'We're not cross, just interested,' I said.

Rebecca sat still avoiding eye contact. Jane turned to look at her. 'Please, Becs.'

'I thought you were going to say you were pregnant, okay.' Her voice rose sharply at the end. I looked at Jane and tears were forming in her eyes. If only. Pulling up on the drive, both cats bounded across the road. Jane got out and headed for the front door. Steven was still asleep and I went to lift him out. He was like a dead weight, his head flopping on my shoulder. I looked into the hall where Jane was checking the phone for messages.

'There are some flowers in the greenhouse,' she said, clutching a delivery note. 'I'll just go and get them.'

'They are from Stephen and Karin. Read the note.'

It said simply, 'We didn't know what else to do.'

JANE

The week that followed involved many discussions. Trying to keep a balanced view, we sought the advice of Luke and Karen.

Sitting on the patio overlooking their garden, our conversation centred round the pros and cons of the treatment offered. The trial would involve chemotherapy, which would allow the doctors to harvest some stem cells. It would be followed by more intensive sessions to suppress my whole immune system. I'd be kept in isolation for several weeks before the stem cells were reintroduced back into my body. With any luck, they would regenerate.

One of my main concerns was that something could go wrong during the harvest and the stem cells would be damaged. There was also the real risk of neutropaenia and scepticaemia, which meant that the slightest infection could overwhelm my body and prove fatal.

My overriding fear was of dying alone in a stark hospital environment without my family around me. Each time I thought about imposing this isolation on myself, the hairs on the back of my neck would prickle, as anxiety overtook me.

The following Thursday, Mike and I returned to Dr Ward's office for the results of the biopsy from the bronchoscopy.

'You have malignant growths in the lining of the bronchials in your lungs,' he said. 'The initial pathology report wasn't able to tell where the cells originated from as they are too malignant. Even comparing samples from your initial tumours, we were unable to identify whether this is the cancer that has spread from your breast.'

I knew this was bad. The tumours in my lungs were aggressive.

'The pathologist has further tests to undertake to see if the cancer cells are oestrogen receptive,' said Dr Ward. 'That would indicate that the tumour biopsies are metastatic breast cancer.'

He paused for a few seconds, allowing Mike and I time to digest the latest news before adding: 'I think we should assume that we are dealing with secondary breast cancer. Have you had time to think about the trial?'

Mike and I both nodded. 'Yes,' I said. 'I've looked at all the detail, and asked advice and I really don't think it's right for me.'

Dr Ward nodded back and reached behind him to pick up some leaflets which he slid along the desk towards me. 'There's another trial for a treatment which is given routinely in America. It isn't licensed over here yet.'

I scanned the first page of the leaflet. The treatment involved the use of Taxotere and Epirubicen. I looked up at Dr Ward. 'You fit the criteria,' he said and began to explain some of the details. 'Can you come back next week? The pathologist may have completed the other tests on the biopsied tissue by then and I'll be able to prescribe the chemo.'

Concentrating on all the information was exhausting. When we got back to the car I noticed that Mike looked drained.

'Shall we drop by Luke's house, see if he's there?' he said.

'Yeah,' I said, knowing we both found it easier to discuss it with someone who was one step away from our situation.

Mike and I took it in turns to describe the appointment with Dr Ward. Luke and Karen listened intently, occasionally asking a pertinent question. I passed them the leaflet and as they took it in turns to read it I got up to wander around the garden.

Luke finished reading the leaflet. 'That sounds all right,' he said. 'You won't be an in-patient and you can spend some time with the kids.'

Mike and I agreed. It sounded like a much better option. It would still be hard, there was still the risk I could end up in hospital with neutropaenia, but it also meant we could plan some weekends away with the children, have some times together that they would be able to remember.

Luke went inside the house and reappeared pointing a silver camera at us. It flashed and then, turning it round, he showed us the photograph he'd just taken.

'Is that a digital camera?' I asked. 'That's amazing!'

He passed it to me and I scrolled through some of the images of their children, Pete, Tom and Sue. There was one of Karen in the kitchen, cooking, a scowl on her face, as she waved the camera away.

'It's our treat,' said Luke. 'We thought the kids might like to use it. Take pictures of all the normal, everyday stuff – you know, you shouting and screaming at them, lying in bed with a hangover, that kind of thing.'

He laughed.

'You know that never happens,' I said in my defence. 'Not often anyway. But Luke, it's too much. We can't accept this.'

'We've talked about it and we've got the pennies,' he said. 'Besides, it's not for you, it's for the kids. They need to make a record for themselves, make a few memories, it's not all about remembering the good times. With this, they can just snap away – it's about the real you, all of the time.'

MIKE

After choosing what form of treatment Jane would undergo, we felt at least a little of the burden lift. It had been a huge decision. The ever-pressing time constraint had made matters much, much worse – already September was rushing by and suddenly February didn't seem that far away.

In some respects, it was as if part of Jane had gone already. When she was told she was dying, her career had come to an end. When you're due to die in six months, there's no point employers investing in your future. It was hard for Jane to bear. Ever since she'd secured a place to study radiography, her work had been part of her very being, something which gave her enormous satisfaction and a sense of worth, so naturally she was saddened to let it go. Although she would continue to work, any career advancement was over.

The previous week, I'd dropped off Jane's financial details to Alan Wood, a friend who was a financial adviser. I returned with Jane to hear his assessment of our predicament.

Alan sat back and grabbed our file out of his briefcase. 'Can I be blunt?'

'I'd rather you were,' Jane replied.

'Jane, you really need to make sure you die in service as it will make a big difference to the amount of money Mike and the kids will get.' He waited and looked at me. 'Without any life insurance you have a major problem, but I'm guessing you know that. The only money you'll get is from Jane's work, so you're still going to be left with a sizeable mortgage and child-care to pay.' My heart fluttered. I knew this, but it didn't make it any more palatable. 'Mike, you should take out some critical illness insurance to ensure the kids are okay if you get poorly.'

'Shit, Alan, I'd never considered what would happen if I got poorly as well. Is there anything else?'

'Not really, Mike. I've written it all down. I've looked at the fixed mortgage options but it would tie you in too much after Jane's died.'

'Thanks, Alan.'

'I've colour highlighted everything in the NHS booklet that's relevant and underlined the salient parts of my document. Have you updated your wills?'

'Yes,' I said. 'A friend I was at university with – Craig – is doing it.'

'Okay, Mike. Are you all right, Jane?'

Jane nodded silently before eventually finding her voice. 'Yes,' she said.

'Careful!'

Jane was sitting next to me on the settee. I never minded her stitching away on her tapestry until it came to changing to a new thread when it would be so long that, with her exaggerated movements, she would nearly take my eye out. 'Watch what you're doing with that thing.'

On the weekend that we had told the kids, Jane had deliberated whether to buy a large William Morris tapestry rug. We worked out that even if she'd dedicated every hour to it, it was unlikely that she'd finish it by February. There followed a 'Should I? Shouldn't I?' debate at the end of which I persuaded her to buy it. As a form of relaxation therapy for her it would be fantastic. Transfixed for a couple of hours each night, she would escape into the realm of repetitive motion of the stitching.

'Why, is it disturbing the football?'

Monday night matches hadn't held the same interest for me since the news and, although I had a book on my lap, I couldn't read either.

'No,' I said. 'But that needle is getting closer to my head.'

'Good,' she smiled.

'I love you too.'

'At least it would save on a messy divorce and everyone hating you.'

'What the chuff are you talking about?'

The strum of Suzanne's guitar upstairs temporarily distracted us. With the GCSE exam year upon her, she'd taken up the novel approach to revising by spending hour upon hour on her six-string hoping to be a female Jimmy Page.

'It's hard on the ears that,' I said.

'Leave her.'

'Ow, it's painful!'

'Do you know divorce rates go up for the terminally ill?'

'You're joking. Don't people pull together? Become more solid?'

'No, that's a misconception. People think, "I've only got a few more months to live, why should I spend it with this tosser?"'

Jane peered over her glasses, an air of menace about her stare.

'Do I need to be worried?' I asked.

'You tell me.'

'Could I just be relegated to the C list for the funeral?'

'C? You think pretty highly of yourself.' We'd been placing people into categories for the funeral. There were several to choose from and how you ended up in each category depended on how you had treated Jane in life. Some people were relegated to the bottom category, irretrievable, beyond redemption. The ultimate surprise for them would be when they got to the church and were barred.

'Buried or cremated?' I said.

'Cremated.'

'Have you chosen the hymns you'd like?'

'The one from our wedding, "I Watch the Sunrise". Then I'll think of another one.'

'Don't take too long.'

'You're barred.'

I looked across and beamed at Jane.

'Get lost,' she said and began coughing.

Jane had chosen to go to Chester because it was close to Liverpool. On Sunday we were to go up to see her childhood home, her primary school and the red squirrel reserve in Formby. We'd booked a hotel, which on any other occasion would have been considerably out of our price range, but we relished the prospect of two days' luxury.

Jane had also lived in Adelaide for three years from the age of eleven and it had always been a dream for her to return. She'd mentioned before the terminal prognosis that if the cancer returned and she was going to die, one of her last wishes would be to visit Australia with us. When I'd asked her if she wanted to go, she'd shaken her head and said: 'We don't have the money. It's people, not places that matter. I have all I wish for here.'

Even so, it became essential for me to piece together her history before we'd met so that I could recount it to the children if required. Going to Australia would help, but first I wanted to go to Liverpool, to see where Jane spent the first eleven years of her life.

*

On Saturday morning we rose late and went into town just before lunch. Tired, Jane immediately needed to rest, so we stopped at a coffee house and sat opposite each other about three feet apart. Jane's shoulder length brown hair looked beautiful. She was wearing a sleeveless olive green polo neck, and no one could have guessed how poorly she was. Unusually for Jane, she had applied some make-up for lunchtime. She looked stunning.

I took some photographs with the digital camera to record the moment for all of us. No one was under any illusion that this would be the last time Jane would have long hair. The chemotherapy would leave her bald and, whatever happened, it wouldn't have time to grow back. My mind flitted back to when I first met her and when she looked very similar to how she did now.

Neither Jane nor I enjoy shopping, so the plan was to have a couple of hours looking around the city walls and buildings, calling only at the occasional shop. We had decided to buy a mobile phone so that Jane could contact me in case of an emergency. With the onset of winter coinciding with her premature hair loss, Jane also thought she'd check out hats. Although there was an £80 allowance for a wig, it was never a serious option as the ribbing would have been too severe. Her features would suit having no hair and her character was strong enough not to be bothered by the potential of inconsiderate remarks.

Jane had been to the town as a child but Chester was new to me. Trailing round is tiring at the best of times but today we were both weary and had to stop every couple of hundred yards so Jane could recoup her strength. We couldn't complete the walk. In just a few weeks she had become immobile, gasping for oxygen, wheezing and coughing like a retired miner. We cut our losses and returned to the hotel.

Returning to Leeds on Sunday under a slate grey sky, we got back home where Mum and Dad – most likely Mum – had tidied the house. We'd never find anything again. All the children were lounging on the settee watching the Sunday afternoon film.

There was no real hint of melancholy, just five people who despite three generations had enjoyed each other's company. It occurred to me how right Jane was – it was people not places that mattered.

JANE

My health was deteriorating quickly. Mike and I managed to spend some time together but we stayed close to home. Too long in the car and my back and shoulder became too painful. The pain would wake me at night. Unable to sleep I would slip quietly out of bed and pad downstairs. I would watch the television with the volume as low as possible, enthralled by the spectacle of the Sydney Olympics.

The enormous tapestry rug I had bought was too daunting to think about in its entirety so I tackled one flower at a time, not daring to hope I would have enough time to see it completed. My eyes would flick from the stitching to the television over and over.

A couple of nights into the games I watched as women dressed in full-body swimming costumes dived into Sydney Harbour, There were dozens of people swimming. Arms flailing, stirring the water of the harbour into a long wave as they swam. Some of the stronger swimmers began to emerge at the other side of the harbour, dripping wet and running barefoot across the ground to bikes with shoes swinging at the pedals. Climbing on to their metal steeds, they set off, pushing their feet into the shoes as they sped down the hill. It was hypnotic to watch. I looked on as they raced back into the transition area, pulling on trainers and dashing out, looking pink with effort but showing no other outward signs of exhaustion

I saw them complete the race, the women sprinting to the finish line near the huge white shells of the Sydney Opera House, their finishing times just over two hours. How was that possible? It was the sport of true Olympians.

The following night, I made a point of getting up to catch the men's race. It was the early hours of the morning, but I watched transfixed as dozens of athletes dived into the harbour, climbed on their bikes and finished with an exhausting run. Our medal hope, Simon Lessing, soon lost touch with the leaders but still came in ninth over all in just under two hours. I was seriously impressed. I couldn't imagine attempting the feat these athletes had and how, after such a punishing event, they could still reach the finishing line with a smile on their faces.

But it was the words of the song which accompanied the review of the day's events at the Olympics which struck a chord. Heather Small's powerful voice singing, 'What have you done today to make you feel proud?'

I thought about it. How many things did I do? I tried to keep active. A walk into Rothwell was an achievement, although it tired me out and I had to stop at several points to rest on the benches that lined the street. And although my illness had meant I was losing touch with friends, I was becoming more proficient with e-mail. I kept in constant touch with my oldest friend, Amanda. She lived in Australia and her first response on hearing how ill I was, was to ask when she could come to visit. I was touched that she would want to drag her family halfway across the world to visit her sick friend. E-mail allowed me to stay in touch, keeping her informed of all the latest developments. 'MRI scan of head is clear thank goodness, start my treatment next week and will go bald very quickly.'

'Did you see Redgrave's race?' I typed into the computer, having watched it the previous night with the whole family. And about the closing ceremony: 'What was all that about? Kylie singing and I'm sure I saw Greg Norman dressed as a shark – please explain?!' As an Australian she had a certain amount of patriotic pride in the spectacle of the games.

Telling people I was dying was difficult as they all wanted to come to spend some time with me and, tired as I was, I tried to accommodate everyone.

Returning from Chester late one afternoon, we'd driven by my childhood village of Crosby and visited an old family friend.

The dull ache in my back had become a constant grinding pain as we drove over the motorway. I felt each jolt in the road, my shoulder throbbed, the pain radiated down my arm and up my neck. My jaw set rigid to try to stop the juddering that tingled and sent spasms through my body.

As I crawled out of the car at home, Mum rang. Uncle Dick was in Leeds and wanted to know if he could pop over. Mike was all for saying no, he knew how much I was suffering, but I didn't want to be the one to dissuade my aunt and uncle.

It felt like visitors passing through to say their farewells. Grimly, I thought I might never see some of these people again. They all wanted to have their chance to visit; some were quiet, unwilling to start a conversation in case they said the wrong thing, others babbled, foot firmly entrenched in mouth – talking of friends who had died as well, some cracking jokes about baldness and wigs. I laughed along with them, disguising my hurt and my simmering anger. Sitting on the dining chair that gave some comfort from the pain in my back, I wondered why people would laugh about the wind blowing my hair off.

Steve's tall frame bent down once more to pull up the overgrown straggling runner bean. The father of Rebecca's school friend Sarah, he'd popped in to say hi and ask if we needed any help. We were all in the garden and I watched as my bed of vegetables was dug up. I bent to pick up the small border spade that I'd used with ease only weeks before, thinking I might be able to help. Even the weight of it sent red hot pain up my back and I had to bend my knees to help me lift the black handle. All I could manage to do was shuffle up the path to hand it to Mike.

I sat on the bench and pulled open the box at my feet. Helianthemums, lavendulas, euphorbias, heleniums and rudbeckias. The small paper-wrapped plants didn't look much, but next year they would grow and flower and fill the garden with colour. I sighed and anxiously watched my small green plants – their fate in others' hands.

We heard the gate clatter open and Andrew, Rona and

Alasdair appeared followed closely by my sister Anne and her husband Bill.

'Hi there,' she called. 'What are you up to?'

'Just finishing off,' I said before introducing them all to Steve.

Steve put his spade down and wiped his hands on his jeans, leaving muddy, black stripes on his thighs.

'Right, we'll see you later,' he said. Sarah collected her bike from the garden and they left.

Back in the kitchen our conversation was slightly stilted. I didn't know what to say to Anne, what help to ask for. We sat and talked, dry-eyed, for an hour, until it was time for them to leave. She hugged me and drew back.

'Keep your chin up, chuck,' she said before packing a confusion of children in the car and setting off.

CHAPTER 9

JANE

Sitting in the corner of the pub, I couldn't help but feel tense as I waited for Mike to return from the bar. My thoughts were of what lay ahead the next day and, sensing my unease, Mike had suggested we take ourselves out for a beer.

I stretched my legs out and looked about the pub. I was glad to be away from the house, the walls had been pressing in on me, the thought of my first chemotherapy session made me shudder with fear.

'How did it go at the gym today?' Mike asked. I smiled as I recalled my efforts that morning.

After our weekend away, Mike had encouraged me to join Oulton Hall, which was a leisure club local to us. The attraction had been the swimming pool, but it had a small gym as well.

On my first day, I was given a schedule. I pulled on my tatty shorts and T-shirt in the dark-wooded changing room. Embarrassed by my appearance, I tied my trainers and joined Neil in the gym, who was going to show me how to use the various pieces of equipment.

He led me to the bikes, adjusting the height for me. I spun my legs slowly round for ten minutes before climbing off to tackle the running machine. Pressing the buttons, he showed me how to set the machine off, how to speed up and slow down. He stood as I ran slowly until my legs started to wobble with the effort. He explained the other machines to me and outlined a series of stretches to finish off the regime.

I was pleased with my accomplishments as I walked back to the changing rooms. I pulled on my swimming costume, and lowered myself into the pool. I managed several lengths of breaststroke before the strength in my legs left me and I couldn't kick any more. I climbed out, clutching the handrail to pull myself out of the water, and headed to the Jacuzzi.

The gentle exercise had helped to relax me and I felt some of the stresses lift as I walked slowly towards home.

'It was good to get out of the house,' I told Mike. 'Neil my instructor couldn't understand why my exercises were so easy. But they tired me out.'

'Good, I'm glad you enjoyed it,' said Mike. 'I'll have to come down there with you some time.'

The truth was, after the chemotherapy session in the morning, neither of us was sure if I'd be fit enough to return to Oulton Hall.

'I'd like that.' We both fell silent as we took sips from our beer.

'What's up?' asked Mike.

'Just scared, that's all,' I replied. I played with the cold drips of water on the side of my glass. 'What if they decide I'm too ill? What if they don't let me have my chemo?' The sick feeling inside made me push my glass further away from me.

'Do you need me to come with you?'

'No. I'll be okay. Mary said she would come with me. At least you can be around the day after if I'm ill.'

The night passed slowly. I finally managed to sleep in the small hours. When I awoke the next day, I dragged myself from my bed, heavy headed, temper fierce with anxiety. I sat quietly, afraid to speak to my family for fear of what I might say.

Mike dropped me at the hospital. Walking up the stairs to the ward I asked a nurse where I should be.

'Ah yes, Jane Tomlinson, it's your first session today, isn't it?' she said. I nodded.

'Just take one of the chairs in that room across the corridor and someone will be with you shortly.'

I waited, watching the other patients. Some were bald and sat laughing with their visitors. One lady was rigid in her chair, her wide eyes flicking nervously to the door every few seconds. Perhaps she was due her first treatment today.

'Hi, Jane, I'm Karen,' said the nurse 'Right, I'll just put a line in and hook you up to a drip while we wait for the pharmacy to bring up your prescription.'

I was shaking as she took my hand and felt for a suitable vein. There was a prick followed by a horrible, sharp sensation that moved in the back of my hand as Karen positioned the needle.

'Okay, that's in,' she said, finally satisfied it was in place.

'It still feels really sharp,' I said, my hand continuing to sting. Karen placed her finger over the end of the line to feel for swellings, then checked the drip, which was already feeding clear liquid down the line into my body. She shook her head.

'No, it's fine,' she said. 'That feeling will wear off in a few minutes.'

She was right. The pain lessened within seconds and I began to relax back into my chair. My sister Mary arrived, gave me a hug and dragged a chair across to be by my side. She soon had to move as Karen returned.

'We'll just get this pamidronate going,' she said. 'It will take about ninety minutes. And then your chemo should be ready.' She started to hook up the large bag of fluid. I put my hand to my brow, to hide my eyes from other patients, who I could see were looking over at me. Tears ran down my cheeks.

'Are you all right?' asked Karen.

'Yes, just scared about . . . all this.'

'You've got every right to be. It's not a very nice thing to go through.' Her sympathy just increased my floods.

'I just want a bit more time with my kids,' I explained.

'I think you're being incredibly brave,' she said. 'It's not an easy thing to cope with. You should be proud of how well you're managing.'

'I don't feel brave,' I said, wiping away the tears with tissues Mary had handed to me. I still felt sick in my stomach.

The morning was long. Mary brought sandwiches with her and we sat deliberating over the crossword in the paper. As one treatment finished another was brought, a syringe of red liquid.

'I need to check you've taken your steroids,' said Karen. I'd remembered. Even after just two doses my eyelids felt puffy, my appetite had increased as well. The red liquid was Epirubicen, I recalled the name from my treatment seven years previously. The memory became clearer as my hand stiffened with a muscular spasm, tears springing to my eyes with the pain. Slowly, Karen eased the syringe's contents into my hand, pulling the plunger back gently so I could see my blood filling the first part of the syringe. Finished, the muscles in my arm began to relax and another bag of saline was hooked up to flush the drugs around my body. Finally, my last bag of solution was brought in, a clear bag of watery fluid containing Taxotere.

Morning became afternoon and Mary and I sat talking as the drugs were pumped around my body. About two o'clock she looked at her watch. I knew she was anxious to pick up her son Jonathan from school.

'I'll have to be going soon,' she said. 'Will you be all right?'

'Yeah. Mike's coming at three. Don't worry.' She began to pack the paper away. 'Thanks for coming,' I said.

'I've not done anything.'

'No, but just being here has helped.' She bent down to hug me and left. I let my eyes close for the first time that afternoon. I could feel a fullness at the back of my nose, forcing me to clench my jaw, and I tried not to swallow as the nausea hit the back of my face.

'Are you all right?' Mike was sitting waiting for me when I returned from the toilet. He looked worried.

'I'm okay, honestly, I just feel sick.'

I unwrapped a mint, hoping its sweetness would alleviate some of the sickness. I had one final bag of saline to go and when that was finished I was able to go home. Karen dispatched Mike to fetch my final prescription and he returned with a bag of anti-sickness tablets and a small bottle full of steroids for my next treatment.

At home, my first thoughts were of bed. I desperately needed to shut my eyes and go to sleep. But when I lay down on the mattress, it was impossible to drift off. I was first hot, then cold. I slept feverishly. When I woke, the bed was damp and cold, my body sour with sweat. The room had become dark, the bedroom door was rimmed with light from the landing and downstairs I could just make out the quiet murmurings of my family.

The back of my neck was damp so I climbed out of bed, placing my feet with care so I didn't trip over the clothes I'd abandoned on the floor only a few hours earlier. Walking to the bathroom, I turned on the light and fumbled for a flannel to run across my face and neck. The heavy floral aroma of the soap on the stand stuck in my nose and mouth. Drying my face, scrubbing it with the rough loops of the towel, I covered myself with my dressing gown and walked to the top of the stairs. Down in the living room I could hear talking, the occasional laugh, and so precariously I made my way downstairs, my grip tight on the banister.

'Hi,' said Mike, surprised to see me. The fire was lit, the room was warm and there was a glow from the small light on the low table. Bright images flickered across the screen of the television. Steven, blue pyjamaed and holding on to his nappy comfort blanket, was snuggled up on Mike's knees. Steven sucked at his fingers, rubbing his nose with his nappy, contented and tired.

'Budge up, Becca, let Mum sit down,' said Mike.

'I'm all right here,' I assured her, moving the small pile of Steven's clothes and sitting gently down on the sofa. I watched the images on the television, not really engaging with any of them or listening to the sounds. Eyes half closed to shield me from the lights, my head heavy rested against the sofa arm.

'Come on, you,' said Mike, lifting Steven off his knee. 'Time for bed. Give your mum a kiss. Tell her you love her.'

Steven ran over to me, laughing, and pecked fiercely at my cheek.

'That's a Becca kiss,' he giggled.

'I know.' I smiled as he leant in and gave me a wet kiss on the cheek.

'And that's a sloppy kiss,' he said.

'Thank you, Steven,' I said, wiping the drool off my cheek.

Mike stood at the doorway. 'Come on, Steven, stop messing around, Mum's not feeling very well.'

Steven came forward again and put his tiny arms round my neck, giving me a smooch on one cheek.

'Love you, Mummy,' he said before running past Mike and thundering up the stairs, trying to reach the top before his dad.

'Don't play on the stairs!' I shouted after them but he was already at the top. Mike returned a few minutes later.

'Do you need anything?' he asked.

'I'm fine, really. I fancy a bath and some clean pyjamas,' I said, but I was unwilling to get either.

'Come on, you two,' said Mike to Rebecca and Suzanne. 'You must have work to do.'

The girls trudged out of the room complaining and went upstairs.

'Don't answer back,' said Mike sternly.

After the children had disappeared to their rooms, I dragged myself up off the sofa and ran myself a bath. Exhaustion made me lazy, but wanting to rid my body of the stale hospital smell I slid down the bath, the back of my head immersed in the warm soapiness. As the water lapped up on to my throat I sat upright, fighting a wave of nausea. I retched but the spasm quickly passed. Carefully, I used the showerhead to rinse the rest of the suds away from my shampooed head.

Climbing out, I dried myself and made my way back to the bedroom. But as I walked through the door, the smell of the shampoo reached me again; another wave of nausea washed over me and, mouth held tight shut, I dashed as quickly as I could back to the bathroom. Horrible, rough retches tore through me, saliva pooling in my mouth. I spat it into the sink and rinsed my mouth with cold water.

Clutching my side against the pain, which came in spasms, I

crouched on the floor, curled round the ache, kneeling there with my head resting on the cool lip of the bath until I could trust my legs to stand and make my way back to the bedroom to pull on clean pyjamas. I buried my head in the smooth cloth. They had been dried on the washing line and smelled of fresh, clean air, no chemicals. I breathed in the smell of out-doors.

I was too tired to spend time with Mike, but climbed back into bed, covering my pillow with a clean towel, to soak up the damp of my hair. I slept heavily and, when I woke, it was still dark. The clock showed 5 a.m. I crawled out of bed and, by the feeble landing light, fumbled in my drawers to find dry night-clothes to replace the damp clinging pyjamas. Mike mumbled in his sleep as I slid back into bed. Tugging at the duvet I pulled the covers over me and faded back into sleep.

Rushed kisses from Suzanne and Rebecca, a half-remembered shout of 'Love you' from Steven as he left the house. The morn-ing routine continued without me. When I managed to shake off sleep, I forced myself to eat. After breakfast, I took my painkillers and steroids, swallowing the bitter pills one by one, washing them down with ice cold milk, which took away some of the burning in my throat.

I sat in the living room and turned on the television, but I did not want to watch it. I took out my tapestry but only managed an hour or so of cross-stitch before my eyes and fingers grew weary and I headed back to bed, where I slept for a few hours, waking just before lunch. The day passed in a pattern of sleep and food. Despite the anti-sickness tablets, I found that if I didn't eat regularly the sickness became unbearable and I would be retching before I could do anything about it.

Monday was even worse. Still weakened by the chemo-therapy, still aching from the cancer, I began to wonder whether I had chosen the right treatment option. Was it the right thing to do or was I just prolonging the agony?

'Give it a few more days,' said Belinda later that afternoon when she rang. Tearful, I tried to explain my fears. 'You're bound to feel like this, it will begin to feel better. Just look after yourself,' she said.

She was right. Over the following days, my breathing began to improve and the pain lessened. But the relief was short-lived and about a week later I felt worse again.

Three weeks after my first chemotherapy I began to lose my hair. I had been brushing it when a huge clump came free. I tugged gently at my long locks and stared in horror at the loose strands.

As requested, Luke called round with his razor and before the children returned from school that day, he had sheared my head. I put my hand to my head and felt the spiky harshness, but even that stubble would be gone soon. Looking in the mirror I saw a woman with a rounded face, her small eyes looking back at me. I didn't recognize myself. I saw a cancer patient having chemotherapy.

MIKE

It was a relief to leave work on Friday night. Work seemed an intrusion into the time I could spend with Jane, hours lost that could never be reclaimed. It was palatable while she was also at work, but when she was at home, it felt as though I should be with her. I'd gone off going to football, stopped going out for the occasional beer and Sunday morning golf – but still the sacrifice didn't seem enough.

Darren and I walked slowly towards our respective cars, which were parked in the nearest free spaces, some distance away. At this time of year, just as the clocks were going back, it was safer to walk in pairs.

'What time are you setting off to London tomorrow?' he asked.

'Kick off's at three so probably around nine.'

'Should be good.'

'Last ever game at Wembley, but if I'm honest, under the circumstances I'd rather not be going and leaving Jane at home. I've no appetite for the game.'

'Does she need any help?'

'No, Suzanne's at home and she's really good with Steven.'

'Is Jane all right? You've been really quiet this week.'

'There's a lot of things to deal with,' I said. 'Mortality's a funny thing when you're staring it in the face.'

'Did I hear you tell Jane that you'd some concert tickets?'

'Marillion. They are doing a small concert at the Bass Brewery in Burton. They'd sold out before I could get through on the phone so I sent an e-mail to their website explaining about Jane. Their PR person, Lucy, replied saying we could have a couple of tickets and just give the money to a cancer charity.'

'That's kind.'

'Yes, it's something for Jane to look forward to.'

We reached the main road and I saw a Fiat Bravo approaching from the right so stepped out in front of it, pulling back immediately. Darren, to my left, was not really paying attention to the traffic and followed my lead but leapt back on to the kerb just as the draught from the car ruffled his hair

'Woah!' he shouted.

'Sorry, I forgot you weren't Jane.'

'You what?'

'It's a game I've been playing with Jane; she's not fallen for it yet. There's a seventy-five thousand pound accidental death policy which we'll collect if she gets killed by a car. We'll get nothing if she's killed by cancer.'

There was a look of disbelief on his face, swiftly followed by a wry smile.

'It's all right, I'd have saved you,' I said.

'Bastard.'

Walking through the door at home, I could smell the aroma of cooking coming from the kitchen. Steven followed me in, throwing his fleece down on the already cluttered shoe rack.

'Hello, Mummy!' He ran through to the kitchen, his uncoordinated feet making him look as though he'd tumble at any stage. 'Dad, Dad, look at Mum.' I walked through and wasn't surprised to see Jane sporting a shaven head. Wearing grey combat-style trousers and a grey round-necked top she looked very slim. Her cheeks were still reddened, swollen from the steroids taken with the chemotherapy.

'You look lovely,' I said. 'It suits you.'

'No it doesn't, there's just no alternative.'

'Where did you get it done?'

'Luke came around with the clippers and did a grade two.' Jane had waited for the hair loss to start. Initially she was able to pick a couple of hairs out. Within twenty-four hours, it was coming out in clumps. To prevent it blocking the bath Jane had visited her local hairdresser's to see if having a shorter style would stop the moulting. Rather than helping, though, it made her look like a mangy dog as the remaining hair started to come out in handfuls.

'No, it looks good, doesn't it, Steven?'

'It does, Mum.' He nodded.

Jane smiled.

Driving home from Wembley, I made a ham-fisted attempt at using the new mobile by calling home.

'Hiya, Suzanne. Is Mum there?' My stomach lurched. At this point I didn't know whether I would be greeted by an angry, dismissive or a cheerful voice. Jane came on the phone.

'Are you okay?' I said.

'No. I'm dying and I spent a day at home, unwell, looking after the kids.' It was clear from her voice that this was not a welcome conversation.

'I'll be home by about ten, the traffic's really bad,' I said.

'Is that it?'

'Yes.'

'Goodbye.'

'Oi, get up!' Jane prodded me just under my ribcage and I was overwhelmed with the immediate desire to vomit. 'Feeling fragile, are we?'

'No.' I turned over and muttered 'Fuck off' under my breath. The glands in my neck felt slightly swollen, my head pounded, my ears still rang from the volume of the gig. The neon light on the digital radio flashed 7.10. I needed paracetamol and I needed them now.

'I'll get Steven ready then, shall I?' said Jane, rising next to me. I didn't move. If I lay perfectly still, I'd be fine. The nausea was only a problem if I moved.

The previous night's Toploader gig had been a laugh, but Jane's friend Jackie and I had both drunk far too much, matching each other pint for pint. In the kitchen, Jackie was eating a piece of toast and sipping at some tea. She looked remarkably well. I grunted a 'Hi' as I bent down to the fridge to find milk for Steven.

Fifteen minutes later I found myself six hundred yards from home, having stopped the car to throw up copious amounts of last night's ale.

Reaching for the phone in my jacket pocket, I phoned Jane, hoping for some sympathy.

'I've been sick,' I said.

'Well, you needn't think you're coming back here so you can mope about all day. I'll see you tonight.'

The last week of the chemotherapy cycle was precious. A time to ensure we partied hard with concerts, meals and plenty of beer. No opportunity for a night out was missed. Ten days from chemotherapy was Jane's nadir, when the white blood cells were at their lowest count so that risk of infection was at its highest. But after missing out on the Toploader gig, she wanted to make every effort to get to the Placebo concert seven days later.

We arrived late deliberately in order to miss the support act, but within ten minutes Jane was tired and weak. The refectory at the university was long and rectangular shaped, which made it difficult to see the stage if you were stuck behind one of the large, solid pillars spaced out across the room. As it was standing room only, I found a chair for Jane, who sat a considerable distance from the stage in the bar area.

'Hi!' I shouted to the solidly built middle-aged security guard standing at the foot of the stairs to the balcony area. He was at least six inches taller than me and looked about as approachable as a Buckingham Palace guard. 'My wife's poorly, is it possible to go upstairs?'

'No.'

It was the answer I'd expected, but I didn't move.

'What's up with her?' he said.

'She's terminally ill with cancer.'

He looked over my shoulder, as if I wasn't there. 'How could I possibly tell?' he said.

'She's bald.'

He pointed to an androgynous young lad sporting lipstick, eyeshadow and blusher. 'That tells me nowt,' he said. 'They're all fucking wierdos in here.'

'You'll be able to tell,' I said.

'If she looks ill, you can.'

I returned to Jane, who was stood leaning against a pillar, look-ing paler than usual. Above the noise, I shouted, 'Follow me.'

The guard looked at us both. 'Up you go, love,' he said and let her pass. I followed and as I passed him he grabbed my arm. 'I've got to be careful. If you need anything, fella, come and see me.' With a smile he patted my back and we were up.

Up on the balcony, the view was better and Jane could sit and watch without fear of being jostled but we were both envious of the swaying crowd below. For us, it was akin to standing out-side a party. As we stood for the encore, holding her from behind, I kissed the nape of her neck.

'I love you,' I said.

'What?'

'I love you.'

'I can't hear you.'

'Forget it.'

Jane was scooping out the seeds from a pumpkin on the kitchen table. Dressed in an old rugby shirt she'd been painting in, the light glistened from her bald pate. She was wearing some make-up to partially hide the effects of chemotherapy and the whites of the eyes stood out like golfballs.

Steven stood next to her on a kitchen chair, a T-shirt and lumberjack-style shirt covering his round shoulders. Remnants of his tea were plastered all around his lips.

'Come on, Mummy,' he said as Jane scooped another enormous spoonful out and deposited the seeds in a large white baking dish. Steven placed a candle in the pumpkin, then carefully the top of the pumpkin was replaced.

With each feast, there was a temptation to think it would be the last one. Christmas, although still some weeks away, prompted numerous people to ask: 'Are you doing anything special?'

'No.'

'Under the circumstances, I didn't know whether you would,' they'd say. I always found it insulting as it was always said in a manner that implied that I should do something special. The knowledge that this would most likely be our last Christmas together was never far from any of our minds, although was only rarely uttered.

Jane bought two big bags of sweets to hand out to the collection of ghouls, witches and monsters that called at the house. With each rap of the door, Steven rose and ran to answer it, closely followed by either Jane or myself, and he'd liberally hand out all the goodies.

'Get the baby bath from the loft, Mike, ' said Jane. Once full of cold water it was placed on the living-room floor and we threw in apples, horse chestnuts and pound coins.

'How do we do it, Mummy?' asked Steven.

'I'll show you,' said Rebecca, already stripped to her baggy Barcelona Olympics T-shirt that Grandma and Granddad had brought back eight years ago.

'Becca!' shouted Suzanne, as Rebecca's face slooshed into the bath, sending a wave of water all over the floor. She emerged, dripping, with nothing in her mouth.

'Here,' said Jane, budging up to take Rebecca's place. Dunking her head down, the water splashed up and over the bald skin and on to the floor. The hair follicles submerged in the bath looked darker, more shadowy than usual and when she sat up her forehead glistened brightly with water. Between her teeth she held a shiny horse chestnut. She dropped it in her hands. 'Easy.'

'Let me have a go,' squealed Steven as Suzanne retrieved an apple between her teeth. Too frightened to get his face wet, I smiled as Jane handed him a pound coin.

With most of the water displaced on to the floor, we packed the bath away and I took Steven upstairs to put him to bed. When I returned, Jane and Rebecca were in the living room quibbling over whose turn it was to make sandwiches.

'I made them two days ago,' said Rebecca.

'But I made them yesterday – and I've got chemo tomorrow so I'd like something nice, please.'

'Well, you'll have to make them yourself, then.'

'Right, well in that case, you might as well go to bed.'

'But it's not time.'

'Oh yes it is.'

JANE

Mike had already set off to work but it was taking me some time to rouse myself to do the same. The pain in my bones was restricting my speed. I outlined my eyes, blushed my cheeks and pencilled in new eyebrows. I didn't usually wear make-up during the day, but it gave my face more definition, more colour, and I thought it might stop people asking how I was once I got to work. My low maintenance, no-hair hair style needed no time at all.

Carol pulled into the drive and kept the engine running while I looped a woolly scarf round my neck and put on a warm hat to cover my ears from the cold. We set off for town. I don't think I was entirely awake. I'd hardly slept and had to get up twice in the night to change because my nightclothes were so drenched in sweat.

I'd dreamt about being locked, bleeding, in a small dark cupboard, shouting to Mike, unable to make him hear me through the shut door. I remembered thinking, 'This isn't how I want to die' as I felt myself fading away, deeper sleep gradually transporting me away from the disturbing images.

'Are you sure you should be going to work?' asked Carol.

'I'll be all right once I get there,' I replied.

The decision to return to work had been an easy one. I'd gone from being an independent woman to someone who needed looking after. I'd found myself existing in a non-place, somewhere in limbo between my old life and the future which held death. At one point, unfit for work, I'd sat at home too weak even to lift Steven and watched as other people mothered him, no longer feeling well enough to look after my own son. My time with him felt like supervised care.

But the chemotherapy had helped, taking away some of the pain and the breathlessness. It was tiring and exhausting and I often wondered whether it was worth it for the short time I had left with my family, but dying is such a hard journey and I wanted to resist it as long as I could.

I reached down into my bag to make sure I'd brought my hat, a royal blue beanie to match the trim of my uniform. I couldn't bear the thought of wearing a wig. I'd tried one on for my sister, Anne, hoping she would boost my confidence. But she took one look and said: 'It might be worth spending an extra bit of money on something else.'

So now I covered my white, bald head with my hat, which stopped many of the inquisitive looks and hopefully wouldn't frighten the children.

Work was tiring but it felt rewarding to be back, doing something normal. My back and shoulder ached when I moved the heavy equipment but when I felt it was getting too painful I would sit in the screening room, where the work wasn't as strenuous. I worked as often as I could, but on my chemotherapy weeks found it impossible to do much at all.

Just over a week after my third chemotherapy session, I'd got over the terrible Monday. That was always the worst day. I was weak from the chemotherapy, still retching on occasions. It was the day I felt most depressed and would retreat to my bed, any optimism swallowed by thoughts of the pain and the bleak future. Covering my head to stop the chill of the air on it, I'd lie there feeling wretched.

Tuesday, however, was only a short day at work. Carol picked me up from home and after work I would walk to Mike's office for the lift back. The bus was no longer an option; the rough, bumpy journey too painful for my sore back.

It was a slow day at work and I had to go to the prep room where all the medical supplies were kept to look for a dressing for a small burn on my right hand. Such a stupid thing to do: I'd lifted a roasting tin out of the oven at home using a tea towel, too lazy to look for the oven glove, and my hand had caught the upper shelf.

'Have you got anything I can put on this to keep it clean?' I asked Helen when she came in and found me searching. I showed her my hand.

'It looks like it's healing all right,' she said, examining the small wound. My hands were bruised from all the needles. I'd resisted having a more permanent line put in because it would have prevented me going to work, the pool or the gym.

'You shouldn't let it get too wet. Allow it to dry out.'

'I know,' I said. 'I'm just a bit worried that it's near one of the veins they use to give me my chemo.'

Mike dropped me off at home after work. After eating, I went through to the living room and picked up my rug. I threaded my needle but only managed the one strand. My face, hands and eyes felt heavy so I headed to bed.

I woke later to the sound of the keys in the lock as Mike opened the front door and called upstairs.

'Hi,' I called back and I could hear him telling Steven to remove his shoes before he came running up the stairs.

'How are you?' he asked, walking through the door, his shape silhouetted against the landing light.

'Fine,' I said, my voice thick with sleep. 'Just a bit tired.'

'I'll leave you to it,' he said, softly closing the bedroom door behind him. I drifted back to sleep.

After a long rest, I ran myself a bath. Luxuriating in the soapy warm water, I looked down at my legs. The one advantage of chemotherapy was that hair fell from everywhere; no need to shave any stubble. I got out and twisted a towel around my body.

It's hard to look sexy when you're going through chemotherapy. I pulled out my green high-necked vest top and grey trousers. The trousers felt a little tight but the top covered the bulge.

I pulled out my make-up case and applied foundation and blusher. Twisting off the top of my mascara, I'd already applied a coat before I realized my error. Looking closely, I only had two lashes left and now, covered in mascara, they looked like two long spider's legs.

'Damn,' I said, leaning in towards the mirror and pulling on the remaining hairs. They came away easily. My eyes looked odd without the lashes so I reached for my dark brown eyeliner, hoping to take away the blank look. I took out a pair of silver earrings and struggled to put them in. I was nearly ready when Mike walked into the bedroom, dripping and naked.

'You look nice,' he smiled.

I scrunched my nose up, knowing how odd I must really look but was grateful for the compliment. I found my dark emerald green hat, pulled it on and looked at myself in the mirror. On reflection, if I pulled my hat low enough you wouldn't notice that I didn't have any hair – it didn't look too bad. I decided against my heeled shoes as my feet were a bit sore and anyway, I'd made enough of an effort tonight.

The Calls Restaurant was at the other side of Leeds. We checked the menu and made our way in. We were seated straightaway at a table overlooking the canal and began debating whether we really wanted a starter or whether that wouldn't leave room for dessert.

The meal was delicious but over far too soon. I didn't want the evening to end just yet.

'Why don't we go next door for a cocktail?' I suggested. Mike agreed, so we paid the bill and headed to the wine bar.

As we sipped our drinks, we watched the waiter flip glasses and twirl cocktail shakers, showing off to his admiring customers. It was a fantastic evening.

I don't know what time we arrived home but as we stumbled up the drive, I was more than a bit tipsy. I struggled to unlock the door and almost fell through. Mike and I giggled like teenagers.

'Hello, you two.' Carol appeared from the living room. 'Did you have a nice time?'

'Yes, thanks,' I slurred, concentrating on enunciating every syllable.

The next morning I woke about 5 a.m., my head heavy with pain, my throat dry and my right arm throbbing. Perhaps I'd slept on it? Rolling over, I groaned as the pain poured through my head; lying still helped, but I needed to move.

In the bathroom, I ran my hands under the cold tap, cupping them to scoop some water into my mouth to slake my thirst. My head pounded, I felt queasy and shivery. I decided I was better off back in bed. I pulled a jumper on over my pyjamas and climbed back in.

'What's up?' Mike stirred next to me. 'You're shivering.'

'I know. I'm freezing.'

Mike leant over. 'You feel like an oven,' he said, sitting up and groaning. 'Oh God, I feel awful too.'

I felt my right arm, still throbbing with pain. It felt hot and swollen.

'I really don't think I'm well, Mike,' I said.

I searched for the thermometer in the bathroom. All the leaflets from the hospital said I had to contact the hospital if my temperature went over thirty-eight degrees. It took it out and read it. It was forty degrees.

'Well?' said Mike as I climbed back in bed, pulling the covers up over me, still shivering.

'My temperature's up,' I said. I rolled up the sleeve of my jumper and looked at my right arm, alarmed. The small burn on my hand looked red and angry, the wound oozing. The veins radiated out from the sore, red and inflamed; it looked like infection from my hand had spread up my arm.

'Oh shit,' I said.

'What?' Mike turned to look at me.

'Look at my arm,' I said.

'That doesn't look too good,' he said, peering closer. 'Do you think we should ring the hospital.'

I had to go to casualty. Mum agreed to come over to see the kids off to school and Luke said he would meet me at Accident and Emergency. My teeth chattered with cold. The nurses, concerned that my body might overheat, had taken my thick blanket away and I was shivering. My head pounded, I was freezing and my stomach was churning.

A doctor came in, holding my notes. 'Hi, Jane, you're not too well, I hear,' she said, leafing through the pages on her clipboard.

I nodded, still shivering.

'We'll need to admit you, the oncology ward are waiting for a bed but the blood results show you're neutropenic. And by the looks of things, you've got scepticaemia.'

She gently examined my arms.

'What does that mean?' I asked.

'The chemotherapy has knocked out your immune system,' she said. 'You've got an infection your body just can't cope with. We need to start you on some antibiotics straightaway.'

I was feeling very fragile.

'How long will I be in for?' I asked, weakly.

'Let's see, it's Wednesday today, you might be out by Monday. Sunday at the earliest.'

'I'm due to go to a concert on Friday,' I said. 'I'd been looking forward to it.' I could hear the childish whine in my voice but felt too ill to stop the tears. I wiped them angrily from my face.

'There's not a lot I can do,' said the doctor softly. 'Listen, you're having the chemotherapy to help with your disease.'

I nodded and sniffled ungraciously.

'If we send you home, you will almost certainly die from this,' she continued. The tears began to flow again, this time because of the gravity of my situation. 'We can treat this very successfully. But it does mean you have to be in hospital with a drip for the antibiotics.'

Hooked up to the drip, there was some debate about which cocktail of antibiotics was best. A porter arrived to wheel me to the ward.

Mum arrived and Mike was able to leave me to go home to fetch some belongings for me. One minute I was freezing, the next, sweat would be rolling down my face. My whole body was drenched, my arm was throbbing, my head ached, pain shot through my stomach.

Mum hastily passed me a bowl and I vomited violently until I felt like my guts were turned inside out. Mum carefully mopped my face with a damp towel, gently wiping my cheeks and patting my brow.

'Thanks,' I said quietly, exhausted from the sickness.

A male nurse appeared, introducing himself as Martin. 'I'm from the IV team. The ward staff are concerned that you're dehydrated. They want me to put another line in so I can give you some more fluids as quickly as possible. It means another needle, I'm afraid.'

By that stage, I didn't care. I was too weak, they could do what they liked. I offered him my left arm wearily.

'Shit!' I swore automatically as Martin plunged the needle in, securing it with some bandages and hooking a line in and attaching me to another drip. I closed my eyes, hoping sleep would take me away from the pain.

I could feel tiredness all the way through me. I looked at the lines in my arms and watched the drips, from the bag suspended above, grow larger and larger until heavy and then disappearing. The pain of cancer, the pain of treatment and now this. I wondered if I should ask them to take the drips out. I wasn't up to it any more, I was too tired of living with death. I should stop trying to live and get the business of dying over with.

A nurse came to take my temperature and I was filled with sadness. Tears ran down my face. I was inconsolable. She pulled the curtains round and passed me some tissues. I dabbed my eyes, she sat and watched.

'What's up, love?' she asked.

'I'm so sorry, I just don't want to do this any more. I'm so tired. I can only feel all the life I've left behind me and dying in front of me. I don't know what the point of all this is any more,' I said, gesturing towards the drips. 'Perhaps it's not right to be carrying on with my treatment.'

'Come on, Jane,' she said. 'You've been very ill. But you've got to stay positive. The antibiotics will help. It won't be long before you start feeling better.'

I knew she was trying to encourage me but everything felt too bleak.

'What about the kids?' she said. 'They'll be in to see you later. They still need their mum, you know.'

It was the right thing to say. This extra time was for my family and maybe I could manage it. I could get through this, spend a last Christmas together.

I pictured us all in bed, squashed tightly together, on Christmas morning for a festive family hug. The nurse opened the curtains and carried on her way.

Mum arrived early and I smiled weakly at her.

'I'll just sit here quietly,' she said. 'You don't need to talk to me, just rest.'

I closed my eyes and slept, tired after my restless battling night. Each time I opened my eyes, I was comforted by the sight of my mum, silently reading or just watching me. As the morning passed, I felt too weak to talk but Mum filled the silence, chatting about members of the family. I let her words wash over me, her familiar voice easing me.

The blood woman arrived mid-morning to check my details.

'She needs her bloods doing now,' said the nurse. 'We can't give her antibiotics until we have the results. We're just wondering how to get around this.'

'If Jane doesn't mind, we could try the back of her foot,' said the woman. I flinched at the thought. 'It's the only alternative,' she said.

'You can have one go,' I said. 'If you don't get in, then I'll wait.'

I clenched my teeth and screwed my eyes tight anticipating the stab in my foot. It was painful. I clenched and unclenched my fists as the dark red blood filled each phial. She took the needle out and placed the plaster over it.

'All done,' she said. 'Sorry about that.'

Mum had been watching my performance and I could tell by the look on her face that she thought I was being daft.

'Well done, girl,' she said. 'Now, I'm just off to shop, can I get you anything?'

I shook my head. I couldn't face the thought of chewing or swallowing.

However, when she returned she was carrying a Tesco bag with fresh French bread and cottage cheese. I tore off a chunk of the baguette and bit into it. It was just what I needed.

Mum smiled. 'Good, I'm glad you're behaving yourself now.'

My blood results came back showing that my white cell counts were coming up. As they did and the antibiotics began to work, I began to feel more myself, less sick and tired.

Dr Perren arrived for the ward round. He was my consultant but this was the first time I'd met him, a tall, slim man with a stern expression on a little-boy-lost face.

'Somebody's told me you've got a concert to go to,' he said, arching an eyebrow.

'I'm trying to get used to the idea that that isn't going to be possible,' I replied.

He looked through the notes, tapping the page as he ran through them.

'If your white cell count continues like this, I don't see why not,' he said and turned to a doctor beside him. 'We can send Jane home with oral antibiotics if she's still improving and there's no sign of infection,' he said.

I smiled but still didn't think I'd be going anywhere.

The following day, I hounded the nurses, asking them to put my antibiotics up. I watched the fat drops of drugs drip down into the IVAC machine, listening to the hum as the machine slowly, slowly pushed the drugs into my arm.

Mike sat with me as I hopped in and out of bed. I was fidgety and twitchy, couldn't keep still – apparently a side effect of the anti-sickness drugs. I was tired but my muscles flicked and I could only stop them by getting out of bed and walking around. But I was anxious to leave, to be ready on time to go to Burton-upon-Trent for the Marillion concert; we just might make it if my drips were all finished. I'd packed my bag ready in case.

At last, the needle was removed and a piece of gauze taped over it. I walked to the bathroom, revelling in the freedom of movement without my cumbersome drip stand to accompany me. I washed my hands and looked in the mirror. My face was round and swollen, my eyes almost shut. The light made me look yellow and I felt my illness lying heavily on me. Looking at my reflection, I could believe that death wasn't far away. My legs wobbled and I held on to the sink to stop them buckling underneath me. Perhaps the drive down the motorway was not such a good idea. Perhaps I should go home and rest.

Mum had other ideas. She was stopping overnight so we didn't have to travel back from the concert on the same evening and a hotel was booked so I could rest afterwards.

'You're going,' she ordered. 'Even if I have to post you into a sleeping bag and tie you into it.'

Her joking encouragement helped bolster me and Mike and I set off down the M1. I sucked sweets all the way. Mike kept looking over anxiously.

'Do you want to go home?' he asked for the third time.

'No, I'm fine. We might just make it on time.'

At the entrance to the brewery we handed in our tickets and were directed in to get our supper of beer and pie and peas. I gave the supper a miss but picked up a bottle of 'Racket Fuel' beer – reassuringly inexpensive – and put it in my bag.

'Have you seen Lucy anywhere?' Mike asked. We wanted to thank her in person for the tickets. Seconds later, a glamorous blonde came running over and enveloped me in a hug.

'I can't believe you're here,' she cried. 'Mike e-mailed to say you were in hospital – when did you get out?'

I looked at my watch. 'About four hours ago,' I said.

'Should you be here?' she asked.

'I'm looking forward to it,' I said.

She showed us to our seats and I looked around, bewildered at all the commotion. It was a far cry from the peace and the routine of the hospital ward.

'Someone wants to meet you,' said Lucy and a small, dark-haired man, who I recognized from previous concerts, smiled at me. It was Steve Hogarth, the lead singer.

'Really glad you could make it, Jane,' he said and hugged me. 'I'm amazed you're here at all.'

It was the best start to a brilliant concert. I cried when they sang a cover version of 'Let It Be', one of my favourite Beatle tracks. Next to us were Steve Hogarth's wife, children, mum and dad. His mum shook my hand as we left.

'You look after yourself,' she offered as motherly advice.

I walked to the car on unsteady legs.

'How long will it take to get home?' I asked Mike.

'Don't you want to stay over?' He sounded surprised.

'I think I just want my own bed,' I said.

MIKE

'Had a good day today?' Jane asked Suzanne as we sat in the kitchen.

'Not really.'

'What do you mean?'

'It's nothing,' said Suzanne, looking down at her plate, moving the food around with her fork. 'Just forget it, okay?'

Jane glanced over at me, then back at Suzanne. 'Okay, but if you want to talk about it, just mention it at any time.'

Rebecca was grinning at her sister on the opposite side of the table.

'I know what it is,' she said.

'Butt out, Becca,' said Suzanne, looking directly at her younger, mischievous sister.

'Okay, Becca, what is it?' asked Jane.

'I'll tell you,' huffed Suzanne, still staring at her plate. 'I ran out of a class today because I was too upset to listen to the teacher any longer.'

Jane and I looked across at each other.

'What was the matter?' said Jane.

'It's nothing,' said Suzanne. 'It was just in RE they started talking about funerals. The teacher asked me and I told her I didn't want to be questioned on it, but she just kept persisting. I just couldn't take it any longer and I had to leave.'

'Had you told the teacher about Mum?' I asked.

'No, of course I haven't. I don't tell anyone, I don't want anyone to know.'

'It doesn't matter, Suzanne,' said Jane. 'It doesn't matter. I'm sure everyone will understand.'

Jane and I had been to see Suzanne and Rebecca's pastoral tutor, Mr White, earlier in the year to tell him about Jane's health. With it being Suzanne's GCSE exam year, we knew how important it was that she settled down and could get on with her work. But we had asked that Jane's prognosis remain confidential. We didn't see why other teachers needed to know and were concerned that Suzanne and Rebecca might be treated differently if it was known that their mother was dying. Clearly, it was time for a rethink. I rang the school the next day and spoke to Mr White, informing him that although we didn't want any fuss, we thought it would be wise to let their teachers know as a way of explaining Suzanne's recent out-of-character behaviour; it should also avoid them any future upset.

Sundays were always quiet, especially in midwinter. Steven and I were playing with his train set, the rather extravagant gift that Jane had bought him last year, while Suzanne studied upstairs and Rebecca watched television in her bedroom. We watched Steven's train circling the living room, chugging away trailing several carriages behind. After a few circuits Steven slowed them by turning down the transformer dial.

'Dad, I don't want to play with it now. Can I watch a video?'

'We'll leave it up, Steven, in case you want to play with it later,' I said. 'I'm just going upstairs to see Mum.'

In the bedroom, Jane was lying on her back beneath the covers, a towel as usual draped over the bedhead.

'How are you, love?' I asked.

'Just the same,' she said, reaching for the towel and wiping her forehead. 'I don't feel very well. My temperature's just below the limit. If it rises any more I'll ring the ward.'

'Don't leave it too late, will you?' I said.

After Jane's skirt with death, we were all twitchy about her developing septicaemia again. But it was difficult to tell whether these symptoms could be a new occurrence or whether it was just the result of chemotherapy. As a consequence of the previous septicaemia the dosage of chemotherapy had had to be reduced, which had worried us at first, but we were assured it would have little effect on treating the disease. Plus, Jane's scans results on Tuesday had shown that the tumour had reduced in size and, with two more doses to go, Jane and I felt we were making progress and that we might have some quality time together.

'I'm going to get up in a minute,' she said. 'Where are the kids?'

'Steven's watching *Thomas the Tank Engine* on Sky, Suzanne and Becca are just about to go and get themselves advent calendars.'

'Oh, so they definitely wanted one?'

'Yeah, they're none too pleased you didn't get them one at the same time you got Steven's.'

'He's three, for heaven's sake.'

'Whoa, nothing to do with me.' I turned to leave the room and murmured, 'Scrooge.'

'I heard that,' said Jane.

With the various sections of the Sunday papers multiplying across the floor and Steven drawing with his washable crayons while Jane and I read, the afternoon ticked lazily over into teatime.

'Mike, I'll just nip upstairs and take my temperature,' said Jane, getting up and throwing her newspaper down on the floor.

Steven had discarded his jumper long ago but he did look a little flushed so I rose, went to the hall and checked the thermostat. It wasn't hot but I turned the dial down slightly and hit the advance button on the heating control, which would eventually turn it off.

Walking back, I noticed Jane was halfway up the stairs, stooping with her right hand holding the banister rail.

'What's up, Jane?' She turned her body to sit on the next step.

'There's nothing up, I just can't climb the stairs all at once,' she said and then for my benefit added, 'Don't worry, Mike, it's just how life is.'

I knew she had been struggling to get around but not to this extent. Frequently, when we were outside, she would have to stop and rest like an old lady but this was different, this was worrying – there were only fourteen steps.

'Go away,' she said. 'I don't need you to watch me.'

Increasingly anxious, I reluctantly skulked back to the living room. Within a couple of minutes she had returned.

'My temperature's gone up again,' she said. 'I'm going to ring the ward. They'll want to admit me. Can you give me a lift?'

My mind whirred. Suzanne was fifteen but I didn't want to leave Steven alone with her. I rang Carol and Jon and, within twenty minutes, Jon had arrived.

Returning home by eight o'clock, I found Steven in his Postman Pat pyjamas sitting on the couch slurping from a bedtime drink of milk. Jon left and it was time for Steven's bedtime. At the bottom step, we both got into our starting positions and raced up the stairs. Steven was still the undefeated champion.

'Have you brushed your teeth?' I asked as he bounced into bed.

'Yes, Daddy.' He grinned, showing me a full set. I sat on the bed next to him, tucking the duvet snugly around his little frame, hoping to make him feel secure.

'Prayers, Steven.'

'I love Daddy, I love Mummy, I love Suzanne, I love Becca, I love Grandma in Leeds, I love Granddad in heaven, I love

Grandma and Granddad in Settle and I love you, you, you, you, you.'

'Goodnight, God, I'm going to bed, work is over, prayers are said, I am not afraid of night, you will watch me till morning light.'

I gave him a quick kiss and crawled across the bed down the four steps of his ladder. I left the door slightly ajar so he could see the landing light. I ran down the stairs, hearing the faint murmur of music from Suzanne's room and the television from Rebecca's. The living room looked odd, it felt strangely subdued. I straightened up the books lying askew on the side table and cleared up the newspapers and mugs on the floor but it still didn't feel right.

Just as the clock in the living room was chiming ten, I heard a scream from upstairs. 'Daddy, Mummy, Daddy, Mummy!' I was on the landing in seconds.

'It's Steven,' said Suzanne, coming out of her room dressed in a long T-shirt, with hair in a towel turban.

Steven was sitting bolt upright in bed, his blond hair sticking up and out, his cheeks red and his eyes wide open.

'It's the monsters, Daddy!' he screamed.

'It's okay, Son, it's okay,' I said, holding his hand.

'Monsters, Daddy!'

I turned to the door.

'Suzanne, please get the Calpol.'

She ran downstairs and returned seconds later with the medicine, which I fed to Steven who was still shaking with fear. I sat and hugged and rocked and soothed, feeling his warm forehead burning through my shirt.

'He's going to be all right, isn't he?' Suzanne, who was still standing in the doorway, asked.

'Yes, his temperature is spiking. You used to get like this,' I said.

'What about Becca?'

'Only once.'

His shaking eventually stopped but I carried on hugging, wondering whether to take him downstairs to sit with me for a while. His eyelids were closing again, it was probably best to leave him in bed. Wasn't it? Releasing him from my arms, I gently lowered his head back down to the pillow. I looked at his bedroom clock, it was 10.30 p.m. Would Jane be awake? I couldn't call her. It was too late, she might be asleep herself. But then, if something happened, she'd never forgive me for not ringing.

'It's probably just a temperature,' she said, in a voice that made me feel as old as Steven. I didn't care, it was reassuring to have her confirm what I already suspected. 'Keep an eye on him and if it happens again control his temperature with some cold flannels. If he doesn't get any better, call the doctor.'

Putting the receiver down I felt better, but slightly guilty. I shouldn't have rung.

An hour later, as I lay in bed, there was another petrified cry.

'Daddy, Daddy! ' I was at his bedside in a moment but he stared right through me.

'Elephants!' he screamed. 'They're coming! No! No! No! Get them away from me!'

Rebecca and Suzanne appeared on the landing, worried expressions on their faces. I held on to Steven's rigid body as he wailed, 'They're coming through the walls.'

'Suzanne,' I said, turning towards the door. 'Run a bath, tepid water, four inches in it, please. Becca, get me a flannel with cold water on it.' I pulled the sheets and duvet from his legs then, with a single motion, yanked his pyjama top off before removing his bottoms. Rebecca ran through and I held the flannel to his forehead.

'Who am I, Steven?' I asked him as I carried him through to the bathroom, trying to determine whether the hallucinations had ceased.

Within a minute of lowering him into the lukewarm water, he was coherent. Suzanne knelt down next to the bath stroking his back and smoothing his hair off his forehead, while I ran downstairs and phoned the emergency doctor. He confirmed what we'd done was correct and that he'd visit in a couple of hours.

Drying him off on the landing, we all sat down together on

the carpet. Wrapped in his warm towel, Steven seemed to improve; he sucked his fingers quietly as he sat on my lap and I held him close.

'Is he going to be okay?' asked Rebecca, huddling next to us.

'Yes, if I can keep his temperature down. He'll sleep in my bed and I'll keep him at home tomorrow. Hopefully Mum will be home in a couple of days.'

It was a relief when night turned into dawn and daylight began to seep through the curtains. Throughout the night, I lay there, wide awake, unable to sleep as Steven slept. His small body looked so vulnerable as he breathed gently, the odd whimper escaping from his mouth as the fever subsided. The doctor came at 1.30 a.m. and was satisfied with Steven. But the whole experience left me feeling distraught. If this was what life was going to be like in the future, they could stick it.

JANE

By Friday morning, my temperature finally remained normal and I was allowed out of hospital. I felt weak and disoriented. The infection had left me tired, but when we arrived home, I packed my bag to travel to Cheadle in Manchester for a long-awaited weekend away with Suzanne and Rebecca. Jack and Alice had agreed to look after Steven so that we could spend some grown-up time with the two girls.

We arrived at the hotel late in the afternoon and Suzanne and Mike carried most of the bags in, Rebecca managing her own holdall. I walked unsteadily behind. The reception desk stood in a large lobby, decorations hung from the walls and a tall Christmas tree was hung with crimson and silver baubles. After the quiet of the hospital, the noise overwhelmed me and I was filled with panic. There were people everywhere, people with cases, people talking loudly. Starting to shake with the assault on my senses, I retreated to a quiet corner. My head prickled with heat from my small hat but, self-conscious of my baldness, I left it on, too fraught to endure the curious stares of strangers.

Opening the door to our room, we saw that it was designed for very close families. There was just enough space between the beds for Rebecca to squeeze down to climb in one side. It would be a very cosy weekend away.

As soon as we had placed the bags on the beds, Rebecca asked to go swimming. Mike looked at me and offered to read at the poolside while the children swam. I pulled the covers back from the bed and lay down, closing my eyes.

Later that afternoon a taxi drove us to a local pub, where we grabbed the last table. Mike and I ordered some beer and we all found dishes we could order.

Rebecca's fish hung over the side of the plate. Having demolished her huge plate of steak and ale pie Suzanne was still hungry enough for dessert but couldn't decide between the chocolate pudding, the lemon meringue or the banoffee pie.

'Why don't you have all three?' I said, teasing her.

'Could I?' She looked at me to see if I was serious.

'I was only joking,' I said, laughing at her face as the eager smile dropped. 'You can't possibly eat all three.' She nodded eagerly. 'Oh. Okay then,' I said.

'Will you be able to bring them all separately so Suzanne has a chance to finish one before the next,' Mike asked the waiter.

The young man arched his eyebrows and joined in the teasing of Suzanne, noting down the instructions as she sat crimson-faced at being the three-pudding glory girl.

Next day, we drove the short distance to Chester. Walking through the park I remembered childhood picnics, playing hide and seek among the trees. We walked along the old walls of the city, passing under the tall clock. Winding down the steep stone stairs we walked round The Rows, two-tiered buildings with windows full of Christmas goodies. We found a small tearoom and sat over coffee and tea.

'You look tired,' Mike said as I sipped at my drink.

'No. I'm fine,' I replied.

'Why don't we go back to the hotel? The kids can go swimming and you can rest.' Suzanne and Rebecca nodded enthusiastically and we headed back to the car.

We went to the White Hart in Lydgate for dinner that evening. Waiting for our table, I sat mesmerized by the open log fire, sending glowing amber sparks up into the chimney. I noted the specials board and checked the desserts, nudging Suzanne.

'Look, you must be able to manage at least two of those,' I said.

'Don't be awful,' she said, pulling a face, and then looked at the board. 'Actually, yeah you're right. At least two, possibly three.' Her eyes opened wide at the prospect of the sweet delights.

I looked at how Suzanne's hair fell across her eyes and gently curled into the back of her neck. She had applied make-up with care and was wearing a shirt that plunged deeply into a cleavage that I'd noted with a small amount of jealousy. She still looked like my little girl but she was growing up into a beautiful young woman.

'Why can't I have a beer?' she said, her bottom lip protruding, her eyes half closed, glazed in temper. The notion that she was a grown-up woman was suddenly dashed. She was still my teenage daughter.

As I ate, I watched and listened as Mike, Rebecca and Suzanne sat giggling and taunting each other, laughing at Suzanne as her drink went down the wrong way and she gave out a very unladylike snort. Rebecca's laugh tinkled and she held her sides, ridiculing Suzanne until she dribbled tea over the table as she poured from the pot. Drink splattered all over the tablecloth.

Mike's mood swung from indulgent father to grumpy old man as Rebecca hastily tried to mop up the spilt tea. However, he smiled as we all started giggling, cheered by good food.

Back in Leeds, I had a few more days left of my good week before I had my next session of chemotherapy. I dreaded those Thursdays of needles, nausea and tiredness. It seemed that with every treatment, the queasiness got worse. Sometimes I managed to get home before vomiting, sometimes I didn't. And even though the doctors had prescribed stronger anti-emetics the nausea was always worst in those first three days.

I loathed the Monday after chemotherapy most of all, it was my lowest point, and this one was no different. I was too frail to do very much, too nauseous to sit still and read. The chemotherapy made me feel empty. On those days I could believe that death wasn't too far away. My illness rested like a heavy grey mantle, dragging me down.

Sitting in the bath, crouched with my knees up to my chest and my chin resting on them, as the water drained away down the plughole I felt paralysed with despair. As the water ebbed further down my body and the cold air chilled my wet skin, I looked at my distorted reflection in the chrome surface of the tap, bald forehead, froggy eyes, hollow cheeks, chin sharpened with weight loss. I stared at the human toad-like image and was overcome with emotions that I could usually keep successfully at bay. 'What's it all for?' I wondered. 'Why the pain? What awfulness was I paying for?'

My buttocks began to hurt against the hardness of the bath but my arms and legs were too weak to move. I couldn't will my body to move. My groin tight, my pelvis twisted and taut, my belly held straight, my chest constricted, still I could feel something wending its way through my body. A great shuddering sob escaped my lips, pain seeped through the strangled half-cry and I sat, my shoulders and body convulsing with grief. My fingers gripped my thighs, my nails dug into my flesh. I sat, rocking and rocking, holding myself tightly letting out silent, unheard howls of deep sorrow at all my losses–my life, my love, my body, my family.

My family – I had another rack of grief, my biggest loss, my family.

Afterwards I stood at my bedroom window, wrapped in my towel feeling tense with anger. I slammed my fist on the windowsill and slammed it again and again and again. Pain shot through my hand, through my wrist, my elbow and my shoulder and I gripped the sill. Straining to scream at the unfairness of it all, my face was distorted, my neck rigid, my mouth open. I screamed silently at the world outside, everything was black, grim, futile, there was nothing more in my life but this, this awfulness. 'I'm too ill to care,' I thought, 'I'm too ill to live.'

I picked up the phone and called Mike at work, sobbing uncontrollably.

'I can't do this any more, Mike, I can't, it's just too awful. I don't want my life to be like this any more. I can't do it any more.'

Mike sounded bewildered on the other end.

'It's all right, Jane, I'm coming home, I'll be there soon.'

'It's shit, Mike, life's just shit, I don't want to do this any more.'

'Don't worry, I'm coming home. I'm coming home.' I heard the despair and anxiety in his voice. I didn't want him to put down the phone but wanted his physical presence more. There was silence at the other end and I cradled the receiver before putting it back on the handset.

Mike was breathless and upset when he got in. Bounding up the stairs, he held me and held me, hoping to take away some of the hurt.

The puffiness began to recede from my face and my eyes were more open, no longer hidden slits. My cheeks became less round, my hair was just showing through, an uneven stubble darkened my shiny white head. I had finished my last course of chemotherapy; the reduced dose had stopped my counts from plummeting and I had managed to stay out of hospital. The sore throat before Christmas didn't brew into anything serious and Christmas Day arrived and we were still all together.

The door opened quietly, the floorboard creaking as Steven crept into our bedroom and stood staring at me, quiet. I opened my eyes and smiled at him.

'Is it Christmas yet?' he asked, smiling hopefully at me.

Mike stirred next to me. 'What time is it?' he croaked.

'Eight o'clock,' I said. 'Yes, Steven, it's Christmas. Did Father Christmas leave you anything?'

Steven's head cocked to one side and he put his finger to his lip. 'I don't know,' he said, 'I didn't check.' He raced out of the bedroom, returning with a parcel wrapped in red paper, and gave it to me. 'Is this for me, Mummy?' he asked.

I checked the label. 'To Steven, love Father Christmas.' Steven's eyes opened wide.

'Father Christmas has been,' he shouted. 'Do you think he's left presents downstairs?'

I pulled the covers back so he could climb into the bed and he pressed his cold feet up against my skin, making me jump.

'Oooh, you're cold,' I said and he laughed, pushing his feet up against me once again. 'Go on, then,' I said. 'Let's see what you've got!'

Delighted, he tugged and pulled at the shiny red paper until the wrapping fell to the floor.

'Wow, Robot Wars!' he said, turning it to show me. 'Hypnodisc – I haven't got him, have I, Mummy?'

'You have now.' I smiled at his excitement.

Suzanne appeared at the bedroom door, her arms up above her head yawning, her flat tummy exposed as her pyjama top rode up. 'Happy Christmas,' she said through her yawn and then came over to give me a kiss, pulling back the covers to get in beside Steven and me. I budged over.

'Hey!' said Mike, being pushed aside. Rebecca bounded in.

'Where can I sit?' she moaned, bouncing on to the end of the bed.

'Nowhere,' we all chorused. Mike's foot moved down under the covers, catching her and sending her off balance. She tumbled, stopping herself before she hit the floor.

'Dad!' she shrieked, clambering over the covers and edging herself bonily between Mike and myself. We moved apart to allow her space. 'Can we go downstairs?'

'Not yet,' I said. 'Let's have a family cuddle.'

We huddled together uncomfortably but enjoyed the closeness. I chuckled as I looked at Rebecca's straw-like mass of hair. 'Have you seen yourself?' I asked her and she looked at me puzzled. Climbing out to see her reflection, she was shocked to see the bird's nest on her head.

'Oh my God!' she said before collapsing in a fit of giggles.

*

Christmas had taken a lot of planning and chemotherapy had given me little time for preparation. I'd racked my brains trying to come up with a suitable item for what would probably be my last gift to Mike and knew it had to be something really special.

But in early December I'd had a moment of inspiration. I'd been stitching a tapestry waistcoat of Arabian Nights' temples. Rothwell had a dress-uniform makers, the windows full of grand coats for parades. They were able to make up a waistcoat in dark blue. I'd mentioned my plan to Suzanne so she knew where to pick it up in case I wasn't around.

Mike lifted out the newly finished waistcoat stitched with gold thread. Constellations of stars glinted in the dark blue of the night sky. He pulled it on, and hugged me, knowing the effort that had gone into it.

It was a huge relief to finish chemotherapy and my scans showed that my disease had receded further. Although my body was weakened by the drugs, I knew my health had improved.

In February, a long-postponed girly weekend away coincided with the date my friend Amanda had given me for coming over from Australia. I hadn't dared to hope that I would be alive to see her and wasn't sure if she would be able to make it before I became too ill to appreciate the time we'd have together.

Mike set off to pick her up from the airport. She was travelling alone with her 18-month-old-son, Tom. Mike had agreed to look after Tom overnight, and Amanda, knowing Mike, trusted her precious charge with him.

We spent a wonderful weekend together in a hotel with two other friends, Jackie and Michelle. It was a girly weekend of indulgence, massage, sauna and Jacuzzi, and good food. No responsibilities, just time to have fun and relax.

MIKE

We reached Watford Gap without really speaking. Amanda's plane was due to leave Heathrow at half past two but the M1 had been surprisingly quiet and I was confident we would be there well on time. It meant I'd easily make it back to Jo's, Steven's childminder, to collect him by six.

Amanda reminded me a lot of a young Anne Robinson, with short, sandy-coloured hair and narrow-rimmed Michael Caine-style glasses that she'd occasionally push up her nose as she was talking. She had that fantastic Australian quality of saying exactly what she was thinking. She was like a breath of fresh air and I was grateful that she'd made the time to come half way round the world to visit. I'd certainly noticed a difference in Jane's outlook over the last few days.

'Mike, do you think you'll be able to look after Jane right to the end or will she have to be admitted somewhere?' she asked.

'I'm hoping she'll stay at home until the end. It'll all depend on how the kids are, especially Steven.'

'I guess it must be difficult, the girls are a big help though, they're so grown up and mature.'

'They have their moments but they are both dealing with it in their own way.'

'What do you mean, Mike?'

'Suzanne's more open than Becca. She doesn't go round telling everyone but if people know, she acknowledges it. Becca's told her three close friends but no one else. When she knew Jane was going to be bald she decided to tell people she'd shaved her head for a bet on a night out.'

'Why?'

'She can't stand people pitying her.'

'Good on her. I wouldn't either.'

'We're proud of them both. It's extremely difficult for them but they're both well balanced. We've got a lot to be thankful for.'

'And Steven?'

'He knows mum's going to die and eventually just Daddy and him will be at home. We joke that we'll just have a two-seater sports car. So he knows on a superficial level but clearly he's no comprehension of the significance yet. I want him to retain his innocence but be aware of what will happen to lessen the shock. What did you think of Jane?'

'To be truthful I didn't know what to expect. The news was just such a shock, I just had to see her. She doesn't look too good though, Mike. She is easily tired. But she managed to keep going when everybody else at the end of the day was flagging. She just kept on.'

'What about mentally?'

'Way better than I imagined. She has her bad times, I guess. I think I'd crack up under the strain she's under, but she's just got some of that Australian guts. Are you going to get her to come to Oz, Mike? You must.'

'I'd come tomorrow. Jane's work colleagues have even raised enough money to cover the airfares for Jane and me.'

'Yeah', she said, 'that's just amazing.'

'I think there was a certain amount of self-interest.'

'Don't be mean.'

'Nah, it was very kind, but I doubt she'll come over. We couldn't afford to bring everyone and Jane wouldn't want to leave them.'

The driving conditions were almost perfect, an unseasonably mild day with perfect visibility. Even though we were moving into commuter distance for London, the roads were no busier.

'You know, you and Steven can always come or the girls if they want to tour. Does Anne know when she'll emigrate to Perth?'

Anne, Jane's sister, had advised us of her family's intention to emigrate when they heard Jane's prognosis. Thoughtfully, they let us know before anyone else so we could arrange new guardians for our children. 'They've got to sell the house in Bolton. It'll be really tough on Jane saying goodbye. When they go she'll never see them again.'

'I know, I was upset at leaving today, it's heartbreaking. But nothing compared to what you're going through.'

'It was a shock, Anne going and finding new guardians is proving more troublesome than I thought. I suppose with one parent dying the chances of being called upon are higher.'

'Surely not? They are great kids.'

'If you think about it, taking three kids into anyone's home would be tough; you've got to think about space, finance, family dynamics – it's not an easy decision.'

'Christ, Mike,' said Amanda. I could see her staring intently at me as I looked at the road ahead. There was a long pause before she said: 'How's the good old National?'

'Fantastic, you couldn't wish for better employers. If you ignore the fact that they're Australians.'

'Get lost.'

'Joking aside, they're brilliant. Jane's employers have been just as good. We couldn't have managed without them. But the flipside is that Jane still goes into work a week after chemo. Who else would do that?'

The conversation flowed from politics to cricket to the bank before we got to the airport. Amanda was travelling to Ireland before going home. Pulling up at the drop-off point, I parked the car. With Tom safely ensconced in his pushchair, Amanda hugged me.

'I don't envy you, Mike,' she said. 'You're going back to have a horrible year. Be brave.'

JANE

The dream of Australia had been held out to me like a carrot on a stick. Now that my treatment had finished I could begin to contemplate a holiday with Mike. Yet the other side of the world seemed too far and I was concerned in case I became too unwell. But I'd always dreamed of returning and showing Mike some of the places I knew from my childhood.

Amanda bolstered my resolve. She'd left me a handwritten itinerary, her ideas for spending the best time down under. Breaking the journey in Singapore, we would travel to Adelaide, where we had an open invitation to her house, follow that with a visit to Sydney and then on to the Gold Coast to relax.

There were many logistics to sort out. Travel insurance was the first hurdle. I spent a whole day on the phone answering intrusive questions about my health. Has your doctor told you your condition is terminal? Did they still expect me to be alive four months after the end of my trip? How often did I see my doctor? Having to spend hours reiterating the fact that, yes, I was terminally ill, yes, I was going to die and, no, it could not be cured, left me feeling despondent. Saying it out loud so many times seemed to make it more real.

By the afternoon, I had found a broker willing to insure us for £400. Later that night, I sat and nursed a large whisky to take away the harsh reality I'd had to face all day.

This would be the first real holiday that Mike and I would spend alone together and I was relishing the thought. We booked it just before my thirty-seventh birthday, at the end of February. As I was starting a new trial for a vaccine which would hopefully boost the immune response to my tumour we had to work round the dates I needed to be in Leeds for the injections. Our flight to Singapore was booked for Wednesday, 28 March, and we would return home on Wednesday, 18 April.

When the big day arrived, Mike and I waited anxiously for the taxi. Our bags were packed, items were shuffled and reshuffled as we checked that we had everything we needed. The insurance documents, doctors' letters and drugs were in my small back-pack. The doctors' letters were another stark reminder of my disease. As well as confirming that I was fit to travel and had a legitimate use for the drugs I was carrying, they were recent let-ters outlining my current condition. Although they only confirmed what I already knew – metastatic breast cancer with bronchial hilar metastases and multiple bone metastases – the terms so familiar from work were hard to relate to myself.

I'd been having a drip of drugs to stop the calcium coming out of deposit in my bones while I was on chemotherapy, but now I was taking it in tablet form. It was the biphosphonate drug, sodium clodronate, which needed to be taken on an empty stomach. I couldn't eat an hour before or after taking it and managing breakfast and an evening meal round the regime was sometimes difficult.

I was nervous about the travelling and we both regretted that the children would be staying at home. I was upset saying goodbye to them before they left for school, but as Jack and Alice waved us off in the taxi the excitement started to build for us both.

We spent two days in Singapore and were bowled over by the entire city, from the vast shopping mall containing the world's largest fountain to the small colonial houses, some of which lined empty sites containing cicadas that shrieked so loudly in the dusk that Mike kept looking round to see what was making the drilling noise. The tastes, the sounds, the heat – it all felt so exotic. We tried some of the local dishes at the buffet, the Malay sweet curries with satay and fragrant rice. Strange noodle soup. Fruit that was fresh and luscious.

The two days felt like four and we were sad to be on our way to the airport once again. I was thrilled by the thought of seeing Amanda again but it meant another long, tiring flight to Adelaide.

Through the queues on arrival, past the passport control, I could see Amanda. We pushed our way through and hugged each other. I couldn't quite believe I'd made it.

We were to spend the next five days with Amanda and her family. Tom had grown so much in the few months since I'd last seen him on their visit. We visited the Barossa Valley to sample wines and drove to Brighton and Glenelg, where I used to swim and sunbathe with my brothers and sisters. The pier at Brighton had been replaced and I looked out towards the blue waves, remembering cold nights threading shellfish on to hooks, casting them far out to catch the silvery whiting. Dropping weighted bait for multicoloured languid squid and meat in nets to tempt crabs.

Amanda and I sat sipping iced coffee, waiting for Mike to reappear, red faced, sweating and breathless after his jog on the seafront.

'That can't be good for you,' I laughed as Mike sat recovering himself.

'You should try it. You never know, you might enjoy it,' he said, when he could talk once more.

Amanda's home wasn't far away from my old school, Cabra College, and I took Mike. We walked up the drive to where the convent stood. It looked so much smaller, the large lawned area where we used to have assemblies was just a small patch of green, scuffed with brown. I traipsed up the covered walkway to the library and the classroom block that housed 10-2, my last class. The shrubs needed trimming, they overhung the path near the science labs. I laughed, recalling failed science experiments. I turned away, walking back towards the gate, leaving my child-hood behind.

On my last night with Amanda, I lay in bed next to Mike, looking through the slit of the blinds at the streetlights, won-dering if Amanda and I would meet again. Neither of us had spoken about my future and I was glad to have visited her, enjoyed the welcome into her family, but now it was time to move on.

Saying goodbye at the airport we were both quiet. I left her, looked back with regret and boarded the aircraft. As we took off, I looked out of the plane window and spotted Tom's blond hair and noticed them waving at us. I waved back, a tear falling down my cheek, knowing they couldn't see my final farewell.

MIKE

We arrived at the All Seasons hotel in Darling Harbour just as Sydney was winding down for the Easter weekend. I turned on the news in our room and saw what seemed like most of Australia's camera crews en masse at Sydney Airport. Some of Ansett's planes had been grounded, sending holiday plans into chaos. We were lucky to get to Sydney, our plane was one of them.

On Friday morning, Jane awoke with a lot of pain in her lower back. She stretched to reach the guidebook.

'We can rest today if you want?' I suggested.

Jane shook her head, opening the book.

'I don't want to waste a day,' she said. 'I'll take some painkillers. What do you want to do tomorrow – it's your day.'

'How lucky does a man need to get?' I said. 'My fortieth birthday in Sydney on Easter Saturday.

'Anything you want, it's your day.'

I raised my eyebrows and gave her a salacious look.

'Get real,' she said and I smiled.

The sun began to beat a little hotter as we made our way over to Sydney Harbour Bridge. At the top we could see a group of people walking along its arc in grey overalls.

'Should we see about booking?' she asked.

When we checked availability, it turned out that Jane could go up today. She was, however, too ill. I left her looking at the available times and the photographs of the rich, famous and Olympians whose climbs were recorded. Jane held her fingernail under the line 'Climbers need to be physically fit.'

'We don't have to tell them,' I said.

'That's not fair on the guides or the other climbers.' We silently pondered the options. 'I don't know how much the overalls or harness will hurt the bone metastases.' We edged towards the reception desk.

'Good day,' smiled the receptionist.

'Hi, I'd like to book a climb for Sunday,' said Jane.

'For one or two?' Jane looked up at me.

I shrugged and shook my head. 'Dunno.'

Jane turned back to the receptionist. 'I'm fit enough to go up but I'm terminally ill with cancer. Am I able to do the climb? I've been really looking forward to it.'

'Oh.' She looked at Jane. 'I'm sorry . . . er . . . I don't know, I'll have to ask.'

Within a couple of minutes, a guide supervisor returned warning Jane that Sunday was predicted to be a hot one, ninety degrees. He did say that it wasn't too tough for anyone reasonably fit. He suggested she tried the harness on the practice steps. I knew that unless they said no, Jane would have a go.

At decision time, I bottled it. But as Jane got her ticket, her face radiated a beaming smile like Steven's after discovering Father Christmas had been.

JANE

I left Mike and joined other members of my BridgeClimb group as we were talked through the safety equipment used during the climb. Each one of us had to pass a breath test before being issued with our BridgeSuit to wear over our own clothes. I stepped into the cubicle and pulled on the grey overalls, emerging minutes later looking like a crew member in Star Trek. My baseball cap was attached by a cord to the back of my suit and, then, a man moved forward and clipped on a belt, pulling on the fastenings to make sure it was secure. He gave us another last-minute talk before directing us on to the Climb simulator. We walked up metal stairs and along a gridded walkway, pulling the harnesses along the cable as we traversed the practice area. We stepped down from the small bridge, practice over, and our group was set for the climb.

We clicked on to a cable one by one and passed through the concrete tunnel of the bridge entrance, tugging our harnesses over the small footbridge that would lead us to the main structure of the bridge. Walking along the narrow catwalk to the pylon, I looked down. The river was a long, long way down; the road beneath buzzed with traffic.

Setting off to climb up narrow ladders through the pylon that would take us up to the eastern arch, I was worried that I would become too breathless to finish the climb. Our leader, Scott, hooked me up directly behind him so he could keep a close eye on me. We started to climb, hand over hand, up the steel steps. I kept my hand on the rail and clenched my teeth to stop the swaying feeling. It started to pass and I concentrated on breathing, slowly and evenly, and was glad when we started on the more gradual ascent up over the brow of the bridge.

I looked around. The sky was blue, the mist at the start of the day had cleared and the sun was just beginning to warm us. As we reached the last part of the climb to the summit I started to relax. I knew that I would be at the top soon.

The view across Sydney Harbour was spectacular. The Opera

House looked diminished from where I was standing, gleaming white against the blueness of the water. We all looked out around us at the harbour, perfect picture-postcard scenery. A red-faced man, bent double with the effort, panted as he tried to get his breath back. The lady behind me gripped the rail tightly, her whole body quivering with nerves. One exuberant couple high-fived their achievement. I looked around me, at the views. Scott looked at me.

'How are you doing?' he asked.

'I'm fine,' I said. 'I'm glad I came, I wouldn't have missed this for anything.'

'See that.' Scott pointed out the coastline. 'And just in the distance up there are the Blue Mountains.' I followed his gaze and could see the purple peaks through the sun haze. Scott took pictures of us with a camera attached to his suit. Couples kissed with the opera house as a backdrop. I raised my arm and cheered, my cheeks pink with effort, and then we were led across the top of the bridge for our return climb.

We started our descent downwards. I could feel myself tiring and I concentrated on placing my weary legs in front of each other, careful not to miss each step. I began to feel light-headed and held on to the rail firmly, edging my foot forward to make sure I would come to rest on the next step down. A boat passed below us and I focused on it, watching it churning up the water white in its wake.

Mike was waiting for me at the bottom, his fear of heights too great for him to make the climb. I had taken some persuading to try the climb, frightened that I would not be able to finish it. Mike hugged me when I had returned my grey uniform.

'I can't believe you managed that. I watched you all the way up. The bloke next to me was looking at me 'cos I was crying.'

I hugged Mike back. 'I'm so glad I let you persuade me. It was fantastic. The views were stunning.'

We stopped for an ice cream and I rested for the return journey back to the hotel. My legs were tired and my head was dizzy with the effort.

*

Boarding the plane to return to England, I sat remembering our excitement on the journey out. All my expectations had been met – and more – we'd had such a good time. Mike was returning back to England a year older – now in his forties. We felt so lucky. Six months ago this holiday was just a dream. Now, here we were, returning from it with a store of happy memories to keep us going over the next few months.

A long, long flight and we were back in Manchester. The same taxi driver picked us up from the airport. We unlocked the door and, startled to see us, Alice jumped.

'I thought you weren't back until this afternoon,' she said.

'What? Aren't you pleased to see us?' said Mike.

In the living room, Suzanne and Rebecca shrieked when they heard us and Steven came bounding out.

'Mummy! Mummy!' he called, hugging my leg. I managed to extricate myself before sitting down on the settee, pulling Steven on to my lap and giving him a cuddle.

Over drinks we distributed our gifts. I'd bought Suzanne a small jewellery case containing a bangle and, as I passed it over to her, I looked again at her, taking in the young woman before me. I'd been carrying a vision of her in my head as a small child but as she took the gift I could see she was an adult. It was the first time I realized just how grown up she had become. She bent down to kiss me and thank me.

Steven held on with his small dry hand gripping tightly round my fingers as I continued to look at Suzanne. I saw again a small blonde girl, hair pushed back with a blue headband, red jumper and a blue denim dungarees. Her small plump hand pumping mine as she marched, swinging her arms and skipping, her other hand held out to an unseen companion.

'Bertha's too tired to walk any further,' she said, looking up at me with earnest blue eyes staring at me from under her ragged blonde fringe.

'Well, we've still got a long way to go before we get to the shops,' I said smiling. Bertha was keeping us company a lot these days, she even had her own place setting at the

table. 'We can't hang around for her, she'll have to wait here for us.'

Suzanne looked aghast at any thought of abandoning her friend. Holding out her hand again she said: 'Come on, up here', and we waited while Bertha shrank in size and leapt on to Suzanne's hand. Placing her in the front pocket of her dungarees, she beamed.

'She's all right now, Mum,' she said and took my hand again for the walk.

CHAPTER 10

JANE

Clearing the dinner dishes from the table, I heard the ring of the phone. Rebecca threw herself down the stairs – as she always did when she was expecting a call from her school friend, Lucy – but then she called from the hallway: 'Mum, it's for you – it's Belinda.' My hand shook as I reached for the phone, my mind racing with possible reasons for the call.

'Hi, Jane.' Her voice was cheery and I felt the sudden tension release from me. 'I've been contacted by the BBC asking if I knew anyone who wouldn't mind talking to them about living with a terminal illness. They've done quite a bit of filming already, but they need someone else and I thought of you.' There was quiet down the phone, and I wasn't sure how to respond. Belinda continued: 'I just wanted to know if I could pass your phone number on to the producer?'

I thought for a brief moment. 'Yeah, go on then – what's his name?'

'It's a she, her name's Jane Beckwith. She'll probably want to come to meet you. You can always say no.'

Jane arrived a few days later and I welcomed her into the house. Sitting opposite me in the living room, with a black notebook on her lap, she asked a series of questions, making her way down the list from her notes. How did I feel about dying? Had it changed my faith? Had it made me want to remove myself psychologically from my family? Her questions were well thought through, searching without being sensationalist. She approached the subject with honesty and wasn't shocked by my openness about my lack of future.

Before she left, we set a date as to when she could come to film. She wanted to film me away from the home and suggested a garden centre so that I could explain how my shortened time meant everything took on a different perspective. I was already thinking what spring bulbs I wanted to plant in the autumn, and I'd potted the forget-me-nots and wallflowers for the borders, despite not knowing if I would see the flowers after the winter. Jane wanted me to talk about this aspect of living with a terminal diagnosis, to show people that it affected all aspects of my life. I didn't know if I would see the vibrant red and pure white tulips, but I could enjoy planting the garden for spring and, as I pinched the young green shoots from the spindly wall flowers, they brought pictures of me and my grandpa to my mind, me as a young girl in a pinafore dress skipping beside him as we bent together to the ordinary yellow flowers with a sweet heavy scent.

I chose a day when I knew Suzanne would not be home studying. Nine months ago, when I'd been told I was going to die, I'd given myself the date of Suzanne's exam results to aim for, maybe even Steven's first day at school. I'd hoped that I would be able to help her through as much of her exams as possible. We'd visited sixth form colleges together, choosing days on which I was well enough to accompany her, and she'd made her choice and was going to study languages at A level. All the months before, I'd hoped and prayed that I would not be too ill; I desperately didn't want to be dying as she studied for her exams.

Jane arrived with a cameraman and a researcher. We drove to a local garden centre and wandered round. I walked between the rows of shrubs answering her questions, feeling as though my answers were clumsy. The sentiment of 'How to plant a garden that you might not live long enough to see bloom' was hard to express without feeling self-conscious, especially with other shoppers watching as they walked by. Finding a low wall, we both sat and the cameraman set up his shot. Jane asked me what my aims were.

'For me, the big goals this year were to get to Australia – which I managed to do – to see my eldest daughter through her exams – which I managed to do – and the next goal is to see her get her GCSE results. One big goal that I really want is to be able to walk my four-year-old to school.' My eyes filled with tears, the sorrow of not being around to see that milestone too much for me to bear. I lived my life without looking to the future, and tried not to dwell on the things I might never experience. Willing the tears to disappear, I looked past Jane at the rows of bedding plants behind her, bright with flowers. I tried to compose myself enough to continue.

'It's hard,' I said. 'I can picture my sixteen-year-old and my thirteen-year-old as grown-ups . . .' I took deep breaths, I wanted to finish the sentence. 'But I can't picture my four-year-old as an adult and I'm not going to see him as a grown-up.'

I bent forward, my chest tight with unexpressed grief. The cameraman searched for a tissue for my tears and, unable to find anything suitable, removed his shirt to offer it to me. That brought a smile to my eyes and I passed him it back unused.

There was another day of filming, which we shot in the garden on a summer afternoon watching Mike and the children playing cricket on the lawn. As Steven bowled out Rebecca he gave out an emphatic cry of 'Yes!' and punched his fists in the air. I stood at the patio door, laughing at their energy and excitement.

'How does it feel to have this time with your family?' asked Jane.

'I don't feel lucky,' I said. 'Sometimes I wish it could be over, it's such a hard thing for us all.' I didn't take my eyes off my family; Suzanne sitting on the bench, unwilling to be filmed, a self-conscious teenager, hiding behind her long fringe; Rebecca crouched over the small cricket bat, laughing, her eyes shining with childish glee.

'I have an image,' I said to Jane. 'It's an image of a shaded wood, with a meandering path disappearing into the darkness. I picture myself following the path; I know what's at the end but I just try and concentrate on this moment now.'

'Do you worry about dying?' asked Jane.

'I try not to. But I know I'm going to get poorly, poorlier and then death. It's not a good way to die and Mike and the children are going to have to go through that.'

'How do you cope with that knowledge?'

'I try to give myself something to aim for,' I said. 'Short-term goals, trying not to think too far into the future. It would be easy to be greedy, to think I might still be here to see Steven finish primary school, but that's very unlikely.'

I didn't feel uncomfortable talking about my mortality, the inevitability of my demise was something I couldn't change, something I'd tried to get used to. Jane asked questions about my faith and how it had been affected.

'My faith hasn't increased or decreased,' I told her. 'It's part of me, just the same. The one thing I do pray for is a calmness, to feel that when the time has come, to know it's my time and to be at peace with that idea.'

I knew they were including Dionne in the programme. We had started treatment at the same time, the year before, and still saw each other when our clinic appointments coincided. She was another of Dr Perren's patients. She was a tall, beautiful young woman in her twenties. They were filming her having scans and going for results.

Like me, her life was regimented into three monthly intervals. We were both on the same vaccine trial, both followed the same routine for scans, results and treatment.

I had only come into the kitchen to pour a glass of milk for Steven, but the sight that greeted me made me bang about the room noisily. The worktops were strewn with crumbs, teabags were mounded up by the kettle. I gritted my teeth as I rinsed the kitchen cloth and wiped away the debris from the evening meal. Rebecca appeared in the doorway, took one look and sidled out – but not quickly enough.

'Becca,' I said, raising my voice as she retreated up the stairs. 'I thought you were tidying the kitchen.'

'I did,' she replied.

'Well I've just finished clearing up after you.' I switched the dishwasher on and turned to face her. 'I could have done with a little help tonight. I'm tired.'

I hadn't slept for the last few nights, but lay awake listening to Mike snoring, disturbed by his shuffling round the bed. I opened the fridge and pulled out an empty milk carton.

'I don't believe it,' I said, as I slammed the fridge door shut and grabbed the car keys from the worktop. As I drove to the local shop I calmed down, but still felt the tension in my body. My neck held tight, my jaw was clenched firmly together to hold in my fear. I was going for my scans tomorrow, CT scan in the morning, bone scan in the afternoon. I was more composed when I arrived home. Rebecca stood in the kitchen.

'Sorry, Mum,' she said. 'I know you're scared about tomorrow, I'm sorry for not helping more.' She looked up at me, her eyes wide with apologies.

'Do you and Dad want to go out tonight? Suzanne can look after us.' I smiled at her attempt to smooth things over.

'No, but thanks anyway,' I said. 'Besides, you just want to stay up and watch *Friends* without us bugging you.'

'As if?' She arched her eyebrow as a grin split her face.

'Go on, take this through for Steven.' I held a glass of milk out to her.

I left my morning coffee on the worktop, remembering that I needed to starve for the CT scan. Instead, I had to drink a jug of foul-tasting contrast solution, which was necessary for the scans, when I arrived at the hospital. The assistant left me with instructions to drink one cup every ten minutes. I nodded, it was a familiar routine, the same contrast to drink, tasting of aniseed, the same form to sign to say I wasn't pregnant, the same amorphous gowns to change into.

I lay on the table, a line attached from my arm to a pump to push contrast into my veins. The round edge of the scanner encircled me.

'When I call to you, Jane, I need you to breathe in and hold your breath,' said Cynthia, the petite radiographer I knew from her training days at the Leeds General Infirmary. The machine whirred into life. I could hear it spinning around the inside of the gantry as the table started to move. The warmth of the contrast as it flushed through my body, the sound of the machine, the holding of my breath for the images, it was all just part of my life now.

Finished with the routine of the scans, it was still hard to relax until I heard the results. Another 'okay' though, and Anne the research nurse took me into a small room where I lifted up my skirt and she injected a small amount of clear solution into the top of my left thigh. It stung, bringing tears to my eyes. I stamped my feet, thundering my heels on the floor.

'Do you want me to wait a few moments before I do the other side?' she asked.

'No.' I gritted my teeth. 'Just get it over with.'

She pinched the top of my thigh and inserted the needle, pushing in the contents of another small phial. I could already feel the hot burning sensation as she withdrew the tiny point.

'Ow, ow, ow, ow!' I stifled my yelp. The pain subsided after just a few minutes and Anne checked the thickened areas on my thighs from previous injections.

'Right, that's all fine,' she said. 'We'll see you in three months.'

MIKE

I replaced the receiver. Mum had been calm as she told me that her sister Margaret's funeral would be on Thursday. Jane had already decided not to attend – not out of any disrespect – she simply didn't know how she would cope.

I walked through to the kitchen, grabbed a glass of water and took a sip to remove the dryness in my mouth. The laces on my trainers felt tight; I crouched down and began tying them again. I just wanted to get out on to the road, knowing that the little enthusiasm I had would soon evaporate.

'Come on, Jane!' I hollered up the stairs.

Jane appeared at the top, slowly descending.

'Do I look all right?' she asked.

'What does it matter what you look like?' I said, nearing the door to leave. 'You're going to look like shit when you've finished anyway.'

'I mean the clothes,' she said, clearly narked. I looked her up and down quickly. Her trainers were pristine, too white, but apart from that she looked like any other jogger. 'You're fine,' I said. 'Let's go. See you later, kids,' I called.

Suzanne came to the door; she had been forced to stop studying for thirty minutes so she could look after Steven.

'Good luck, Mum,' she said.

I followed Jane out of the door, turning to Suzanne to pull a face. 'Should we warm up?' Jane asked, her concert T-shirt hanging over her leggings.

'Are you taking the piss?'

'Why?'

'At the pace you're running, the run will be the warm-up.'

She ignored my remark. 'Which way?'

'Left at the bottom,' I said. We'd discussed what level she should be training at beforehand. Although it was called the Race for Life, it was a walk or run, whatever anyone could manage. But Jane didn't want to turn up on the day and just walk around, there would be no sense of achievement for her.

She'd never done any running before apart from a little on the treadmill at her new gym, so it was difficult to gauge how far she would be able to go and the training pattern was worked out on a best-guess basis. Thirty-five minutes for five kilometres seemed a realistic goal.

Setting off, we ran painstakingly slowly down to the park and turned left on to a flat path. I wasn't convinced Jane had the heart for it, so to test her, after only 600 metres I turned on to the biggest hill in Rothwell, 400 metres up a 1:6 gradient. At its start, I was fifteen metres ahead.

'Mike! Wait!' Jane called. I turned round to see her gasping for breath, doubled-up on the pavement.

'What's up?' I said. 'You can't be tired.' Thinking Jane's fledgling running career might already be over, I pulled up. We'd barely started. There was little point in continuing the charade if it was the best she could do.

'I'm struggling to get my breath,' she said, leaning against a wall. 'Give me a minute.'

I shook my head and tutted. 'Let's go home, save any embarrassment.'

'I'm all right,' she snapped and with that set off again slowly before getting another fifty yards and stopping again.

'Jane, this is pathetic. There's no shame in calling it a day. The key is to keep going, however slowly.'

Her stride pattern was extremely short. It was painful to watch her uneasy running action – head down, shoulders hunched. Within yards, she had to stop again, rasping and wheezing to get her breath back. I stood with my hands on my hips, looking round to see if anyone was watching. After a few minutes she set off again. It was agonizingly slow, anyone walking up the same hill would have overtaken us easily. Back on the flat, her run became more of a lurch but she steadily picked up momentum and got slightly faster as we started the descent back down the hill. She was looking extremely uncomfortable. When we finally arrived back home twenty-five minutes later we'd covered two and a half kilometres. I congratulated her.

'Piss off,' she said, massaging her sides as though she had stitch. While she stayed outside to cool down and stretch, I went in, where Suzanne greeted me.

'How did Mum do?' she asked.

'Don't ask.'

'Really?'

'She did okay, she's all right.'

Jane walked through the door. 'What's he saying?' she said. 'Nothing,' said Suzanne.

I felt sure that would be the last I'd see of Jane running. All next day she complained how her calves felt tight, her hip hurt and her knees felt sore. I'd warned her about the stress that road-running places on the joints but she'd ignored me. Her most recent bone scan had showed a further reduction in her bone metastases and she was confident she could complete the run, even if it was in a slow time. I wasn't so sure. Time was passing quickly and, even in our most optimistic moments, we knew this was Jane's last summer. I didn't want her doing anything that might shorten the time we had left.

'Where are we going?' asked Jane, who had donned her trainers again and was ready to come out on her second run.

'Same as Sunday,' I said. I'd initially been reluctant to take her out again but as she was determined, I felt I should be with her in case anything went wrong. 'But instead of turning right by the cemetery. We're going to the stepping stones.'

'What's the point in doing the hill? Roundhay Park is on the flat.'

'It's not. It's a fair drag from the lake to the mansion. Plus, if you can do more than the distance with hills, you'll be more confident on the day.' Jane strode out, a little more relaxed, but after 400 metres she tailed off. Reaching the hill, I shouted back to her.

'No stopping! Go as slow as you want but don't stop!'

Monotonously, she ground out the climb with short strides, grimacing in pain as each foot hit the ground. I stopped half way to encourage her.

'Come on! Come on!' I yelled 'Work! Keep working!'

I ran alongside her. We were barely moving but she kept going relentlessly to the top. I patted her back, which was damp from the effort.

'Well done!' I said.

'Get lost, you patronizing git,' she said.

We got home again in twenty-five minutes but had covered an extra 600 metres.

*

Considering he'd spent most of his life avoiding churches, it seemed odd to see Dad in one. Today, although dressed professionally as if on pall-bearing duty, he was here to say goodbye to my mother's sister.

I sat beside my parents as if reeling back the years. I looked around me; childhood memories came flooding back; all the faces were familiar if a little older. My parents' generation was suddenly looking fragile. Illnesses were affecting each family to some extent. It would have been easy not to come.

My mind wandered. Would the next time be Jane? Looking at the coffin, the future became virtual reality. Would the next time I saw all these people be in St Mary's church in Rothwell? Visions of sitting with the kids made me well up and I sat looking at my feet trying to think of football, work, our forthcoming holiday in Italy, anything but the service. Dad sat next to me stony-faced, as mum sniffled.

It was a short car ride to the cemetery. Walking past the headstones, I chatted to several cousins I'd not seen since we buried our grandparents over a decade ago. For me, the weather felt like it was November – damp and miserable. I stood away from the plot, head bowed as the last elements of the service took place.

Later, at the wake, picking at remnants of food left on the trestle tables, my Uncle Frank walked over. How could I greet him? We embraced hard and pulled away.

'Michael, it's really tough, much harder than I thought it would be. My heart goes out to you,' he said. I remained silent. I didn't need to hear any more.

Jane was on my case about fundraising. When she'd told me she planned to do the Race for Life three weeks earlier, I somewhat rashly said that raising £500 would be a cinch, but so far we were exactly that amount away from achieving it. Imperial Cancer Research provided us with a sponsorship form and guidelines as to how to maximize fundraising. But handing round a form wouldn't even scratch the surface. Equally, I didn't want to press-gang people into supporting Jane. There were so many sponsorship forms doing the rounds that I didn't want to add to them.

The bank had a bulletin board and I considered putting something on there. This would get the message across. If people wanted to support her they would have to be proactive.

I sat at my computer and typed out a notice but reading back the words they seemed too powerful. I'd just written from the heart – with a touch of added angst. I saved it as a draft and would come back to it later. But then I heard Jane's voice in my head, telling me to get on with it.

I didn't want the message to go out in my name. I'd been at the bank seventeen years and knew lots of people and hadn't got round everyone to tell them Jane was dying. The last thing I needed was more conversations and breaking the news to people. So I asked my colleague Richard to put the message out for me.

A Matter of Life & Death

Mike Tomlinson's wife was diagnosed terminally ill with breast cancer last August. Originally given only a short time to live, by November she could not walk up a flight of stairs without taking a rest. After chemotherapy she believes she is fit enough to run the Race for Life in Leeds for the Imperial Cancer Research Fund on 03/06/2001. The prognosis is still terminal and the cancer is in her spine and so every step will be extremely painful. She is still determined to run the whole way with no walking.

Needless to say this is a one-off event. For Jane next year will definitely be too late.

Many people have asked Mike if there is anything they could do to help, well now is the chance. This is a one-off attempt to raise money for Cancer Research so that in future this doesn't happen to your wife, mother or children.

Minutes later, Richard called me over to his computer. 'Mike, you've got to see this,' he said.

I stepped over to his screen and began reading an e-mail reply. 'Shit. A hundred pounds. That must be a typing mistake. You'd better drop him a note.'

But it wasn't. For the rest of the morning, e-mails flooded Richard's inbox with promises of sponsorship money. The message had only been posted at 11.16 a.m. but shortly after lunch the spreadsheet Richard had designed was full of names and amounts.

I'd not thought through the mechanics of what I'd done until e-mails started asking: 'Where do I send the money?' 'Where do I get a form?' I'd not predicted anyone would respond. We quickly revised the original note twice.

'Mike, we've got two hundred and thirty-five pounds already and I've sent out forms to five different departments,' said Richard.

'We're nearly at the target already,' I said. 'We might be able to get one thousand pounds.'

'It hasn't even gone on some of the servers yet,' he said.

At the end of the day, more and more offers had come in from people throughout the bank. Grabbing my coat to head out of the door I turned to thank Richard for his help.

'You're welcome,' he said. 'That's been the most enjoyable day at work for ages.'

JANE

Mum walked alongside Karen and me, down the stone steps outside her house and along the tree-lined street to Soldier's Field. We turned left and made our way towards the main gate of Roundhay Park, where we could already hear voices echoing across the field from loudspeakers. Mum held my hand and kissed my cheek.

'Have a good run, then,' she said.

'Thanks.' I watched as she turned to stroll home, then Karen and I joined a group of women collecting on the park.

'Perhaps this isn't such a good idea,' I said to Karen.

'Well you got us into this, so don't be going having second thoughts now.' My sister-in-law chuckled, then laughed harder. I joined her. Helpless with laughter, we looked at each other in our T-shirts and leggings. A most unlikely pair.

I was amazed by the sight of so many women of all shapes and sizes arriving for the Race for Life. My neighbour, Cynthia, power-walked the five kilometres every year, and each year as I handed my sponsor money over to her I vowed that I would take part in the next run. This year, I had finally met my promise, and stood looking around me at the huge numbers willing to give up a Sunday morning to raise funds for charity. There were some vested runners, but most of the women looked like fun runners and walkers like Karen and me. As well as the racing numbers on their fronts, I noticed many women wore notices on their backs. 'For Mum,' said one. Another said: 'For my friend Joanna' – it seemed everyone had a reason to be there.

The loudspeakers announced the beginning of the warming-up exercises and we rose to our feet. Forests of arms stretched up and down in a rhythmic beat as the instructor ordered us to bend and stretch. After ten minutes of synchronized movement, we were told to make our way to the starting line. We walked, hustled by lycra-clad women, towards the bannered start. I felt a finger poke me in my back.

'What are you doing back here?' I turned and saw Cynthia behind me. 'We're walking, you know,' she said, pointing her thumb at a couple of friends with her. 'I thought you were going to run it? You need to be near the front.'

I was about to reply when the sound of a loud hooter pierced the air and the mass of women moved forward, slowly at first then quickening to a brisk walk. Finally I started to run as the groups of women stretched out, leaving gaps to jog through. Karen was by my side but waved me on.

'I'm much slower than you – you go on, I'll see you at the end.'

'Have a good run,' I said as I upped the pace and let my legs roll, feet falling one after the other as I concentrated on the rhythm of my footfalls. My chest felt heavy, the pain in my right side harsh, as I drew in breath through my mouth and nose. At my left shoulder, a triangle of stabbing. I eased to a more comfortable tempo, the pain became less persistent and I looked around me trying to enjoy the experience.

I made my way to the opposite end of the park, then I turned to run up the same path, passing people still making their way. The path started to rise, the incline heavy on my legs, my head went down, my eyes on the ground as I concentrated on running, passing women who were already walking. My pace slowed, as my ribs sawed against my side, making me clasp it to ease the ache. I nearly stopped to join the pedestrians but I would never live it down if someone saw me walking and the thought of not reaching my own personal goal spurred me on. I gritted my teeth, breathing shallowly to stop the stitch keening in my side, pushed against the burning pain in my thighs, ignoring the rubbing sensation at my heels.

'Come on, Jane, keep going, you can do it!' Carol and her girls, Holly and Sophie, were yelling at me from above on the grassed verge. I smiled as I passed them, still climbing, and came to the gates where the runners escaped on to the road. With the hill behind me, I pushed myself along the slight decline, allowing my breathing to slow. My legs rolled out before me and I picked up speed as I headed for the corner. A large smile broke out across my face as Peter called my name. He and Tom sprayed me with jets of cold water from two powerful waterguns. The woman next to me grumbled as she was splashed by a misdirected arc of water. I laughed and left her moaning.

At the last corner, I began to tire. On the road back to the finish I could feel the slight incline pushing up into my legs and my breath became laboured once again. Just at that moment my stomach decided to turn. I could taste bile as the finish line came into view.

'Come on, Jane, put your foot down!' I glanced to the side – it was Carol's husband, Jon. 'Come on, sprint finish!' he shouted.

My stomach lurched but I urged myself onwards, trying to pick up the pace. I could see the finishing line, crowded with other women already done, bent double with their effort. I forced down again and my legs felt lighter as I ran towards the blue-bannered end of the race. As I passed the finishing line I tilted my head back to take in the time on the overhead digital clock. Twenty-eight minutes. I'd broken my target by two minutes.

I didn't have time to celebrate. The elation of finishing the race disappeared rapidly as the bile surged up into my throat and I spun round desperately searching for a quiet spot, away from the hordes of women, where I could throw up. Pushing my way urgently through sweaty bodies, I bent over and retched, vomiting noisily on to a patch of grass. I wiped my mouth on the edge of my T-shirt and hobbled to where teams of organizers were handing out small medals. I grabbed a bottle of water and, sipping from it, I scanned the faces of the crowd, watching and waiting for Mike. I started to cool down quickly, rivulets of sweat were running down my back and sticking to my T-shirt, blanketing me in cold cotton.

Carol sat down next to me and pushed her glasses up her nose on her perfectly made-up face. Her hair was neatly groomed as always. I lifted my hand up to my head to feel my hair sticking up and out like a bristled yard brush.

'Well done,' she said, smiling at me, delighted. 'I can't believe you did that!'

I grinned at her, unable to believe it myself and carried on looking for Mike.

'Have you seen Mike and the kids yet?' I asked.

'Yeah, they were here earlier, they'll be somewhere around.' She stood up to get a better look at the crowd. 'You wait here, I'll see if I can spot him.' I stayed sitting, watching her walk to the finishing area.

'Mummy!' Steven appeared out of nowhere. Mike was with him.

'Where have you been?' he asked.

'Looking for you,' I answered defensively.

'Look who I've found,' he said. I could barely miss Phil, Mike's friend from work, towering over Mike, shoulders broad, his hair blond and peppered with grey.

'Well done, Jane.' He leaned forward to kiss me and then drew away quickly. 'Ugh, you're wet!' he said in mock disgust. Louise stood next to him, her expectant belly huge with their second child. She was holding hands with her daughter, Hannah, who stood shyly behind the bulk of her dad.

'Thank you,' I said. 'You didn't have to come.'

'There's no way we would have missed it,' said Phil. 'We'll have to go now, though, I'm afraid. Lou's tired and I've promised I'll take Hannah out on her bike.'

We walked slowly back with them to their car before heading back to my mum's.

The support and encouragement of friends meant a great deal to me but Mike and I decided that renewing our wedding vows should be a private event with only Jack, Alice, my mum, Suzanne, Rebecca and Steven present at the weekday morning Mass.

Mike and I sat together quietly throughout the service until Father Pat called us out to the front and we stood to restate our vows.

I was first. I struggled with the line about in sickness and in health, my voice dropping away with the impact of the words. Then Mike's turn. My eyes were silvery with tears that held until Mike's voice broke, unable to continue. I nodded as Father Pat completed the words 'until death us do part'. We stood together tearfully, my hand on Mike's ring finger as I handed him a small silver band engraved with the words 'On and on and on', a symbol of my love for him. Mike's ring to me was plain with a small groove deeply furrowing the surface all the way round. Fingers entwined, we listened to the prayers and I stood thinking of the first time we uttered the words. We were filled with hope and happiness, anticipating a life together. A smooth ride, working as a team. We chose the same readings we'd listened to when we first made our vows. The first seemed so poignant now, so vital. Our time together had been a time of turmoil, good and bad, happiness and sorrow, a bittersweet togetherness. The reading: Paul to the Corinthians, 'Be ambitious for the higher gifts and I am going to show you a way that is better than any of them.' The reading continued: 'Love is always patient and kind, it is never jealous, it is never boastful or conceited, it is never rude or selfish, it does not take offence and it is not resentful. Love takes no pleasure in other people's sins but delights in the truth. It is always ready to excuse, to trust, to hope and to endure whatever comes.'

We sat and listened and I thought of all the love that had endured throughout our marriage. We had the one hymn we had chosen and Father Pat led the small congregation at the end of Mass, without any instruments, his voice ringing out clearly. As we came to the chorus, my voice broke and tears slid down my face.

> For you are always close to me,
> Following all my ways,
> May I be always close to you,
> Following all your ways Lord.

MIKE

The sun was relentless and queues snaked around the Piazza del Duomo. Jane passed a bottle of water to Steven, who gulped down half the bottle thirstily. Suzanne had left the poolside for the first time since arriving in Italy to come to enjoy the splendours of Florence. Rebecca was walking round with her little bag full of her life's essentials: water, Lipsil and purse.

I was surprised that Jane seemed to be handling the heat well. I'd noticed that, since she'd started running, her zest for life had flourished. Her renewed vigour and greater energy had given the whole family an extra impetus. However, her trainers had been conspicuous in their absence since the Race for Life. But to see her tanned, toned and happy was pleasing on the eye – especially now her hair had reached a respectable length.

On entering, we immediately headed to the dome steps, spurred on by Steven's enthusiasm. Each step to him was a huge rise but with nappy in hand he picked off the 463 steps at a pace, closely followed by Jane. When we got to the top, the view was spectacular. Steven and I looked down on to a marble pavement on the church floor, trying to follow its path.

The views over the city were exhilarating. Steven hung on to the iron railing, his feet scuffing the floor. 'Wow!' he said, thrilled. Jane and I looked at each other. Our holiday to Italy was our way of making it up to the kids for them not going to Australia. It wasn't the same experience, but the best we could do.

Oulton Park was on our left as we pulled in and made our way to the car park. Suzanne looked round to her brother.

'This is better than the flower show, isn't it, Steven?' she said. 'We can even listen to Jeff Buckley without Mum moaning.'

Steven was enthralled by the chequered flags at the entrance. As I turned off the engine we could hear the booms of the motorbikes rippling like thunder.

'Too noisy, Daddy!' said Steven. I'd forgotten how sensitive he was to loud sounds. This was going to be a long day. It was great to be able to spend some time with Suzanne. Family life meant that we rarely got time to spend together without Jane and Rebecca.

'When do you start school?'

Suzanne said, 'It's September, isn't it, Steven?'

'I was referring to you, not Steven.'

'It's not school, it's sixth form college.'

'Whatever. When do your O-level results come out?'

'GCSEs. Last week in August.'

'It doesn't matter if you don't pass, you know,' I said. 'We'll still love you. Failing never did me any harm.'

She shook her head. 'I don't want to talk about it.'

'You'll be fine.'

'When are Anne and Bill going to Australia?' she asked. I was unsure. In all likelihood, when they left the country Jane would not see her sister and family again. Anne had not been in touch with us and when the potential opportunities had arisen, they had been shunned. I wondered what I could do. I came to the conclusion that, as it wasn't my family, I was best to stay out of it. Even so, it was difficult to quantify the level of Jane's distress. I presumed it was easier for Anne not having to confront saying goodbye.

Walking up to work on what the radio had said was Yorkshire Day, I was feeling queasy. The results of Jane's scans the day before had been inconclusive. When she had been desperately ill, I hadn't been in fear of the scans at all, knowing that the situation was so dire that bad news couldn't have made the situation any worse.

But the run up to this second set of scans since chemotherapy had finished and the treatment started had been dreadful. We knew that if the disease became more active Jane would be taken off the trial. So these results at best would mean a continuation, at worst uncertainty and a shortening of Jane's life expectancy. But what was clear was that there were inflammatory cells from the breast to the abdomen. Her radiologist was convinced it was a tumour but Dr Perren thought it was caused by a silicon leak. I had the utmost confidence in Dr Perren's views but the uncertainty was driving me to distraction.

A dog jumped up at a flimsy garden fence; on its hind legs it was as tall as me. Startled, I jumped back. My brain reminded me that this happened every day. As I bollocked myself, the sudden lurch set off a chain reaction. I ran quickly to a ginnel, leant against a wall and retched. It hurt my throat as my stomach emptied.

'Concentrate, Mike. It's just stress, compose yourself,' I said. For the first time, we'd not told the children so it was vital I showed no weakness at home. 'Onwards, Mike. Deal with it.'

Three days later, sitting behind the goal at Burnley, I tried to focus on the game. John Bird turned to me.

'I never thought I'd see us losing at Burnley,' he said. It was only a pre-season friendly but Steven's first ever Chelsea game could not have got off to a worse start. Mick sat back in his chair, smug, making the most of our discomfort. Jane was enjoying every minute – not of the game – but of the constant ribbing Suzanne was dishing out to John.

'I never want to see another game sitting anywhere near her,' he said in all seriousness.

Three sharp drills of the whistle indicated half-time and Stephen Whiteside and I went down on to the concourse to go to the toilet.

'How's Jane bearing up?' asked Stephen. 'She looks okay.'

'It's dreadful,' I said. 'The kids don't know.'

'I figured as much, what are they going to do? You said in your e-mail something about a biopsy?'

I nodded. 'They'll have a look at some of the cells. I'm eighty per cent sure she's going to be fine. But it's shaken me up. I've got used to her being okay. Don't get me wrong, I know she's going to die. I just don't think this is the right time.'

'Is there anything we can do?'

'No, we're on our own. I know we've had nearly a year, but I want more. A lot more.'

Stephen looked at me.

'We'd better go,' I said to him. 'She'll think I've gone for a pint.'

Concentration in the second half was impossible and I was glad of the distraction of Steven, for whom the ninety minutes were dragging. Stephen asked if we'd all like to stop by as Karin would make tea, but we decided if we got to Settle for six we could get to Mass and therefore have a lazy Sunday morning. Jane's condition had taught us to appreciate those days where nothing much happens.

JANE

A year on from my diagnosis and the August Bank Holiday weekend loomed ahead. My thoughts returned to the Friday afternoon when our lives had changed and my future was taken from me. Almost twelve months on, I knew I should feel happy, relieved that the things that had seemed so important back then were now in reach. Suzanne was due to start sixth form, taking the courageous step to follow her career and not her friends. She'd opted to attend the language college to study French, German and Religious Studies. I admired her maturity and drive; stepping out on your own isn't easy at any age and I hoped she would make the transition smoothly.

Steven's first day at school approached. I'd taken him shopping for his uniform – small shorts, black blazer, blue shirt, grey jumper and grey socks. The socks had been difficult to find in his size and we'd hunted high and low throughout Leeds for some small enough for his tiny, narrow feet. I'd bought him a blue tie on elastic cord and smart black shoes with shiny polished toes. He'd bounced alongside me, full of questions, as we turned into a shop to look for some black pumps.

'I'll need my name on my pumps bag, won't I, Mummy?'

'Yes, Steven.'

'I need a purse for my bus fare, don't I, Mummy?'

'Yes, Steven.'

'How much is the bus fare, Mummy? Is it a ten pence and a twenty pence?'

'Yes, Steven.'

As fortunate as I was to be still around, I wasn't feeling particularly lucky. Death shadowed everything. All summer I'd hoped that I might be able to walk with Steven to his first day at school and all summer I'd dreaded the dream disappearing with a rapid decline in my health. Each morning as I rolled out of bed, the aches in my bones still made me stiff and sore. It would take a while for the pain to fade as I got on with the business of the day, which distracted me from the constancy of the pain.

The bright September morning arrived. Steven leapt out of bed when I called him, all excited and raring to go.

'Come on, sleepy head, it's time to get dressed, it's your big day.'

Rubbing one eye and peering up at me through the other he said: 'Is it school today?' and was then surprised by a yawn which made his eyes close and arms stretch out. I touched his tongue and his arms sprang back; he opened his eyes.

'Mum!' he snapped crossly.

'What? Did I spoil your yawn?' I said.

'Yes!' he said and he laughed. 'I need a wee!'

Returning to get dressed in his uniform he struggled with the last two buttons on his shirt, his tiny fingers unable to force them through the crisp, new fabric. I knelt down and finished buttoning them for up him.

'Keep still for just one minute,' I said. He stretched his neck up and lifted his chin high.

'But you're hurting me!' he said as he twisted away from me.

'I'm sorry, gorgeous boy,' I said, tapping his nose with my finger.

He looped the elasticated tie over his head, grimacing as it pinged over his ears and caught on his chin. It looked comical, stuck halfway down his face. He pulled it further and folded his collar over it. I helped him into his little grey jumper, watching as his blonde hair blossomed through the stretched grey neck. His arms stretching into wool, he stood in front of me, the V of his neck to one side. I pulled him towards me and straightened him up.

There was a knock at the door. Jane Beckwith had arrived to film my much dreamt of goal. The cameraman loomed large in our kitchen, as we bustled around the small room. Steven sat on his chair in the corner looking sleepy.

'Do you want some breakfast?' I asked. He shook his head.

'What about some milk and a yoghurt?' I said.

'Yoghurt!' he nodded and I passed him a pot. He dipped the teaspoon in, ignoring Jane's questions.

'Mum,' he asked. 'Can I take some fruit? We're not allowed biscuits.' I turned to look at the serious expression on his face.

'What about a banana?' I said. He nodded vigorously, his top lip covered in raspberry yoghurt. I placed a banana and an envelope of dinner money in his small backpack. Jumping down from the table, he found his shoes to put them on and wriggled his arms into his black blazer. He pulled it to one side, checking that

I'd sewn his school badge on in the right place. It was a rite of passage, the moment when my little boy became a 'big school' boy.

Mike, Rebecca, Steven and I set off down the street. Steven stepped out purposefully, holding my hand, his backpack on his shoulders. We walked into the school grounds and round the path to the playground. Steven's grip tightened on my hand as he looked round, frightened by the strange faces everywhere. He clung to me, scanning the playground for any of the bigger boys he knew. The bell rang and Mrs Reynolds stepped into the playground.

'Class One here, please!' she shouted loudly, gesturing with exaggerated movements as to where to congregate. Small boys squirmed from their mothers' embraces, I hugged Steven and he left me to join them. Standing at the front, the other children towered behind him, his year group mostly boys, the three girls bunched together.

'Right Steven, lead us in,' said Mrs Reynolds and Steven marched off towards his class. I waved at him and as he marched past he lifted his head, acknowledging me, raising his hand in a small gesture.

Mike turned to hug me as we made our way out of the playground. Rebecca held my hand and I looked at the other mums who were tearful at the goodbyes. It was a big day for Steven – and for me – I'd achieved something that meant so much to me. I wouldn't cry, though; Steven was at school, his small boy days were over, and I was there to witness it.

Jane Beckwith accompanied us back home. She wanted another interview before we finished off. She wanted to know how it felt for me to see Steven at school.

'I'm pleased,' I told her. 'Overjoyed, in fact, that I've been able to see him start school. It means I've met all the goals that I set a year ago and now I've got to find a way to move on.'

My health had stabilized. I was sick at night sometimes with bouts of acute pain now and then and the dull ache in my back, shoulder and ribs had become constant, sometimes bad, sometimes very bad.

Suzanne was at college, Steven was at school, Mike's work trundled on, Rebecca was settled. But there was still a huge cloud hanging over us. Every three months we had scans and results, then another three months of waiting. How long could this continue?

I lay in bed staring up at the darkness, pushing up the covers to block out the small slit of light showing through the chink in the curtains. My mind wanted rest but sleep eluded me. My shoulders and hands were cramped with lying awake, not moving so as not to disturb Mike. I woke again before it was light and my thoughts turned once more to the future. The constant physical reminders of my illness made it hard to be positive. The alarm shrilled and dressing for work I felt weary, my limbs ached. My eyes were dry, my head tight.

At work, X-raying children, it was an effort to cajole them into keeping still and I was glad when I was able to leave. I almost fell asleep on the bus home, jumping up out of my seat when I realized I was about to miss my stop. I dragged myself wearily home, kicked off my shoes, hung up my bag on the banister and crawled up the stairs to my bed. I longed for sleep; my whole body ached with tiredness and my legs felt heavy and tense under the cover. I shut my eyes and fell into a heavy sleep. Roused awake, the room was still lit by the late afternoon sun, My face felt numb, my mouth dry. I looked at the clock. I'd only been in bed a few minutes.

I placed a pillow behind my back to help ease the pain and closed my eyes but sleep had gone. I should get up, I thought, to read, garden, sew, anything positive but I felt too tired. My mind darted around, unfocused, slipping from one thought to the next, returning to one thought over and over: 'Why am I still here?' I'd done all I could, what good was it to still be here? My family had lived through this for a year, wouldn't it be best if I died now? The strain on us all was immense, I shouldn't still be alive. I felt a burden, stopping the people I loved from moving on with their lives while I was frozen in my dying. I couldn't bear the sadness, the illness, the pain, the lack of future. I was distraught at how much it was hurting my family.

I couldn't lie down any more but was too tired to sit up. I couldn't shake the sad thoughts from my head. I stared at the curtains, trying to chase the bleakness away. I threw back the covers and sat up. I found leggings, T-shirt and towelling socks, changed, and walked downstairs. I grabbed my trainers from by the door and bent to lace them. Hunting for my house keys in my coat pocket, I unlocked the door and stepped outside. If I couldn't sleep, maybe I could chase the bad thoughts out of my head.

I set off running alongside the park, past the vast old horse chestnut trees, their branches spreading across the path and split cases on the floor. The odd brown conker shone among the leaves on the ground. Running down the small hill, my calves hurt and my shoulder screamed with pain at each jolt. It was nearly ten minutes before I reached the end of the road. I stopped, brushing the beads of sweat from my forehead with the bottom of my T-shirt. Ten minutes seemed to have gone on for so long. I walked across the four lanes of traffic and set off up Leeds Road. The hill stretched out in front of me, lampposts punctuated the rise, and my pace slowed so that I was barely moving. I didn't want to stop, didn't want the hill to rule me. I concentrated on the grey poles in front of me, imagining a heavy rope stretching from my waist and attached to the next lamppost. In my mind, I hauled myself hand over hand towards the pole ahead and, reaching it, pictured the rope round the next lamppost. I steadily pulled myself along and ploughed on up the hill, ignoring the pain in my legs, back and shoulder and narrowing my vision to concentrate on just me, the hill, the footpath and the grey posts.

The top of the hill came into view and I forced myself forward to reach it. My breathing heavy and laboured, I recrossed the busy road and walked a couple of paces before setting off running again, past the graveyard and then up another small hill. My legs carried me on onwards. Then there was a long downhill stretch. My feet bounced away from the ground, I tipped my body forward and stretched out the length of my pace as I accelerated. The steepness stopped and the flat forced me into an upright run. I pushed down, not forwards, as I continued on for the next few yards. The park was in sight and I ran the last few yards up towards the vet's. Stopping at the war memorial I allowed myself to walk the short distance home. The restless feeling was still there and, as I stood by the door to stretch my calves, my neck and shoulder still ached. It seemed to have lessened, my mind distracted by the stiffness in my legs from the short run. I peeled off my damp kit, ran water into the tub and sat soaking my limbs in a deep bubble bath.

MIKE

Jane leant over and hit the big round button on the car radio, silencing the music.

'What you doing?' I said.

'I'm not listening to the Black Crowes.'

'Who are you all of a sudden? The music police?'

'I'm not listening to that first thing in the morning,' she said.

I put my foot on the pedal, tailgating the car in front. Although the clocks had gone back, the mornings were still miserably dark. I turned left and the acrid smell of the landfill site swamped the car. It was particularly pungent today. Carrier bags that had escaped from the site were snaggled on branches, tip debris – deflated footballs and cushions – littered the road.

'Will you get some bread and milk when you get Steven tonight?' she said. I gave an exaggerated sigh. 'Or I tell you what,' she continued. 'Why don't I get it? Let the cancer in my shoulder have an extra reason to be painful.'

'For God's sake, shut up, woman!' I said.

'No, I won't. You've been miserable like this for weeks. Everything's too much of an effort for you.'

'Oh, shut up.'

As we stopped at the traffic lights near her work, Jane jumped out without the ritual morning pleasantries. Hunched up like a little old lady, rucksack over her shoulder, she turned back firing a dirty look. I hit the button and 'Stop Kicking My Heart Around' continued.

Walking through the ground-floor garage at work, the stench from the sewers was worse than normal. Our basement was off to the left. The artificial light made it feel like a nuclear bunker, only not as plush. Keeping my head down, I grabbed my laptop from the cupboard, put my headphones on and ignored everyone. I didn't want a petty conversation or to answer any banal questions, I just wanted to be left alone. What did it matter? I was just killing time until Jane died.

I tapped my foot impatiently. How long was it taking to log on? When I finally did sign on, the number of e-mails in my inbox only added to my despair.

At eleven thirty, I grabbed my gym kit and headed off to the gym. After the first door out of the dungeon, Darren tapped me on my shoulder.

'You okay, Tommo?' he said.

'I'm fine, just a little flat,' I said. He didn't need or deserve the truth.

'Why don't you go home?'

'That's not the answer,' I said.

As I changed into my gear I realized I needed some new kit. A faded T-shirt and cropped shorts were not the ideal running gear for the November rain. Running past the hospital, down Kirkstall Road towards the abbey, I joined the canal. Suddenly, the wind was face on. The driving rain stung my legs. Runners coming from the opposite direction seemed almost to be floating past, making no effort. I came off the canal at Crown Point Bridge and was spent. I walked up past the Playhouse and back to work.

Jane had started training a little bit harder and had made a passing reference to doing the marathon. I was a little disappointed that I was so unfit. Only thirteen days to my first road race and visions of coming last haunted me. What had I got myself into? Bloody Jane.

*

Pulling into the drive that evening with Steven, I suddenly remembered Jane's instructions.

'Damn,' I said.

'What's up, Daddy?'

'We need to go to the shops.'

'Oh,' he said, sharing my lack of enthusiasm.

We returned from the supermarket and Steven ran up to the door and tapped on it noisily. There was no answer. He rapped more loudly as I came up behind him, arms laden with carrier bags. I could see Suzanne sitting in the living room watching television but she didn't move a muscle.

'Come on, Suzanne,' I said irritably. She wasn't going to move. I placed the bags down, fumbled for my keys and let us in. 'Thanks, Suzanne,' I called.

She came running to the door. 'Sorry, I couldn't hear you.'

'If you didn't have the bloody television on so loud you might be able to – anyway, have they stopped giving out homework for A-level students? Where's your mum?

'Upstairs,' she mumbled.

I put the bags on the kitchen worktop and discarded my fleece over the banister. I went upstairs and I heard the beats of the latest boy band emanating from Rebecca's bedroom.

'Turn that racket down,' I barked, opening the door to find her half-dressed. Yet another change of clothes. 'And draw the curtains if you're getting dressed.'

'It's not a racket,' she snapped and I slammed the door.

My frustration was unsettling me. I went into our bedroom where Jane was sitting on her heels, with the contents of her chest of drawers strewn all over the floor.

'What are you doing?' I said.

'Just sorting out some papers.' She didn't even look up.

'I can see that. What are you doing in particular?'

'There's loads of correspondence here, Mike,' she said. 'Some of it going back years. I'm going through it and chucking it away.'

'Why?'

'It needs to be done.'

I took my shoes off and shut the curtains. I'd been sweating most of the day since my run and was desperate to change my clothes.

'It's like you're preparing for death, Jane,' I said. 'Is there no end to this?'

'That's exactly what I'm doing. If I don't do it, it will be left to you when I'm gone.'

I ripped off my shirt and threw it towards the laundry basket.

'Oh, for fuck's sake, does it matter? Can't we just live for a day without the spectre of bloody death. It's all right for you. I'll be the one who's left on my own.'

Jane stood up, aghast. 'All right for me? All right for me?' she shrieked. 'Don't be so bloody condescending. I'm dying. Do you think I want to die?'

By now our row was full throttle. Steven opened the door.

'Mummy, can I have a gispit and a drink?' (Steven hadn't got the hang of pronouncing 'biscuit'.)

'Yes, I'll be down in a minute, Steven. Go downstairs.' She continued to look at me. 'Stop thinking about yourself, you selfish prick. You're not the one who's suffering.'

'Come on, Jane,' I said. 'Michelle and Jack will be here before long to go to the bonfire.' I had felt a pressure building for a while that I couldn't release.

At her mum's the following week, Jane had not settled all morning. The Race for Life had been different. This was a competitive five-mile road race and it was clear she was nervous. We set off walking half a mile to the start. I was shivering in my shorts and top; Jane had wrapped up a little better. The race numbers pinned to our vests, there was a small amount of nervous excitement in the air. The closer we got to the start, the more of our fellow competitors we saw. Some were even running up and down the road to warm up.

'What's that about?' Jane asked. 'Isn't five miles enough for them?' We were due to meet two of Jane's friends from work, who were also running. The air smelt of liniment oil. Looking around the hundreds of athletes I suddenly felt very unprepared.

Some of them had bodies like whippets, their muscles defined and taut. I looked down at myself, my gut slightly hanging over my Lycra shorts, and immediately felt out of place. Then I looked at Jane and felt slightly better.

At the start line, we stood watching the faster runners jockeying for position. Jane found Gill and Doranne and she stood chatting to them. She was obviously excited. Her arms gestured wildly, her speech was animated. Over the last few weeks, I'd noticed how important running had become to her. The marathon had been dropped into the conversation on several occasions. Would her body hold out? Fracture? Would she become paraplegic? Was it worth it?

The hooter sounded and the front of the group took off. After about thirty seconds we began to move, slowly, slowly, until finally we broke into a gentle jog. We descended the hill and the runners began to disperse but the pace was too slow for me. I looked at Jane making steady punchy movements, keeping pace with Gill.

'See you, Jane, I'm off,' I said.

At the finishing line, I walked through the funnel, collected some water and a T-shirt and was walking back to the final straight when I spotted Jane approaching the end. Her hat was in her gloved hand, her T-shirt was wet with sweat.

'Come on, Jane,' I yelled. 'Come on, you can do it!'

Her grimace turned into a smile. I looked at the clock on the leading car, forty-seven minutes.

'That was bloody fantastic,' I said, leaning over the barriers to try to get to her when she'd finished. She was too out of breath to answer. Gill and Doranne followed minutes later, with plenty more runners behind. What a confidence boost.

'That wasn't too bad,' she said, when she finally regained her breath. 'At least I wasn't last.'

JANE

'Jane, it's Karen . . .' I tried to recall who Karen was. '. . . from the BBC.' Now I remembered.

'Hello, how are you?' I said.

'Fine, how are you?'

'Not bad, my last scans were okay. I'm getting more pain but there was nothing to see in any of the tests, so life is just carrying on.'

'That's good. The schedulers have told us that the documentary will definitely be going out in December. We've had some good response from the media we've contacted. *You Magazine* want to interview you, if that's okay?'

I was surprised that I'd been chosen to be featured. There were other people who seemed to be getting on with their lives in a way I admired – Dionne, with her matter-of-fact approach to death, Jeff who was making the most of the time he had left to share with his wife and son.

'You don't have to do the interview,' said Karen. 'But if you decide to, I'll come along to make sure you're not on your own.'

'That should be okay,' I said. 'As long as they can fit in around work.' I was relieved that I had some kind of buffer between myself and the journalist. 'I'll get back to you with some dates.'

'They'll want some photographs as well,' she said. 'Are you sure you're up to it?'

'Yes, I'll be fine.'

Karen arrived early on the day; a make-up artist had already arrived and was tidying up my unruly eyebrows and hair. She offered to put some colour on Rebecca, who shook her head. There was a knock at the door.

Karen showed a dark-haired woman into the living room. I felt a little strange, the make-up was heavier than I would normally use but the colours were browns and pinks so at least I didn't look too false. I stepped through to the living room and the woman stood to greet me.

'Hi, I'm Catherine,' she said.

'Has anyone made you a drink?' I asked.

'No, I'm fine, honestly. Shall we get on with the interview then when Charlotte, the photographer, arrives we can stop for a while?' I nodded and she reached down into her bag to retrieve a small dictaphone. She placed it beside me.

'Is it okay if I use this?' she asked. 'I'll make notes but it's just for my reference for later.'

'Yes, that's fine,' I said as she started the tape recording and began her questions. She mentioned Ruth Picardie, the journalist who had died of breast cancer. I'd read her book and had admired the courage she'd shown and the stark way she had approached death. There were queries about my background, my childhood, my parents and then we talked through my initial diagnosis, the recurrence and when I was told my disease was incurable. As I talked about the experiences of twelve months before, I still felt the same sadness, the same horror of living without a future. I tried to answer her questions honestly. What it was like living with the knowledge that I might not be around six months from now. How planting up the garden for spring seemed like wishful thinking, but allowed me to focus on next year and kept some of the dread at bay.

She asked about Mike and how he was coping. I tried to explain how the nature of the illness separates you as a couple. Mike had to cope with my illness and watch me become unwell. He would be there to pick up the pieces when I was gone. I was struggling to stay well enough to see Steven at Christmas, spend another festive day with my children. I was unable to comfort Mike over his loss, neither could he make me better nor take away the pain. We could only continue our lives and enjoy the time we had left together.

The interview stopped when Charlotte arrived. She wanted some pictures of me with Steven and Rebecca. She brought an assistant who passed her films, which she loaded up into the back of her camera. A flash and then a Polaroid film was pulled out of the camera. The back ripped off, within a few minutes the picture was checked and everything was okay. She started clicking away. I smiled into the camera and played with Steven. Outside, she placed me under my garden arch, standing next to golden marigolds and dark cabbages. Finally satisfied with her shots, we went back inside and Charlotte started packing up her equipment. Catherine and I sat in the kitchen to finish off the interview.

I described the episode of septicaemia and tried to explain how it was possible to go on with life knowing that death was near.

'None of us know what is going to happen,' I said. 'We all feel slightly indestructible, that's how we get on with life.'

She asked if I had any plans for the next few months and I laughed and told her that's not what my life was about. Planning was dangerous, it meant that there were things you could miss out on. It was best to aim for small things – Halloween, Bonfire Night, Christmas perhaps?

Not being able to look ahead too far is hard. Jogging eased some of the distress of time running out. I started to run a little further on my outings, with the aim that I would compete in a ten kilometre race at the end of November. Only a little further than five miles but my thighs and my calves would scream in pain and tell me otherwise. The idea of running a marathon was a dream; I didn't think for one moment that I would be well enough to complete the distance, but it gave me a reason to carry on running. The vague hope that it might just be possible made me don my trainers and run on even the most foul of days. Mike didn't take me seriously until the end of October when I rang the Imperial Cancer Research Fund to enquire about a Golden Bond place for the London Marathon.

Mike's reaction was one of concern.

'Do you realize how far twenty-six miles is?' he said, his eyes searching mine to check if I was serious about this idea. When he saw I was, he laughed loudly. 'You couldn't run that distance if you weren't ill.'

Twenty-six miles was the distance from Leeds to Skipton, and the thought of running that far scared me, but if I didn't try for it, how would I ever know if it was possible? Mike's implication that I could never have run a marathon was like a red rag to a bull.

The form arrived and I worked my way down it, filling in the reasons why I deserved one of their coveted places. Having raised £3,500 already for completing the five-kilometre 'Race for Life' in May, I hoped that I might be able to raise £5,000 for a marathon. Mike tried to put me off, but I filled out the form, signed it and posted it off before I had second thoughts.

By mid-November I was running about fifteen miles a week and I looked up a schedule for my marathon training in a *Runner's World* magazine. The distances and training regime looked incredibly tough. I tried not to worry about running fifteen and eighteen miles, as I struggled round a four-mile loop near home, but focused on the next race, the Abbey Dash, ten kilometres from Leeds city centre to Kirkstall Abbey and back.

Mike was apprehensive as he waved me off at the start. All week, my calf had been cramping and I'd not been able to get any further than across the park and back.

The smell of deep heat and muscle rubs filled the air; the steam from everyone's breath rose above us. Lean, athletic men stood in doorways stretching their legs, easing them behind them on steps and stretching their calf muscles. Others held their foot behind them, stretching their hamstring. People jogged from the International Pool to warm up, sprinting then slowing. The road was massed with vested club runners. I stood at the back, out of the way of all the jostling. I set off slowly, trying to avoid being bumped.

A man in a black bin liner, arms held to the side, kept pace with me. The thudding of his feet was uneven as he fell more heavily on one foot than the other. The bin liner rustled and crinkled; he stayed on my shoulder, looming closely and breathing on the back of my head. I slowed and watched as he lurched forward beyond me. The distraction over, the pain in my calf stabbed, reminding me of the stiffness in my legs.

Nearly three miles into the race, people started clapping and cheering. The leading man loped out alone, other groups of runners further back tried to catch up with him. There was a huge cheer for the first woman. I had watched with envy at her easy running style, long strides quickening her passing as I ran slowly onwards.

At the halfway point, I knew I could finish and paced myself faster, making my steps shorter and quicker. I even began to pass people, which lifted me on the long straight back to Leeds. Ignoring the cramps and spasm in my legs until they refused to take me any further, I stepped to one side to stretch out, watching the runners I had just passed run by, and then set off again. I kept the same few words going round in my head and kept stride for stride with them: 'Come on, Jane, you can do it. Come on, Jane, you can do it.'

With this mantra, the road disappeared behind me and I came to the bottom of the small hill towards the finish. At the sidelines I could see my friend Gill calling out to me: 'Come on Jane, good run!' It was what I needed to spur me on for the last few minutes.

I crossed the line in just under one hour.

I was pleased with my finishing time; it gave me confidence to continue my training. When my legs were sore, I swam, if my shoulder ached, I cycled at the gym. Gradually, I was able to increase my distances and my speed.

'Can I speak to Jane Tomlinson?' said a voice on the phone.

'Speaking,' I said.

'Oh great. Hi, Jane, it's Helen from the Imperial Cancer Research Fund here. I just wanted to let you know that you've got a marathon place.' The enthusiasm in her voice bounced down the phone. 'How's the training going?' she asked.

'Slowly. But I'm getting further and further each week. I ran my first *10k* last week in under an hour.'

'That's fantastic,' came her bubbly reply. 'I'm running the marathon as well. I've just been too busy to get out training for the last fortnight.' We swapped running tips before finally she said goodbye.

'There'll be a pack in the post for you,' she said. 'Good luck with the training.'

'And you!'

I phoned Mike, elated to have got a place, but then the reality kicked in.

'Oh my God, what have I done?' I said.

'There's no going back now,' said Mike. I felt despair and

euphoria, glee at success in gaining a place, horror at the notion of running twenty-six miles with only one *10k* race under my belt. I had a lot of mileage to cover over the next four months.

'I still can't believe you're going to run a marathon,' said Mike.

'Why not?'

'It's ridiculous,' he said. 'You might hurt yourself, fracture a leg or your back.'

'I know,' I said, 'but that could happen anyway.' I'd been living with extensive bone disease and knew of the risk of fractures through weakened bones. The running might put too much pressure on the cancerous areas, causing my bones to break, my spine to collapse.

'Well,' said Mike that evening when he returned from work, 'if you're going to go for it you might as well apply for this.' He waved a white leaflet topped with the picture of a monkey in front of me. It was the entry form for the York Half Marathon at the end of January. A cold, windy, flat run. The winter run gives it its name – the Brass Monkey.

'You've got eight weeks to train for it,' said Mike. 'If you can finish that then you might just be able to finish the marathon.' I nodded enthusiastically, taking the form. There was one for me, one for Mike. We would run together so he could make sure I got round safely.

'Oh Jane, what have you done?' he said raising his eyebrows at me.

MIKE

We came out of the tube and turned left to the hotel. Jane wasn't looking too well. Our late arrival due to work commitments had left us both feeling weary and dejected. Although it was only six days before Christmas, you'd never have guessed it from the cheerlessness of Shepherd's Bush.

We were in London to promote the *Everyman* programme. With Jane's back and shoulder being so sore, I'd questioned whether it was a good idea, but because she had agreed some weeks previously, she wouldn't go back on her word. Although it wasn't particularly cold outside, it was the kind of damp that permeated every pore of your body.

As the car was supposed to be picking us up at seven-fifteen the next morning, we agreed to go to the studio for the interview and have breakfast when we returned. At six-thirty, Jane was having a shower. Hearing the water turned off, I rolled over to avoid her gaze. It didn't work.

'Aren't you getting up?' she said.

'There's plenty of time,' I said sleepily. Her voice sounded tense and agitated. I heard her opening the wardrobe and getting dressed.

'Do I look all right?' she said after a few minutes.

'Perfect.'

'You've not even looked,' she said moving to my side of the bed. 'Come on.'

I rolled over and within seconds was up and getting dressed into a shirt and black trousers. Jane was peering into the mirror at her face.

'You won't need any make-up,' I said. 'They'll do it for you there.'

'I'm not turning up there looking like death.'

I knew I wasn't required for the TV interview but Jane had wanted me there. I was quite looking forward to it, a new experience and one which was unlikely to be repeated.

The car turned up promptly at 7.15 a.m. and drove us for the surprisingly short distance to Broadcasting House, where we were dropped off outside the main reception. Within seconds we were escorted to the greenroom which appeared not to have been decorated in living memory. There was an eclectic array of guests. Pam St Clement who plays Pat in *Eastenders* said hello to me. She was the only one. Professor Richard Wiseman was in to talk about the world's funniest joke as voted for on the internet. It was instantly forgettable but apparently popular in Germany. The Conservative MP Julie Kirkbride, who asked in the House of Commons whether Tony Blair's son had had the

MMR jab, was giving her toddler a drink. Jane was whisked off to make-up. A black coffee was slapped down in front of me and soon the joke-collecting professor and the MP were shunted out of the greenroom and taken to the studio. Pam disappeared outside and I was left alone with Julie's young child. I sat anonymously in the corner observing the comings and goings.

Things started to get frantic because Eddie Izzard was a guest, and by all accounts was running late. A trailer appeared about Jane so afterwards, as soon as some BBC staff returned, I got up and walked out. I couldn't be doing with people sympathizing with me when they saw what the interview was about.

I heard Jane's voice coming over the TV screen. I went to a closed café area near by. I waited a respectable few minutes before returning to the greenroom, where I noticed Eddie being fussed over by several luvvies. Jane was just getting back from the studio.

'What did you think? Was I all right?'

'Dunno,' I said. 'I didn't watch it.'

'Why not?'

'Just didn't fancy it. Especially not in there.'

By 9 a.m. we were back in the hotel. The whole experience had been hollow. I'd noticed there had been a definite pecking order as to who was looked after. Because Jane was unwell, it had been arranged that we would stay overnight in London and travel back the next day. So the day stretched out before us. Although Jane was tired she suggested we go to a new multiplex cinema which had just opened near the hotel. The first part of the *Lord of the Rings* trilogy, *The Fellowship of the Ring*, had just opened. Our tastes didn't coincide. I'd not enjoyed the book; I'd only got to about page 140 and after three attempts had given up. Jane, meanwhile, had loved it. There was little else on and I thought seeing the film might make the book more accessible to me.

As we left the cinema she looked wistful. She'd really got into the film, I'd used most of the three hours to catch up with my lack of sleep.

'What's up, love?' I asked.

'I won't get to see the second or third part,' she said.

'You don't know that,' I said. I couldn't cope right then with one of those introspective conversations where we zoomed in on the darker side of death. We held hands and tootled off to catch the tube to central London. Drifting down Oxford Street the pavements were packed so we decided to seek sanctuary in a coffee shop.

'Go get the *Guardian*, will you, Mike?' she said. 'We can do the crossword.'

There was no better way of idling away the hour. When I returned, I handed the paper to Jane, which she now guarded jealously, I didn't get a sniff until she was desperate for clues.

'Here you go,' she said, handing the paper to me, four clues left, all beyond me. I was about to put it in my bag when I noticed something.

'Jane, look here!' I said, handing back the paper
'What?'

'It's you and Rebecca,' I said. It was a beautiful picture taken for the *You Magazine* feature with a preview of the programme that was showing that evening. Jane read it out aloud.

'"A Modern Way of Dying" – what a crap title,' I said. I went to check the other papers. There she was again, in the *Independent*, the *Express*, *The Scotsman*. In the *Financial Times* it read: 'saddest of all is the story of Jane, a 37-year-old mother who is desperate to live long enough to hold her 4-year-old son Steven's hand on his first day at school'.

Reading about Jane's death unexpectedly made me feel depressed and I wanted to be far away from the Christmas lights on Oxford Street. Jane was seriously flagging; the constant dodging, weaving and bumping of London had made her extremely sore. We grabbed a pizza and a beer and were glad to get back to the hotel.

Arriving home on the Friday night, the house looked amazing; warm, clean, tidy with all the Christmas cards on display. Mum had done a terrific job. As we walked into the living room, Mum stood up.

'You were brilliant, Jane,' she said. 'We all cried last night, it was lovely.'

'Aye, it was, Alice,' said my dad. 'Rebecca didn't half sob.'

My mum turned to me. 'What did you think, Michael?'

'I didn't watch it, Mum,' I said.

'Why ever not?'

'It's bad enough living it, Mum. I don't need to be reminded.'

CHAPTER 11

JANE

I stood on the kneeler on tiptoe, to give myself some extra inches of height, and strained to see the children gathered at the front of the church. Due to refurbishments at Steven's school, there had been no nativity play for Class One parents to attend. Instead, the children were invited to be part of a tableau at the children's Mass on Christmas Eve. Steven was a shepherd, in a class of twenty-five boys and only three girls – there were a lot of shepherds.

I glimpsed his tea-towelled head and pushed myself higher to catch a better view. His eyes were searching the church and opened wider as he caught sight of me. I smiled at him and he raised his hand to his waist and gave me the smallest of waves, smiling back at me. He turned his attention back to the group surrounding the small crib, but I carried on watching him.

After the Mass, he joined his dad at the altar, each lighting a candle and kneeling to pray, then bounded down the aisle to join me in the pew. I stood to walk from the church, following the rest of the congregation, saying hello to friends. It was bitterly cold and as we walked home Steven swung on my arm excitedly.

'Look at the road, Steven,' I pointed.' It's all sparkly.'

'That's because it's Christmas,' he replied. We pulled coats, gloves and hats off and I chased Steven upstairs, helping him into his pyjamas.

'Downstairs, now,' I said. 'It's time to put the pillowcases out.'

We all placed our pillowcases around the edges of the room for Father Christmas, each one of us with a different patterned sack to be filled with presents.

'How will Father Christmas get in?' asked Steven. 'We haven't got a chimney.'

'Father Christmas has got a magic sparkly key to open the door,' Rebecca said.

'Really!' said Steven, eyes opened wide, his face pink with excitement.

'Come on, drink your milk,' I said.

'What about Father Christmas?' asked Steven. 'He might be hungry.'

Suzanne fetched a mince pie, a carrot and a small can of beer and Steven placed them on the stool by the large tree hung with lights.

'Come on, bedtime,' I said.

'Aren't you forgetting something?' asked Suzanne. I looked at her, puzzled, unable to think what she meant. 'You need to read us "The Night Before Christmas". Christmas isn't the same if you don't.'

'I don't know where it is,' I said.

'I do,' said Rebecca and raced from the room. She rushed back with the picture-book version of Clement Moore's classic Christmas poem. I opened it and read the inscription in the front.

'"Love to Suzanne from Grandpa, Grandma, Sara and everyone."' It was dated 1987. Mike sat on the settee and the three children sat around me as I turned to the first page and read:

'Twas the night before Christmas, when all through the house
Not a creature was stirring, not even a mouse . . .

'Now, Dasher! Now, Dancer! Now Prancer and Vixen!
On, Comet! On, Cupid! On, Donner and Blitzen!' . . .

'Happy Christmas to all,
And to all a good night!'

I closed the book and looked at the faces turned towards me, all
glowing, lit by the bright lights on the tree.

'Come on, bed time.'

The spell broken, the children moved. I stood and opened the
door and followed Steven up the stairs.

'Have I been a good boy, Mummy?' asked Steven.

'You're the best little boy in the world,' I replied, and bent to
kiss him.

'When will Father Christmas come?'

'When you're asleep.'

'What if I can't sleep?'

'You'll sleep,' I said and I smiled at him as I tucked the covers
around him.

The week before the Brass Monkey Run at the end of January
was busy. On the Tuesday afternoon I had another appointment at the hospital, the hours passing by as we sat waiting for
results once again. I knew from the increasing pain I was in that
I was not going to be hearing good news. The only question was
how bad the news would be.

As my name was called, Mike and I followed the doctor into
the consulting room. My hastily gathered coat was trailing on
the floor in our rush. It was Dr Jeffers – we'd not met him
before. He smiled and read through my notes before finally
swivelling back to us.

'I'm sorry to tell you that the last scans show a new area of disease in your back,' he said. 'There's also an area of increased
activity in your shoulder.' I nodded in agreement, knowing myself
that my shoulder was becoming problematic. 'The radiologists
have reported this as progressive disease,' he continued. 'So I'm
afraid this means you're no longer eligible for the Theratope trial.

Only women with stable disease are eligible for the injections.'

I breathed deeply, opening my mouth to ask, 'What next', but Mike broke into the silence.

'Is there any other treatment you can offer Jane?' he asked. Dr Jeffers looked down at my notes, checking what treatment I'd been prescribed in the past.

'There are several options available but you have to understand that it's like looking in a medicine cabinet. We've only got so many drugs to offer you and once you've removed another from the shelf to take it, that's one more gone, until we reach the end.'

We sat silently, taking in the information.

'The good news is that the scans of your lungs and liver show no new areas of disease,' he said, tapping the sheet in front of him. 'There are treatments such as Herceptin, which we can offer, plus other chemotherapies. But as you've no disease in your viscera . . .'

He noticed Mike's quizzical look.

'Sorry, viscera, that means your internal organs. As there's no disease there we have the luxury of time.'

'The luxury of time.' The expression jarred in my mind. We were sitting discussing how I might keep my disease at bay and the doctor was talking about the luxury of time. There was nothing luxurious about my time. My face must have given away my thoughts because he hurriedly continued and ran through some chemotherapy options.

'I think we should start by changing your hormone therapy,' he said. 'And if that doesn't help we can start you on Herceptin. Then we can always add Vinorelbine later, which is tolerated quite well by most women.'

I held my printed prescription in my hand and passed my appointment sheet to the clerk. One of the nurses stopped us as we were leaving the department.

'Jane? Are you okay?' It was Anne, the research nurse who usually gave me my treatment. 'I heard you were out of remission?' I nodded and sighed. 'Nothing I wasn't expecting,' I said. 'I'm fine, I just need to get my head around it.'

Anne looked past me towards Mike for confirmation.

'Listen,' she said, 'I'll ring you tomorrow. If there's anything you need to know you can ask then.'

'Thanks,' I said and Mike and I left, walking past the painting of an autumnal tree that had become so familiar after our many visits.

I had little time to worry. My portfolio for my postgraduate study needed final labelling and the index needed checking. A couple of days later, Mike drove me to Sheffield to meet with Christine Ferris, my tutor. I handed in my folder, thick and heavy with a year's work of papers, and waited for my receipt from the office staff, then walked down the college campus towards Christine's room. She cleared books from the chair and shifted folders.

'I can't believe I've managed to finish all the work,' I said as she sat down next to us. 'Thanks for the encouragement. It's means a lot to me that I've been able to complete my studies. I couldn't have done it without your help.'

'That's what I'm here for.' She smiled as I handed her a bouquet of flowers and a card. Fifteen months earlier, Christine had persuaded me not to give up the course but to defer my studies. I never dreamt that I'd finish the course. It was a big milestone and a huge effort to push myself professionally while being so ill.

Christine could talk for England but glancing up at the clock we realized we needed to dash. Standing, she walked us to the door of her minute office and we hugged.

'See you at the graduation ceremony,' she said.

'I haven't passed yet,' I said.

I woke early on the day of the York Half Marathon. As we drove to the racecourse, I noticed white frost patches on the pavements. The parking area was boggy and the long grass dampened our trainers. Some runners were jogging gently and others were stretching out. I scanned the area and found Mike was standing with our friend Delia, who was jumping up and down on the spot to keep herself warm, laughing nervously at the morning ahead. We were all half-marathon virgins with no great hopes of a good time; we just wanted to finish in under two and a half hours.

The horn sounded. We trod carefully, afraid of tripping over people's feet on the rough track until we got on to the road and we could start running in earnest.

Mike, Delia and I began to relax into the race and as we did so I found myself pulling away from them. My shoes started to rub, I tried to distract myself – there were miles and miles of road ahead with figures moving steadily into the distance. My ankle began to chafe where the tongue of the trainer had slipped and it was already beginning to feel sore and uncomfortable.

I stopped to relace my shoes and Mike and Delia overtook me. I started running again and tried to catch up, only to find that when I reached them, my legs were too tired to keep pace with them for long. The icy patches on the road had mostly turned into slush thanks to the many feet before us, but there were still times when I had to concentrate on the small pockets of frost that the sun hadn't yet melted.

Passing each mile marker, I checked my watch and saw that we were managing a little over ten minutes per mile. At mile six, I started hoping the drinks station would appear soon. Finally, I arrived at the trestle table laden with paper cups. I lifted two and began to walk so I could drink.

'Come on, Jane,' shouted Mike from up ahead. 'Don't walk, you'll stiffen up.' I threw my cups to the side of the road, already littered from other passing runners, and began to run again. My hip was hurting, the small of my back was a pinpoint of pain. As I passed mile eleven, I knew I could finish. Mike slowed up ahead and I was able to catch him. He urged me up the hill. As we ran, I found myself overtaking straggling runners. Struggling with the small incline as we returned on to the familiar roads we'd run on earlier that morning, I pushed myself harder, ignoring the rub in my ankle, the pain in my hip. My left knee was screaming at me. Delia and I sped on, breathless, unable to talk. I smiled as I heard her swearing at Mike as we tried to stay with him. Finally, we could see the clock tower of the racecourse ahead of us. Ignoring the pain, breathing open-mouthed, my chest heavy, we gained more ground on the other runners, pulling them in, pushing ourselves on.

We made it to the racecourse, forced ourselves past the car park and on towards the finishing line, our legs and lungs screaming. I glanced at the clock. We'd finished in just under two and a quarter hours. Delia turned to Mike.

'Bloody hell, that hurt, you bastard,' she panted.

MIKE

Jane's confidence was boosted considerably by her finishing the York Brass Monkeys Half Marathon. While her time of two hours fifteen minutes was respectable, there were only eleven weeks to go before the London Marathon and she needed to do a lot of work to increase her stamina. The length of runs and the intensity of training required were daunting.

For a while we'd talked about joining the local running group, the Rothwell Harriers, then, when we'd sobered up, decided against it. We'd seen runners from the club in their vests at the Roundhay Five, Abbey Dash and York. Training for the marathon would be a boring, lonely experience, especially on the longer runs, and there was no doubt Jane would benefit from having some company. The Harriers' pace would push Jane to a speed outside her comfort zone, escalating her training, and would force her out on those nights when she just wanted to curl up on the settee.

After vacillating for several weeks, we decided to attend the club one night during February half term when the kids were in Settle. Parking the car, we could see all manner of shapes and sizes making their way to the sports centre entrance.

Lycra running trousers, yellow fluorescent jackets and well-used running shoes seemed to be in fashion. Looking down at my crappy trainers, baggy shorts and faded concert T-shirt, I thought at least they won't be expecting much from me. All the runners looked lean athletes and I wondered whether they had a session for fuller figures like myself. Within seconds Jane was in conversation with the secretary.

As the time reached seven, there were a few quick words and then we were off. I moved close to Jane. 'Are you okay?'

'Yes.'

I dropped off to one of the bunches at the back, where a gentleman called Malcolm introduced himself. He must have sensed my discomfort. 'Don't worry, Mike, they won't go any faster that this.'

'I'm not very good, I'm afraid.'

'We all have to start somewhere.'

'Oh, I've been running for years. I'm just rubbish.'

There was a sense of well being and safety in being surrounded by up to thirty runners, something I'd never experienced before. Several came up to say hello but by mile three I was in no position to reciprocate. Jane, on the other hand, looked comfortable, chatting away to a woman at her side, clearly enjoying the run. Her fitness had improved even in the three weeks since York.

We ran the first five miles as a group then, for the last mile, everyone ran at their own pace. No one ran at mine.

Arriving back at the sports centre, I was the last to return together with Paul the secretary, because someone stays with the last runner. My calves were pounding, knees creaking, saliva dribbling from the sides of my mouth as I gasped for breath.

As we got in the car Jane asked: 'What did you think?'

'Friendly people,' I said. 'It wasn't like I thought it would be.'

'It's just what I need,' she said. 'They force me to run faster. Just before the marathon they do longer runs. I'd welcome the company.'

Jane and I looked forward to the school holidays, which gave us a period of welcome respite from the day-to-day responsibilities of parenthood. This year, however, only Rebecca and Steven were up with my parents in Settle. Suzanne was working as a cashier at the bank. Although she didn't need looking after, it meant the house was not our own.

On Friday, Jane went down to London with Jackie while I went to pick the kids up from Settle. I also went to buy Jane a birthday present, a unique experience, having never booked a holiday by myself before. I was unsure as to what Jane's reaction would be, after all, we'd already been to Australia and were due to go to Lanzarote by ourselves, so would a weekend in Paris together be too much of an indulgence?

Once the marathon was over, it would leave a huge gap in Jane's life which we'd struggle to fill. She always enjoyed having small goals to achieve and if I booked the trip to Paris just afterwards, it would help cushion the blow.

There was a balance between allowing Jane and me to spend some precious time together and being away from the kids. Jane and I knew we wouldn't have a long marriage and wanted to discover things about each other that we wouldn't be able to do later in life. That sense of spending individual time with her also extended to the three children. It was important to us that Suzanne, Rebecca and Steven had unique memories of their mum, away from those shared with the others.

But just as important to Jane was to retain as much independence and freedom as possible. Although family time was precious, Jane still had a life outside it. Since we'd been married – as a result of financial constraints, family and me – she had not enjoyed anywhere near the freedom she would have wished. Now that time was limited, we had to go some way to redressing the balance, even if time was short.

For some months, we'd contemplated having some kind of party. Jane would be forty in 2004 but the likelihood of her reaching that age seemed remote and the previous year it had been out of the question, she had only just finished chemotherapy. We discussed it with the children. They thought it was a wonderful idea. Others weren't so sure.

'Alice, why do they want to waste their money on a party?' asked Dad.

'It'll be great,' said my mum. 'Are you inviting your cousins?'

Jane's mum said: 'So what's it all about then, Jane?'

'It's a a chance to say thank you to all the people who've helped over the last year,' said Jane.

'Oh, I thought you'd get us there to ask us to sponsor you.'

'No, we just hope everyone enjoys themselves.'

As usual, we left the arrangements until the last minute. I'd managed to book Dave Sounds, the DJ from our local pub – along with his humorous taste in shirts – but as the day approached I was a little alarmed by the number of responses we'd had. Although I'd booked the clubhouse of a local golf club, which held 200, I'd reckoned at the time that about 30 per cent of people would decline. In fact, only eight people couldn't attend which meant 250 guests were due to arrive.

I was worried it might be an anti-climax. Mum and Dad had arrived early to check into a hotel. It was unusual for them not to be staying with us but we'd felt certain Dad would find it difficult to cope with the revolving door of people at our house.

We didn't have access to the room until late, preparing it was somewhat rushed, and together with my cack-handed approach it meant everyone was running around. With just a handful of us putting up banners, balloons and trimmings it looked like we'd booked too big a venue. Rebecca and Suzanne stood on chairs at either side of concertinaed double doors, placing a long banner across. Some of my aunts and uncles laboured over filling balloons. Dave Sounds was setting up in the corner and Steven was being introduced to relatives he didn't know he had.

Planning a birthday party in February was risky but luckily the snow, ice and fog stayed away. We'd decided there would be no speeches, no formalities. Many times in life it's better to say nothing and we were aware everyone knew the significance of the party.

By seven o'clock, the room was dressed and I sat with my mother's brothers and sisters at a table in a room away off the main dance floor/bar area discussing the missing decades. There was a sense, and not just because of Jane, it would be the last celebration we would attend all together.

The whole atmosphere began to develop as more and more people arrived, staking claims on chairs and tables around the room. Within an hour the room was full of friends re-establishing old relationships. Jane flitted from person to person, delighted to be seeing so many friends.

My nephew Jack ploughed around the dance floor, shirtless, entertaining everyone with his dance moves. Like the Pied Piper, others joined him, including a normally reserved Steven. The two cousins gyrated in front of the DJ's speakers. Two huge, and very cheap, cakes were brought in. Jane said thank you. An hour later, her work colleagues had her on a chair in the middle of the dance floor while they sang 'Simply the Best.' We'd tried desperately not to make it a sentimental evening. Jane's death was never far from our thoughts, but now the tears flowed.

JANE

I met up with other runners from the Rothwell Harriers most Wednesday evenings to join in the club runs. One night, after we had already covered about four miles, I decided to tag on to the dedicated group of runners who were all training for the marathon. I needed the extra miles. We set off towards Leeds Road, and I was soon straggling behind. A more experienced runner called Steve stayed with me as I pushed my body hard to force myself the extra three miles.

I found a second wind and eased myself faster, managing to close the gap with the small number of runners ahead. Panting as Rothwell Sports Centre came into view, I raised my face to feel the cold rain lash against it.

'Well done, Jane. That was a good run.'

'Thanks for that,' I said and turned to Pete, another Rothwell Harrier. 'How many miles was that tonight?'

'About nine,' he said. 'You were running well there at the end. You must have been running at eight-minute mile pace.'

'Really?' I dug out my keys and I headed for the car. 'See you next week.'

Driving homewards I smiled, pleased with my progress. When I had joined the Harriers I had struggled to run a mile in under ten minutes.

'You look cold,' Mike said as I pulled my sodden trainers off. 'So how many miles have you done this week, then?'

I counted up the runs from the previous seven days. 'Must be about thirty-five this week,' I said and headed up the stairs for a long, relaxing bath.

MIKE

When Jane told me she was definitely going to run the marathon, I'd said I could raise £5,000. With the marathon less than a month away that boast seemed rash.

We'd already promised to raise at least £1,500 for Imperial Cancer Research as part of the deal for obtaining a Golden Bond place. In among the literature they'd sent were guidelines as to how to maximize the fundraising. Getting the wealthiest person to sponsor you first was one suggestion, the thinking being that it would set a figure that others would feel obliged to match. But that wasn't how I wanted to approach the fundraising. I felt that if people wanted to contribute, it needed to come from a desire to help rather than an obligation.

Having lived with Jane's diagnosis for so many years – especially over the last eighteen months – I wouldn't have wished it on my worst enemy. If I could raise money to help prevent other families and other women suffering what we'd been through, then all the better. I just wanted to raise as much money as I could but I wanted the donations to be by altruistic gestures.

We realized that what Jane was about to do was unique and there would be some parts of the media that would be interested in her story. On reflection, we decided not to let anyone know. Jane didn't want to see herself in the papers or on television. Although the experience of *Everyman* had been okay, she had no desire to repeat it.

Sitting at work I contemplated whether an exception could be made for the local press. On the basis that regional papers often ran stories of local people pounding the capital's streets during the marathon, I thought of sending an e-mail. Unsure how Jane would react, I didn't. An hour later, in a rare quiet second, I momentarily took leave of my senses. I bashed out a note, hitting the send button before I'd really thought about the consequences. I immediately felt embarrassed. I picked up my gym kit and went downstairs for a run, cringing at the thought of the news desk opening up my e-mail. They'd all have a laugh and then delete it straightaway.

Returning to my desk, the beads of sweat were running down into my eyes making them sting. Jane's training efforts had proved to be a catalyst for me to make a bigger effort. I unlocked the laptop. I had new mail. I was surprised to see one so quickly from Eric Roberts at the *Yorkshire Post* saying that he'd written the *Everyman* review and he'd be delighted to do a follow-up. Now I had a problem.

For the second time that day I acted rashly and phoned Jane to check if she'd meet up with him. With some persuasion – 'I need to raise fifteen hundred pounds somehow' and 'your efforts deserve a decent fund' – she agreed.

Walking into The Cube, a stylish minimalist bar in Leeds, my furtive glances around the room must have attracted Eric's attention. He came over.

I explained Jane would be along in a minute. No sooner had I spoken than I noticed the familiar rucksacked figure hobbling over Millennium Square towards us.

'I'd like to write a small piece to tie in with the marathon, if that's okay?' he said.

'It should be fine,' I said. 'But is there any chance you could print it at least a week before the race so it will help our fundraising?'

'Shouldn't be a problem. Have you mentioned this to any other paper?'

'No, we weren't going to.'

'That's great, if we could leave it like that?'

'Sure.' I doubted anyone else would be interested.

'You'll be on with Harry and Christa on the day of publication,' he said.

I looked at him quizzically. 'Who are Harry and Christa?'

'Harry Gration? Christa Ackroyd? BBC1, *Look North*.'

I recognized Harry's name from his commentaries on BBC Sport but had never heard of Christa.

'We don't watch the local news,' I explained.

He asked if a photographer could come out to take some pictures and then, with an assurance that he'd let us know when it came out, we said goodbye. Frantic phone calls were made to Cancer Research UK, who had changed their name from Imperial Cancer Research Fund, to get a logoed T-shirt for the photo; it arrived at the last minute.

Two weeks later, an e-mail arrived from Eric telling us that the article would be published the following day. It came as something of a shock. Easter, Steven's first school concert, not to mention more hospital appointments, had distracted us and we'd assumed the article would have been 'spiked' for another, more interesting story.

I dropped Suzanne off in town at work. Jane had gone to the gym for a quick session. With only ten days to go, her training was tapering. I called at the newspaper kiosk and was stunned to see Jane as a banner headline on the regional broadsheet. 'Miles and miles of courage – why this Yorkshire mother dying of cancer is running the London Marathon, Page 13.' I opened it up to see a huge picture of Jane running.

'Oh shit,' I hadn't been expecting that.

As I walked into the office, my colleague Andy shouted across the office.

'Mike, we've had an e-mail from a recruitment agency, they want a sponsorship form.' We'd only set the e-mail account up yesterday afternoon and never anticipated it would be used so quickly. I put the paper inside my drawer thinking I'd read it later.

About forty minutes on, I answered my phone.

'I'm Danni from *Look North*, is Mike Tomlinson there please?'

'Yes, speaking.'

'I'm trying to get a number for Jane Tomlinson. Do you know where I can contact her?'

'Er, what's it for?'

'We wondered if she'd like to come to the studio this evening to talk to Harry and Christa about the marathon?'

'Er, I'm not sure, can I get back to you?'

I rang home and left a message, then rang Oulton Hall to see if I could get someone at the gym to contact Jane. Oh Lord, what had I started? No one at the gym could find her, but an hour later Jane called.

'Mike, there are some journalists parked down the road. What shall I do? I'm scared.' She sounded as though she'd been crying. 'I spoke to the man from the *Sun* through the letterbox.' A vision came to mind which led to an involuntary smile. 'He's saying they'd like some photos. I've tried to reason with him but it's no use. They are going to run a story whether we like it or not. The BBC are going to be here in five minutes and I've had a women's magazine parked outside and a freelance journalist ringing me as well. Please can you come home?'

'Why are the BBC coming?'

'To do some filming. Listen, I need you here.'

'Okay, okay, I'm on my way.' I arrived home just in time to see a large blue BBC van pull out of the estate. As I walked into the house, I noticed Jane was still wearing her running kit. We hugged.

'Are you okay?' I asked.

'Yeah, I'm fine.' She sounded a little shaky.

'What happened?'

'I spoke to Alasdair, the *Sun* journalist,' she said. 'He was nice enough but a bit insistent. There was nothing I could say to put him off.'

Later that afternoon I rang Danni at the BBC to find out what we needed to do that evening. She asked us to wear something sober as the presenters were wearing black out of respect for the Queen Mum who had died only five days previously. I phoned the freelance journalist and the women's magazine and kindly declined their offers. Ground down by their persistence, I agreed that they could call back when everything was a little calmer.

I sat on the stairs, contemplating what to do. Instinctively I picked up the phone in an attempt to appeal to the *Sun* journalist's better nature. The futility of our position became clear when he advised that there was nothing we could do about it. They were going to run the story whatever our thoughts.

After a long walk, we had decided there was no alternative but to cooperate. If they were going to print the story, at least I could ask that the charity details were included. I phoned Alasdair again and asked for the piece not to be too sensational. When everyone else had forgotten it, there would still be our kids' memories. Losing their mum was bad enough to deal with. He explained that he would do his best and provided there wasn't a major news story in the next couple of hours it would be in tomorrow.

Jane had insisted I went on to *Look North* with her that evening; her retribution, I thought. In any case, it would make a good comparison: a dying woman who looks great, sitting next to a healthy man in need of a diet. The interview went well. I tried to be funny. I wasn't. Jane had stumbled over a few words at the beginning but seemed to find confidence in my discomfort and was word perfect for the rest of the interview.

Within the week, we found ourselves in yet another greenroom, this time in the studio for GMTV. I was surrounded by beautiful women and couldn't help but grin.

Jane looked at me.

'I feel a bit out of place,' she whispered.

'Thought as much,' I said.

The room was cramped but we squeezed in, quite snugly, I thought. Jane was scrunched up. The night before she'd been in pain and was wondering if she would be able to run at all. She'd asked me to mention during the interview that she was unwell and might not be able to complete the course. GMTV had brought us down to London and with only three days to go it was something of a risk. It had come off the back of the *Sun* story and originally I'd been tempted to turn it down. But I'd been seduced by the money. Only two days after the *Yorkshire Post* article had been published, the fundraising account stood at £500. With a national television interview, the fruit machine in my head was hitting jackpot.

A producer and researcher walked over. I stood up to give them more room to chat to Jane. A smartly dressed man was hovering by the door, obviously waiting to go to the studio.

'Hi,' I said. 'What are you going on for?'

'I'm addicted to eating pens,' he said.

I pondered whether to ask any further questions but it was too weird to leave alone. 'How many do you get through?'

'About fifty a week.'

'Is this the first time you've been on television?'

'No, I was on *Blind Date*.'

I looked across at Jane, who was looking weary. Her eyes were tired, her cheeks puffy. The last time I'd been out running with her was ten days ago and she'd been awesome. Accompanied by Gill, another runner from the club, they'd sped off at such a pace I could barely keep up with them. It was so bad that at one point a police car, noticing I'd been following them for so long, pulled up alongside me and kept pace. The two officers eyed me up suspiciously, clearly thinking I was some kind of pervert, lagging behind two women. Then they realized I was harmless and I was just being shown up.

Escorted into the wings of the studio, we stood next to Shaznay Lewis and Parminder Nagra, two girls from *Bend it Like Beckham*.

Mr Pen-Eater was being interviewed by Lorraine Kelly and he proceeded to choke on one while demonstrating his habit. For someone who admitted to eating fifty a week, he wasn't half making a meal out of this one. During the break, we were seated on the sofa and miked up. Lorraine said to the crew: 'Who booked that wazzerk?'

I sat in trepidation; Jane was growing in confidence. When asked what I thought about her doing the marathon I made some comment about her health and how risky it was. I knew by the look on Jane's face I'd said something wrong.

'I'll finish,' she said determinedly. 'I'll finish.'

I'd not fall for that one again.

JANE

I lay on the bed in the London hotel for a rest, unable to sleep for worrying about the next day. My friend Caroline looked over at me. She'd agreed to travel down with me for moral support. The enormity of my undertaking when I could hardly walk made me close my eyes to try to blot out the awful mistake I had made coming here. I doubted that I would see the three-mile marker, the *Cutty Sark* seemed only a remote possibility, the finish an unlikely dream. After telling so many people I was going to run the 26.2 miles, after all the months of training, I didn't know if I was ready for this. I reined myself in. 'You can do it, Jane,' I told myself. I pulled out the map of the course and studied the route again, trying to memorize where the Lucozade points were. I took the timing chip out of the envelope and struggled to interpret the cryptic instructions before finally attaching it to my laces.

I laid back down again to rest. Closing my eyes, I visualized the course, imagining my legs pounding the road as I approached the finishing line. I'd made it all the way round to Birdcage Walk, the clock was in sight, arms aloft triumphant, I could see my goal achieved. All these months of cold lonely runs were all for this one moment. This was my challenge, could my body take five hours of pounding on the roads? Would my back and legs make the distance?

I pulled down images of my family, a circle of guardian angels around me. My dad's face smiled at me, his eyes crinkled with encouragement, my gran, round-cheeked, hair curling, eyes flashing, had determination in her looks. I looked round at the group of faces in my head, taking encouragement from them. They lifted my spirits. I drew them in and pushed away the pains.

I set out my running kit, pinned the number to my T-shirt and checked my socks. I packed some warm clothes in the kit bag for when I finished, remembering I would need clean underwear. Everything was ready.

The next morning, I woke to the persistent beeping of the alarm. It was 5.30 a.m., time to take my bone strengthening tablets. My mind was buzzing, my stomach bubbling with nerves. I drew back the covers, the room was dark. I peeped through the curtains to where the streetlamps were still glowing orange and the sky was just turning purple.

I pulled on my running vest and blue T-shirt, my running number crackling as I eased the blue material over my head. I looked down at my name stencilled in black across my front. Stretching my knee supports up my calves and over my lower thighs, I smeared Vaseline liberally along the seamed edges to stop them rubbing. I rubbed more into my heels, and then rolled my socks on, using more Vaseline on them before pulling on my shoes and lacing them. My stomach heaved, my back felt clammy, my mouth was dry with nerves for the day ahead.

MIKE

'Steven, come on, it's time to get up.'

The clock next to Steven's bed said 03.45. It was little wonder I couldn't wake him. I gently shook his shoulder but he didn't stir so I slid one arm under his knees, one behind the back of his neck and lifted him out of the bed. Placing his feet on the floor, he wobbled unsteadily like a newborn foal before straightening up and opening his eyes.

'Come on, Steven,' I said. 'We're all off to see Mum.'

The five of us were heading down to London. Dad was staying in our house being looked after by his sister Margaret. It had been a heartbreaking decision not to take him, as he loved the marathon and seeing Jane run it would have made him so proud. But he was too unwell.

As I reversed off the drive I reset the trip mileage to zero. We were on the A1 bypassing Doncaster, thirty-five minutes later, when it read 26.2 miles. She'd never do it.

Steven was still snoozing as we drove through the Blackwall Tunnel and pulled into the car park of the hotel in Greenwich. At this early hour, London was deserted, its normally packed streets eerily quiet. As we climbed out of the car, my phone went.

'Hello?' I said.

'Oh, hi,' said the voice on the other end. 'I was hoping to speak to Jane Tomlinson.'

'This is her husband, Mike. Who's this?'

'It's John from BBC Sport. We were wondering if it would be possible to interview Jane before the start? Is she running?'

I'd given Jane's details to Helen at Cancer Research. She'd said the BBC might ring. 'Yes. Where and when?'

'She's on the red start. At the bottom by the park gates there'll be a camera crew. We could do it at eight forty-five.'

'No problem,' I said.

It was barely seven o'clock but the entrance and the breakfast area of the hotel were heaving with track-suited runners, their relatives and friends. We couldn't see Jane so Suzanne went up to her room. Within a few minutes she was back down again.

'Watch out, Dad, she's in a foul mood.'

'Why? What have you said?'

'Nothing,' said Suzanne and joined me, my mum, Rebecca and Steven at a table. 'She told me to get lost and she'd be down in a minute.'

About ten minutes later, the lift doors pinged open and Jane emerged. The newspaper article that morning had described her as 'small and frail' and she looked exactly that. Her face was grey and tired.

'Hiya,' she said. 'Sorry I snapped, Suzanne. I'll get some breakfast.'

'I've got some sandwiches here if you want some,' said Mum, holding up one of the many packs she'd prepared.

'No thanks, Alice. I'll get some cereal and toast,' said Jane.

'They're ham. I got it fresh from the butchers. You'll like them.'

'No,' said Jane, more firmly. 'I'll sort myself out.'

We watched as she disappeared towards the breakfast bar.

'Told you,' said Suzanne.

Rebecca piped up, 'When are you going to tell her about the interview, Dad?'

'I'll do it in a minute.'

'Rather you than me.'

We ate our sandwiches in silence, waiting outside the dining area for Jane. 'Good breakfast?' I asked as Jane bent down to kiss Steven.

She shrugged. 'It was breakfast, nothing special. I'll just get my stuff. The start is about a mile away, we'll have to leave in about an hour to get there on time.'

'Actually . . .' I began and Suzanne turned away quickly. Rebecca and Mum started their own little conversation. 'Could we possibly set off a little earlier? The BBC wants to do an interview with you at eight forty-five and ITV are going to meet you up there at eight thirty.'

Jane's face turned to thunder and, Hulk-like, I could have sworn she grew six inches. I cowered.

'I told you on Friday,' she hissed. 'I've got a marathon to do. I'm aching, Mike. I don't need any more shit.'

My phone rang. 'You'll be fine,' I said, picking it out of my pocket to answer it. 'Hello? Mike Tomlinson. Yes. No problem. Eight thirty? Yes, that's fine. Okay.'

Jane looked at me, puce with anger: 'And?'

'Yorkshire Television are going to be at the start in fifteen minutes.'

She turned on her heels and stormed off, turning round to say, 'We'll talk later.'

'Well done, Dad!' said Rebecca.

'What? I don't know why she gets so upset over nothing.'

'You wouldn't like it,' she said. 'You know she doesn't like doing those interviews.'

Suzanne and I both turned round and in unison said: 'Shut up, Becca.'

Fifteen minutes later we joined a trickle of people making their way down Blackwall Lane towards Trafalgar Road. I said to anyone listening: 'Aren't you forgetting something?' Jane turned, looking puzzled like a child doing some complicated mental arithmetic.

'No, I think I've got everything.'

'Not just you, Jane. Suzanne, Becca, Steven?' There were more frowns before Jane piped up.

'What?'

'Well, if you can't work it out I'm not going to tell you.'

'Mike, stop playing games, it's not the day.' Jane's limited patience was showing.

'Oh, but I think you'll find it is.'

'What?'

'The day.'

'For Christ's sake, Michael.' Jane was becoming completely exasperated as she dodged out of the way of a man errecting a metal crowd-control fence. We could see the yellow and green balloon gantry of a mile marker ahead.

'You've all forgotten.'

'Yes, yes, yes we have,' Jane snapped.

'It's my birthday.'

My mum laughed. 'Oh so it is, happy birthday, Son.'

The kids looked a little sheepish but Jane barked: 'No I haven't, there's a present waiting for you at home.' But it didn't stop me from taking the moral high ground for a while until Jane told me to shut up. We turned into Maze Hill and the crowd began to thicken. Twenty minutes later, we reached pen nine. I could see the Yorkshire Television crew, partly because their reporter was 6 ft 5 in. tall and was standing on a box. I asked him if he'd seen the BBC crew anywhere.

'No, there's some park gates about half a mile away. You

can't see them because of the crowds. See the camera crane,' he pointed ahead, 'try ringing them.'

I looked at the phone. 'Network's busy.'

'It always is at the marathon start. I'd go to that crane, there'll be someone manning it.'

Jane was fussing with her laces.

'I need a pee, Mike,' she said.

'Okay, I'll go and find the BBC crew,' I said.

'Here, take my bag.' She pushed her bum bag to me, I lengthened the strap and fastened it around my waist.

Aware of the time constraints, I ran slowly down the outside of the pens but it was impossible to get anywhere fast in the congestion of runners. When I finally got to the gates, the crane with the camera on top of it was unmanned. I'd got the wrong place.

I asked a policeman who suggested I ran across the park to where there was a selection of TV trucks. Checking my watch, I realized it was reaching the designated meeting time. I picked up my mobile – network busy. Should I find the crew or return to Jane who I knew would be fretting? But there was plenty of time to the start. I started jogging again, hindered by my jeans and heavy pockets full of Steven's paraphernalia. Slowly picking up speed I could hear feet behind me. I tried to increase speed but a quick draught blew across me as a group of elite Kenyans made me feel motionless. They were warming up.

I reached a large van emblazoned with the BBC logo on the side and knocked at the door. A man wearing headphones opened it.

'Yes?' he said.

'Hi. Mike Tomlinson. My wife is due to be interviewed at eight forty-five, where do we need to be?'

My heart sank as the man pointed over to the gates I'd just come from. 'You need to find Hazel Irvine. She's over there by the park gates,' he said.

'What does she look like?'

'Small, blonde, you'll recognize her from television.'

'Sorry, that doesn't help.'

'She'll be wearing a green jacket.' A slight pause before he said, 'The only one with a camera crew.'

I set off back again, my heart pumping, beads of sweat forming on my forehead. I checked my watch. This was going to be tight. I retrieved my mobile phone and started dialling. 'Network busy.' Shit.

I got to the gate again and immediately recognized Hazel. She was in the middle of an interview. I hung around at the side getting my breath back and as soon as she'd finished I caught her eye.

'Hi. I'm Mike Tomlinson. You're due to interview my wife.'

In a soft Scottish accent she said, 'Jane? Yes, is she here?'

'Not quite. She's at pen nine,' I said.

'Can you get her here in two minutes?' she said.

'No chance. It'll take at least twenty.'

'We really want to interview her,' she said, then pointed up to her head to indicate someone was talking into her headphones. She talked back into her headset and then announced, 'Come on, guys, let's go for it.'

Hazel, the cameraman, soundman and myself took off through the massed runners to where Jane was waiting. At that minute, my mobile rang.

'Mike, where are you?' It was Caroline. 'Jane's really upset.' Like a car sliding on a greasy surface, I felt an impact was inevitable. There was a rustle, crackle, then Jane came on the line.

'You ignorant git! Where the hell are you? You've been gone for forty-five minutes and you've got my bag with all my things. We'll be starting soon, I need them now. I'm really fucking mad. Get you're arse back here now.' Her voice started to shake, unable to hold back the tears. 'I can't believe you've been so fucking thoughtless.'

She passed Suzanne the phone. 'You'd better get back here, Dad,' she said quietly. 'I've never seen Mum so mad.'

I put the phone back in my pocket and carried on running.

'Everything all right?' asked Hazel. 'Is she still okay to be interviewed?'

'Yeah,' I said. 'Of course she is.'

As we ran, Hazel said, 'Can you give me some background on Jane?'

'She's dying of cancer.'

The soundman interrupted. 'I've got no signal.' Above us, the canopy of foliage was blocking out any chance of a transmission, but ahead was a clearing where the signal might be stronger.

'We'll have to do it here,' said the soundman as we reached pen five. 'Is there any chance you can get her over here? We haven't got much time, the women's elite race has already started.'

'Yeah, no problem,' I lied again. 'I'll be about five minutes.'

I dashed off and got to the spot where I'd left Jane fifty minutes earlier. The kids were all sitting with their backs to a large tree trunk, wearing the weary expressions of people who had already been up for six hours.

'Where's Mum?'

'Over there,' said Suzanne. 'Be careful, Dad, she's really mad.'

I turned and saw a solitary figure, surrounded by discarded clothing, bin bags, foil blankets and empty liquid bottles. She looked desolate, standing there sobbing, her body rocking gently. I stood silently while taking the verbal beating, waiting until her sting had been drawn.

'Jane, the BBC are in pen five waiting to interview you,' I said.

'Well, you'd better tell them I'm not coming,' she replied.

'Don't be unreasonable.'

'I'm tired. I've got to run a marathon and you've got the audacity to call me unreasonable. There's a TV crew there and then you with the bloody camcorder.'

'It's just one interview—'

'No.'

'Look,' I tried to reason. 'Your mum, my dad, everyone we know is watching the telly right now waiting for the merest glimpse of you. And here you are with a chance for them to see you. Don't be selfish, think of them, you know what it would mean to them.' I put my arms around her. 'Come on, you know it makes it sense.' I winked at Suzanne, who shook her head. 'We'll need to run, though.'

By the time we made it to pen five, I thought we would be too late. But Hazel and her crew were waiting patiently. Jane's eyes were red, her face blotchy, she looked highly emotional. Hazel waited for the signal to start the interview and she turned to Jane.

'There are many different reasons for running a marathon. Some have something to prove to themselves, others for other people and for Jane Tomlinson I suspect it's a bit of both. How important is it for you to finish this marathon today, Jane?'

'I think it's immensely important from a personal sort of point of view but I want to show people. I'm terminally ill with breast cancer. I want to show somebody who might have a similar prognosis that you can set yourself goals, that it doesn't matter if it seems a bit impossible, set yourself a goal and aim for it and get on with it. I'm here to raise funds for Cancer Research UK because I'm not going to actually survive my disease and I am hoping to raise funds for others in the future who might get a better chance than myself.'

'When were you diagnosed, Jane?'

'I was diagnosed twelve years ago, but eighteen months ago I was told that I was terminally ill. I had perhaps only months to live and following treatment, I've got myself gradually fitter and fitter. I've been training full on for the marathon since October now.'

'Jane, we're all very much on your side, willing you round this course today. Our very best wishes to you.'

'Thank you very much.'

When she had finished the crew stood silently before saying good luck. Jane nodded and said thank you before walking back to me. I moved forward to hug her.

'And you can fuck off,' she said.

JANE

I squeezed through the barrier and made my way towards the back of the pen, away from the crush at the front. There was

silence as thousands of people stood in remembrance of the
Queen Mother. The only sound was the buzz of the helicopter
hovering in the distance.

The murmurings of the crowds started again. People stood
stretching, and the noise increased as onlookers shouted to
loved ones. My throat constricted with anxiety. I clutched my
arms to my body.

I turned to kiss Steven leaning over the barrier towards me. I
looked back as the runners started to move forwards, waving
before I turned to face the start. Carried along with the runners
and walkers, there were so many T-shirt-clad people all declar-
ing allegiances to different charities. A blue-haired man passed
me; there was red, yellow, blue hair in the crowd. A blue, round
Mr Bump, long limbed, moved alongside me. Many other runners were running for Cancer Research UK – a greeting of
comrades as we wished each other luck. The crowds ebbed forwards. Some runners leapt over the barriers heading for the
toilet blocks, now absent of queues. My bladder felt heavy and
I made the dash with the others. I sat and relieved myself one
more time before returning to the streams of people heading for
the start.

Passing under the tall yellow crane, everyone lifted their
hands and faces towards the camera and waved. Rupert Bear
jogged past me in yellow checked trousers. I could see a huge
white and red hot air balloon, stationary on the field to our
right. Then, finally, we reached the start, after nearly fifteen
minutes moving, and we were running underneath the yellow
Flora banner announcing the start of the 26 miles, 286 yards.

I was part of a mass of over 30,000 runners taking part in the
twenty-second London Marathon. It was a sunny day, there
were so many runners and yet such a long and lonely run ahead.
I passed under the banner to the strains of Abba's 'Dancing
Queen'. My legs felt strangely light, the pain in my tendons was
forgotten, my shoulder at peace. Fuelled with the excitement, I
clicked the button of my watch and started the count of the
hours and minutes towards the finish.

The streets were lined with cheering onlookers. My legs were stiff. After the initial euphoria, now there was just the hard slog of running, mentally keeping my feet falling in front of me. Step by step I passed groups of people.

'Go, Jane, go!' I waved, thankful for the encouragement. A group of young lads took our pace and ran alongside us for a few minutes. When they stopped, one drew a whistle to his lips, shrilling us on. I looked at my watch as I passed each mile marker, pleased with the steady ten-minute-mile pace I was keeping to. After thirty minutes I passed under the three-mile marker. The distractions made the time pass and I kept moving past the children holding out their hands for high fives. Outstretched hands held drinks and oranges. I shook my head and passed on watching for the next drinks station. I grabbed a bottle, unscrewed the lid and took a few sips, slowing my run to stop me gulping down air. Screwing the top back, I kept the bottle in my right hand and picked the pace back up.

As I approached mile six, I searched the sea of faces in the crowd for Mike, straining to hear his voice above everyone else. No familiar faces, my head swung from side to side to see if I could catch a glimpse of him.

The white masts and black riggings of *Cutty Sark* came into view and the runners in front slowed to almost walking as we made our way round the narrow paths surrounding the ancient ship. A kilted band piped us round, the steely rap of the accompanying drums keeping time with our footfalls.

I lifted my head as a photographer snapped at all the passing runners. With the ship to our left, the runners began to span out and sped up. The muffled musical booms of a steel band were setting a cheering rhythm. A clown with a blue wig pushed back on the crown of his head sidled past me, then came to a halt as he brought his phone to his ear.

'Yeah,' he was shouting. 'I'm just coming up to the seven-mile marker. On the right, okay, yeah, I'll see you there.' I cursed him under my breath, avoiding falling by changing my stride and running around him. As I ran on, I heard his group of friends, all waving and shouting his name. I kept scanning the crowds hoping to see Mike and the kids.

A DJ dressed as Elvis uh uhed us along as he belted out 'Hound Dog'. I smiled at the middle-aged impersonator as he yelled, 'Come on, Jane, keep going!' He curled his lip and flicked his black quiff at me.

The smell of fried onions hung in the air, making my mouth water as I passed a hot dog stand. Another pub, another DJ and 'Ride Sally Ride' boomed out of the PA. My hips swayed to the music, buoyed by the sight of the twelve-mile marker.

Five, six, seven minutes beyond the twelve-mile marker I was passing under the high grey arches of Tower Bridge, the blue swagged support overhung with many faces all yelling encouragement. I could make out a stream of runners making their way out of the Tower, along the carpeted cobbles.

'You'll be there soon,' I cajoled myself as I was carried along in the stream of people across the bridge. I scanned the crowds again, searching for Mike, convinced I'd see him, but there were no familiar faces. Tears of disappointment fell down my face as I ran away from the crowds, towards the Isle of Dogs over-looked by the mirrored tower at Canary Wharf. The noise and excitement of the first few miles was gone, now I was on a dreary drudge past thousands of runners coming the other way. How I wished I was there, nine miles further on and nearing the end. The toilets came into view, nestled under the railway bridge near mile fifteen, and my bladder full, a balloon of discomfort at the bottom of my belly, I stood behind other shuffling runners, feet moving involuntarily as we stood waiting to relieve ourselves in the small, smelly, plastic cubicle.

The crowds had thinned out as we made our way past the fifteen-mile marker through a red-brick estate, its narrow paths meanly edged with grass. There were groups of people lounging around on deck chairs, leaning forward and sneering encouragement as they cracked open tins of beer. My legs felt heavy, they were screaming at me to walk. There was little distraction. I glanced at my watch, peered into the distance willing the next arch of green, white and yellow balloons into view so I could mentally tick off another mile. I felt as if I'd been running for hours but only five minutes had passed. I willed myself not to look at the time so I lifted my head and looked over the heads of the other runners, breathing in, breathing out, counting the breaths – one and two and one and two and – another set of hoardings and then another mile marker before I was heading back towards the tower and forcing my legs forwards. I wasn't going to stop. I would make it.

'Come on, Jane, you can finish,' I repeated to myself, a personal mantra to keep me running, as I descended on to the cobbled stretch just outside the Tower of London. The thin green carpet laid out for the runners and the wheelchairs did nothing to ease the jarring of the uneven surface beneath.

My back throbbed, my knees shuddered with every step and my thigh muscles were knotted with pain. I was too sore to run and slowed to a walk with my legs screaming at me to stop but my head willing me to run.

I pushed down, ignoring the agony, and kept running. I pulled the faces of people I loved in front of me, holding the familiar smiles of my dad and gran in my mind, counting the seconds, making the minutes, passing the yards. A shout came from above:

'Jane! Up here!' I lifted my head wearily and saw Dave and Andy from Yorkshire Television, their camera following my slow progress from the bridge ahead. I passed under and glanced back and saw the tall figure of Dave, his hand cupped to his mouth yelling encouragement. The crowds thickened and there were many yells of 'Jane, you can do it!'

My exuberant wave of those early miles to acknowledge their cries of support was now barely a nod of the head. I had to concentrate on keeping my legs moving as I made my way along The Embankment. An orange-faced caterpillar made its way past me, many legs moving under its orange and purple body. A small antenna bobbing comically above its large eyes. If I'd had the strength I would have dug deeper to find the pace to keep up with it but I couldn't. But as I watched it crawl further and further ahead of me I knew I'd have to suffer the indignity of being beaten by a multicoloured larva.

The huge wheel of the London Eye turned slowly to my left

and ahead of me was the clock tower of Big Ben. Finally, I was on Birdcage Walk, the green of St James's Park to my right. I could see a camera up ahead; the railings were decked with yellow banners. I turned right for the final 300 yards to the finish.

Mike was there yelling himself hoarse, Steven clutched firmly to his side.

'Come on, Jane, come on.'

I raised my head, lifted my legs and ran steadily towards the finish. It had taken nearly five hours but I'd made it – twenty-six miles all around London. Tears rolled down my face, tears of joy, tears of pain, tears for all those miles of training, all those races run in my head.

I finished. I stopped, turned and fell into Mike's arms with Steven by our side.

MIKE

Pall Mall was heaving with people standing five to ten deep lining the course. With no grandstand ticket, the chances of me getting anywhere near the finishing line were remote. But I had three props: Steven, a letter from the BBC saying I was filming a video diary and a battered old camcorder with a BBC sticker on it that looked like it had been made from a child's activity set.

BBC *Look North* had entrusted me to film a video diary of the weekend. Well, it was cheaper than sending a crew down to London. So far, though, my footage was non-existent. I'd hoped to get some shots of Jane before she set off but she'd refused to be interviewed by me.

Cameramen Andy and Dave from Yorkshire Television were marathon veterans and advised that just after the seven-mile mark would be a good place to catch her as it was easy to get to from the start. We'd stood, cameras poised at the apex of a road traffic island and waited.

The male elite had just gone through and now the remaining

field started trickling by. Before long, it was a stampede. Thousands of runners surged towards us and parted like the Red Sea as they came to the traffic island. We studied the collective, with numerous false sightings of Jane. The Cancer Research T-shirts were of no help whatsoever, their colours were everywhere. I'd suggested she put her name on the front.

Suddenly Andy yelled, 'There she is!' and left us, matching a female athlete pace for pace and holding his camera inches from her face. Within a couple of minutes, he was back.

'Wrong one again,' he said. 'I saw the Jane T on her T-shirt.' Dave and I both stifled laughs.

'What?' said Andy, looking bemused.

'It wasn't Jane T,' said Dave. 'It was Janet.'

Even so, it was the closest we got. After two hours, even the slowest runners had passed us – at least they had as much space at the elite. The deserted streets heightened my sense of foreboding, a solitary trainer lay in the gutter,

Heading to Tower Hill, it was pandemonium and certainly no place for Steven. We separated from Andy and Dave – clearly I couldn't blag six of us into the grandstand – so I set off to gain entry with just Steven.

The security guard looked with some disdain at my letter. We had a frank and robust exchange of views, while a queue began to form. I wasn't about to budge and with Steven I felt there was little likelihood of someone moving us with any ease.

'Come on,' I said to the guard. 'You're going to look very silly if a senior BBC guy has to come down and sort this out.'

He looked flummoxed and then opened the barrier. 'I didn't let you in, right?' he said.

'I've never seen you before,' I replied.

We went round the back of the grandstand until we were on the road with the finishing gantry just thirty yards ahead. A security guard came over.

'Where's your pass?' he said.

'BBC,' I said, flashed him the camera and strode purposefully over to where Sue Barker and her crew were filming. I stood as close as I could to them without being classed as a weirdo stalker. Steven and I stood patiently as hundreds and hundreds of runners passed by. The celebrities filtered off to the left by us for their post-race interview. Every couple of minutes I kept checking my watch, concerned that we'd not heard anything about her in over four hours. The tension was unbearable. My phone rang.

'Mike, it's Dave. We've just seen her at mile twenty-three. She looks fit. We're on a bridge, she waved to us.'

'Fantastic, thanks Dave.'

'We're coming to the finish, we'll see you there.'

I told Steven and we did a little jig, then I phoned the girls. We figured she'd been running for just over four hours. Suddenly, down the home straight came a streaker. I averted Steven's eyes and then thought about filming it for the BBC. Perhaps not. I didn't want to encourage streaking.

We waited . . . and waited . . . and waited. A multipersonned caterpillar came into view, we'd seen it at the start. She'd never live this one down – outclassed by a caterpillar. As the minutes ticked on, my concern grew. It had been fifty minutes since Dave phoned so that was seventeen minutes per mile to the finish. What had gone wrong?

The tannoy announced someone special would be coming along in a minute. I daydreamt that it could be Jane, but that was frankly ridiculous as no one knew who she was. We waited. After so many false sightings, I thought, 'It's Jane. Yes, it's Jane', one hundred and fifty yards away on the opposite side of the road, moving at granny pace.

I grabbed Steven's hand. 'It's Mummy!'

We ran, weaving between runners, desperate to get across. I grabbed the camera and started to film as some people in the crowd began to call her name. She waved, palms sky high, tears starting to flow. She passed us with no acknowledgement, running to the line. Steven and I passed underneath the finishing gantry. A small, grey-haired middle-aged woman wearing a white marathon top grabbed my elbow.

'You're not allowed in here,' she shouted. 'It's for runners only.'

'I need to get to my wife, she's poorly,' I said.

'I don't care, you're not allowed.'

Jane was only two yards ahead, crying uncontrollably. She turned and grabbed Steven's hand. Sobbing, she collected her medal. Hazel Irvine, cameraman and soundman appeared and Hazel hugged Jane like a long-lost friend, making sure she was all right. Then she ran off to get her a foil blanket.

'Do you need any medical help, Jane?' she asked, worried over Jane's tears.

'I'm just in an immense amount of pain, the last two miles were awful.'

Two minutes later, she'd stopped crying and did another interview together with Steven. The phone rang.

'Where are you?' It was Suzanne.

'Mum's here,' I said. 'She's finished.'

'We know! She was all over the big screens all the way down the finishing straight!'

'We'll see you in a minute at Buckingham Palace.'

Jane hobbled over after her interview.

'Mike, I need to get changed,' she said. 'Let's get my bag.' She looked at me as I fumbled with the camcorder bag. 'What on earth are you doing?' she asked.

'Looking for the lens cap,' I said.

'It's on the camera.'

'Shit.'

'Don't worry. It serves them right for not sending a proper cameraman. We told them you were a joke.'

It was a relief to be back in the car, heading north. The A1 was quiet. Steve Ridgeway phoned us to tell us that he'd heard Brendan Foster call her the heroine of the marathon and they'd make a big fuss about her on the highlights programme.

We walked into the living room and Jane threw her arms in the air.

'I did it!'

Aunt Margaret, who had been looking after Dad, came over and hugged her. 'You were unbelievable, Jane, well done.'

My dad came across and shook her hand. 'I've never seen 'owt like it, you should have seen the TV, fantastic Jane, just fantastic.'

Steven trundled through wearing Jane's finisher's medal around his neck. Within a couple of minutes Suzanne arrived in a taxi after travelling up from London with Caroline on Jane's return ticket.

'Becca, get some champagne, will you?' I asked. She rushed off to the kitchen. I fetched the champagne flutes, a wedding present being used for the first time.

'We don't need to do this, Mike,' Jane said.

'Get lost, Jane, this is the greatest achievement of your life. Let's celebrate the moment.'

'Here, Dad.' Rebecca handed me the bottle, we popped the cork and filled the glasses.

'To Jane and the bravest marathon ever run,' I said.

An hour later, with everyone preparing for bed, I grabbed the camcorder. 'Any chance of that interview now?'

She mouthed something I didn't catch, but I got the gist.

CHAPTER 12

MIKE

'Mike! Mike! What's wrong?' The voice sounded like Jane, but it couldn't be, she was dead. Attempting to fight him off, I threw a flurry of punches in his direction.

'Stop! Stop! What are you doing?' My mind raced. We're in bed. The man. Oh Lord, it's a nightmare. I woke, sat bolt upright in bed and saw Jane and Rebecca staring at me. Feeling embarrassed, I feigned confusion.

'Where am I? Who was that screaming?'

'What's happened?' asked Rebecca, alerted by the noise.

'Nothing, love, your dad's just had a nightmare, go back to bed.'

'Ha ha!' she laughed and disappeared to her bedroom.

I fell back on to the pillow, exhausted by the dream, then reality hit home harder than the nightmare; Jane's death.

Despite the fact we'd had eighteen months to share together as a family, our situation remained the same. Jane was still going to die and in all likelihood it would be soon. Reflecting on the last two weeks they seemed as surreal as the nightmare.

The day after the marathon we were already committed to go back to *Look North* and to appear on *Calendar*. Driving between the two, I saw a newspaper billboard saying 'Courage of Cancer Mother'.

'Did you see that, Jane?'

'What?' I pulled over to the side of the road.

'Becca, nip in the newsagent's back there and get an *Evening Post*.'

'Can't you do it?' she said from the back seat.

'Becca!'

'There you are.' I opened the front page out.

'Who's that, Steven?'

'Me and Mummy.' Jane reached across and grabbed the paper.

'Oh, that's an awful picture,' she said.

'Did you see it, Becca?' I asked.

'I saw it earlier at school.'

'Why didn't you tell us?' Rebecca shrugged her shoulders, ambivalent. 'Did anyone see Mum on the telly at the marathon yesterday?'

'All the teachers.'

'What did they say?'

'They were like, "Isn't your mum brilliant, can't believe your mum did the marathon."'

'Do you mind your mum being in the papers and on the telly?'

'No, I'm really proud. I just need to get home, I've got loads of homework to do.'

Arriving home from work with Steven, the *Daily Mirror* journalist was already sitting on the couch talking to Jane. Part of Jane's scepticism towards the press meant that she always wanted to be chaperoned during interviews.

'There's a photographer coming in an hour for a family photograph,' I told Suzanne, who had just arrived from school.

'Do I have to?' she said. She'd always been camera shy and I knew it would be a big sacrifice for her to be in the pictures. As she disappeared into the kitchen, I left Steven playing with his toys on the carpet and followed her.

'It would be nice,' I said quietly. 'I'm not too happy about it either, as everyone will know I'm married to her.'

'Yes, but that was your choice. I'm lumbered,' she smiled.

Jane's voice shouted from the living room, 'Oi, you two, we can hear you.'

The phone in the hall interrupted the exchange. It was Leeds City Council wanting Jane. The four of us listened in to the conversation. 'Yes, I'd be delighted,' she said, and after a few minutes returned back to the room. 'They've asked me to run the last leg of the relay and give the baton to the Queen.' She looked rather startled.

'I always thought you were a republican,' I said, teasing.

'Yeah, Mum,' said Suzanne. 'Since when have you become a royalist?'

Seconds later the phone rang again.

'Ah, that'll be them coming to their senses,' I said.

'Yeah, they got the wrong person,' said Suzanne.

This time I went to the phone. 'Mike Tomlinson.'

'Hi, Mike, it's Paul at the *Yorkshire Evening Post*. We've just heard about Jane and the relay. Is it okay to do photographs and an interview?'

That was quick. I was slightly flummoxed. 'Yeah, is in an hour all right?'

The afternoon began to take a surreal turn. By 4.30 p.m., Rebecca was also home and the house was filled with two journalists and two photographers.

The car headlights lit up the street. I'd bargained on John being prompt.

He knew no other way to be. It had been eighteenth months since I'd had a day to myself – the Chelsea FA Cup appearance had been the catalyst.

As I approached the car, I felt uncomfortable about going but Jane had been insistent.

'Well,' John said, in his usual sardonic tone as I buckled up. 'I feel humbled to have the pleasure of a TV star in the car.'

'Don't,' I said. 'It's not funny.'

'You must have had quite a couple of weeks. I've seen more of Jane on the telly than Posh and Becks. We watched the marathon, she was fantastic. You must have been so proud.'

'Jane was a little disappointed with her time but it was just good to see her safe. I'd been a bit worried beforehand with all the bumping at the start but she was all right.'

'Has she got any other plans?'

'Yeah, Brendan Foster's company have invited her up to take part in the Great North Run in October. She's got us both doing that. She's also doing the Great Women's Run in Manchester with Rebecca and Suzanne.'

'It's all right for some. You'll have to lose some weight, though,' he said, looking across at me.

Cardiff was a fair distance away and by Sheffield I was asleep. We cruised down some Welsh country lanes to avoid the M4 corridor and reached our destination by nine.

After a bright start, the day went down hill. My prophetic words of 'It's only Ray Parlour', preceded the first goal by a nanosecond. We didn't stay to watch the cup being lifted. I was welcomed home by Suzanne chanting 'two nil, two nil' as she jabbed a finger towards my head.

There was a sense of a return to normality. It was Steven's fifth birthday on Friday, his birthday party the day after, twenty kids at Rothwell Sports Centre for a football party. Seven days later it was Rebecca's confirmation, another family celebration.

One thing had changed irrevocably: the little goals we'd set on the horizon as a family – weekends away, concerts, nights out – were being replaced by things in Jane's new life, which seemed to be stretching out across the summer.

JANE

Rebecca and I walked across Roundhay Park heading for the start area of the Race for Life, where thousands of women thronged together. My legs were still heavy, weeks after finishing the marathon, but along with Rebecca, I was looking forward to the run.

Standing near the tape, Tracey Barraclough, a local supporter of Cancer Research UK, was invited to sound the horn to set off the runners. That was the last I saw of Rebecca, her blonde hair disappearing among all the bodies. I dashed after her but quickly realized I'd no hope of catching her slim figure.

A year on from the last Race for Life, I still felt the same excitement running with thousands of women of all shapes and sizes. Jack and Alice found us at the finish and we sat chatting on the grass before heading for home.

The race took my mind off my scan results but by Monday night my nerves were fraught. The house was its usual mess, and I found myself snapping at Suzanne and Rebecca, demanding that they move their own articles of clothing up to their rooms. Suzanne picked up her coat and shoes, stony-faced, silent, and headed for the door. Rebecca crashed around the room, muttering under her breath and pointedly closing the door behind her. I sat alone, knowing I'd been unreasonable but too agitated to apologize. I gathered up toys and books, clearing the carpet in the living room, and struggled upstairs with my arms laden. Dumping the array of plastic in Steven's room, he turned and looked at me.

'I thought you were asleep,' I whispered.

'How can I be when you're in my room?' his voice rang out clearly, his cheeky tone cheering me. A smile flashed at me as he rested his head on the pillow. I leant over him, kissed my hand and placed it on his forehead.

'Settle down now or you'll be too tired for school.' He started to say something and I shushed him. 'Go to sleep.'

He sighed and turned over and I made for the doorway, tripping over the toys I'd deposited there myself. Cursing, I left the room but not before I heard Steven saying: 'Well, you shouldn't have put them there then.'

I turned. 'Steven, cheeky baggage, go to sleep.'

Downstairs, I began picking up the cushions strewn across the living room. Some had been used for goalposts, others just dropped on to the floor. Folding the blue and yellow throw, I rested it over the back of the tall-armed pine rocking chair and sat letting the pictures on the television roll in front of me.

The tension made me weary, my sleep had been disturbed, the tiredness had stayed with me all day. I sat on the edge of the settee summoning the energy to stand up. Rebecca's videos were on the floor. I piled them and carried them up to her room, knocking on the door and entering. She was sitting, huddled in the corner of her room, scribbling away at her homework.

I put the boxes down. 'Sorry I shouted at you, it's not your fault I'm just a bit grumpy.'

'No, it's all right.' She looked at me. 'You're off to the hospital tomorrow?' She raised her eyebrows quizzically.

'Yeah, we might be late home, we'll have to wait to speak to Dr Perren about some treatments. I was going to make some hot chocolate,' I say. 'Do you want some?'

'Yes, please.'

I walked over and gave her a hug. 'Love you. I really am sorry.'

'So am I. love you too.' She looked up at me, her blues eyes open and earnest.

Suzanne's door was ajar and I tapped on it before pushing it further. Music drifted quietly and she was sitting surrounded by books. 'Sorry for being grumpy,' I said.

'Don't worry about it,' she said, raising her head from her books. 'It's results day tomorrow, we're used to it by now.'

'I know, it doesn't make it right though,' I said.

'No, it doesn't,' she said, not letting me off the hook lightly. I shifted a book and sat down next to her. She rested her head on my shoulders and I put my arm round her.

I had a big decision to make. My disease was still showing signs of progressing and I was starting to be much more uncomfortable with small foci of pain in many areas of my body. I could start a relatively new treatment called Herceptin, only available to women whose tumours have a greater amount of HEr2 receptors – the growth hormone receptors – on them, and it would stop them working, hopefully slowing down the growth of the tumours.

Dr Perren closed the door to the office and sat down. 'Congratulations on the marathon. What was it like?'

'A painful experience,' I replied.

'You've not come back a couple of inches shorter, have you?' He arched his eyebrows and peered down at me.

'No, I'm not too bad, but the pain in my bones is getting worse, and I have more bad days than good days now.'

'It's probably time to start some further treatment then.' He checked my notes. 'Dr Jeffers discussed Herceptin with you at your last appointment. Your heart scans were normal, so we could start you on that. I don't think we need to think about chemo just now. We can add that later if we think it's necessary.'

'When would I start?'

'There's no point in hanging around. If that's what you decide to go for I'll prescribe it today and you can start next week.'

Mike and I had talked about this. I knew I needed to start the treatment, but the drug was only licensed for weekly treatments which meant I would have to attend clinic every Wednesday. At that stage, I really was not sure I wanted such a regular reminder of my disease but the pain was starting to intrude into every aspect of my life. I was finding it increasingly hard to move the equipment around at work, and by the time I arrived home, the pain meant I had to ask the family for more help with small jobs round the house.

'I'll need you to sign the consent form.' Dr Perren started to fill out the long yellow form. 'We'll start you on a larger loading dose. It might leave you feeling achy afterwards, but it shouldn't last more than a day or two.'

I signed the forms and handed them back to Dr Perren. 'As you are going to be having treatment regularly I'll prescribe the biphosphonates to be had by infusion instead of tablet form.'

I nodded my understanding. It would be a relief to be free of the twice daily dose that made meal planning so difficult. I left the hospital feeling drained, relieved at having made a decision.

After dropping Steven at his childminder's the next morning, Mike and I continued into town. 'Don't forget Rob Spedding from *Runner's World* is coming after work,' Mike said.

'Oh, yeah. I'm glad you reminded me. You won't be late

home, will you?' I turned to kiss him as he pulled up near my work.

Rob Spedding was prompt and brought the latest edition of *Runner's World* for me to look through. I came across an article outlining the first training principles for the London Triathlon in August. I read it, intrigued by the idea of a triathlon. The swimming sounded all right but cycling – I was not sure I could cycle forty kilometres let alone run ten kilometres straight after.

'You should have a go at that,' said Rob.

'Actually, it sounds really interesting but I'm not sure I can manage it.'

Rob pulled out a notebook and started to run through some questions. Mike arrived just as we were finishing and pulled up a chair, listening in. He picked up a magazine and flicked through it. He saw the piece on triathlons. 'So you reckon you could manage that?' he said, eyebrows raised questioningly.

'I'd need to work at my swimming. The run's no problem, it's the cycling that's the issue.' I turned to Rob. 'I haven't even got a bike.'

'You're mad, you know that, don't you?' said Mike.

I laughed at the look on his face. 'I only said it looked interesting.'

'Yeah, I know that look,' he replied.

Rob picked up his bag. 'If you do decide that you're interested in the triathlon and need any help with it, any kit, and any other bits and bobs, let us know,' he said as he headed for the door.

The idea of the triathlon blossomed in my head. It would be such a fantastic event to take part in, but I was due to start my Herceptin the following week and had no idea how that would leave me feeling.

The day before my first treatment I was invited to a lunch at the Queens Hotel to honour the women of Yorkshire. Mum, Mary and Alice met Rebecca and me in the foyer of the art nouveau style hotel. We made our way into the ballroom. Each round table was bedecked with flowers and balloons, and on each chair was a bag filled with samples from the many sponsors of the event. The noise in the room was deafening, the voices of all the women raised, so I had to lean into my mum to hear her as she spoke.

'Thank you for coming,' I said. 'It's a shame Suzanne can't make it.'

'I'm delighted to be here. Was Suzanne busy?'

'Yes. She had a French oral exam late this morning, and couldn't get here in time.'

Although I knew I'd been nominated for an award, when I was announced as the Woman of Courage I stood bemused, overcome with emotion. Alice stood to take a photo as I made my way to the stage to receive a framed certificate.

'Well done there, girl,' said Mum as I retook my seat and watched and applauded other award winners. Faye Banks, a young woman who had overcome a difficult childhood to become a successful engineer, was given the business award. Carol Maddox, easily recognizable from the local papers having had an argument with the prime minister on *Question Time*, received the *Yorkshire Evening Post* readers award for her outspoken bravery.

The room was full of Leeds lunching ladies, but amongst them were others who were there to have their achievements recognized. Real people, with stories of courage and hardships overcome, women without wealth and status, not celebrities. The applause for each recipient was rousing, the welcome warm as each woman honoured was escorted to the stage.

I was led to the stage again as I was announced the overall winner, the Yorkshire Woman of Achievement 2002. I turned to Rebecca, who had followed me, and clasped her hand in mine, leaving Alice trailing us, anxious to get a photograph of the two of us. I stood before the audience, glad I was partially hidden behind a lectern to hide the fact I was shaking.

'I don't think of myself as having done anything extraordinary,' I said. It was the first thing that came into my head. 'I ran the marathon because I wanted to do it and because I wanted to raise some money.' I paused, realizing there was something else

I should add. 'Maybe, also, because I wanted to say to people that if I can do this, as I am, just think what you can do. There is only yourself stopping you.'

As all the recipients of awards stood together for a photo, Faye Banks turned to speak to me. She was a runner and fancied taking part in the marathon.

'What about a triathlon?' I said jokingly.

'Why? Do you fancy doing one?' she said earnestly.

'I'm thinking about it but I'm not sure if I could manage it.'

Faye's eyes shone brightly. 'Well, if you decide to do it, let me know and we'll do it together.'

I nodded. 'It's a deal.'

Even though Dr Perren had warned me that I might feel a bit achy after the first dose of Herceptin, I was unprepared for the first two days of pain. I ached everywhere. My whole body felt as if it was being pummelled. My shoulder was exquisitely painful, pinpoints of pain shot through the ball joint. My fingers, toes, even my eyes hurt. I climbed into bed, curling myself round a hot-water bottle, and tried to find some comfort.

By Friday morning the pain had started to subside. I no longer felt bruised and sore, more like I was recovering from a bad bout of flu; I was a little feverish and my throat felt a bit raw. On Friday night I felt the pain ease and by Saturday I felt better. My head was clearer, my concentration span increased, my clumsiness lessened.

It was six o'clock. It had been a long day. I had been to Leicester for a paediatric study day and I just had time to pick up my bag before we travelled to Manchester, where Rebecca and I were going to take part in the Great Women's Run. Although we had been training regularly, I wasn't sure how the Herceptin would affect my performance and was nervous. Rebecca and I were both capable of running the five miles in under forty minutes, and were looking forward to competing together.

It didn't take long to drive to Manchester and, after checking into the hotel, we met up with some of the people from the

Cancer Research UK events team, who had been responsible for our invitation to the race. Helen and Nicki we already knew from the marathon but there were a few new people, too.

A familiar face appeared at the bar, and Helen introduced me to Peter Elliott. I've only ever seen him on television, his red hair was short and the colour faded, but he looked little different to when I used to watch him running on the track. As I lifted my pint to my lips I heard another voice, this one extremely familiar to me. Brendan Foster appeared.

'Ah Jane, it's great to meet you at last.' He leant forward and kissed my cheek. Standing back he noticed my drink. 'What's that? A pint?' he asked. 'Aren't you running tomorrow?'

'Yes, it's only the one. I don't think it will endanger my performance.'

Brendan laughed. 'Well done there, girl. I'm really glad you're running.'

'It's great to be here. I can't thank you enough for what you said about me at the marathon. It made a huge difference to the fundraising.'

'Ah well, it was truly deserved. What you did that day was extraordinary.' He patted me on the shoulder. 'Enjoy the run tomorrow.'

Lining up the next day with thousands of women, some in costumes, others in club vests, the serious runners and fun runners were all setting off together. I quickly lost sight of Rebecca as she stormed off ahead. I ran a slow steady race and about a mile from the finish caught her up. She was holding her stomach.

'I've got a stitch,' she said, pressing her hand into her side. I took her free hand and urged her on as she slowed to a walk.

'Come on, it's not far now, only another few minutes and we'll be finished.' I pulled her forwards and she gritted her teeth and set off running again. Her cheeks were pink and her brow creased as she kept pace with me and we headed towards the finish in front of the town hall. We raised our arms and crossed the finishing line together. I looked at the clock. We'd run the five miles in just under forty-one minutes.

MIKE

I'd promised both mums that if we had the opportunity, while on holiday in the Dordogne, I'd take Jane to Lourdes. When Jane awoke on Tuesday feeling better again after severe pain in her shoulder had threatened to shorten our holiday we decided to make a visit. It would be a three-hour drive mostly by motorway. Although Catholic, my primary reason for wanting to go there was the fact that it was in the foothills of the Pyrenees and as a Tour de France devotee I fancied going up a couple of the climbs. In the car, obviously.

But there was also a small part of me that wanted to see Lourdes to find out what the fuss was about. If I'd have believed there was any way Jane could be healed by going there, I would have taken her years ago. But I didn't.

Pulling into the Hotel Campanile at Lourdes the backdrop was breathtaking. The high Pyrenean peaks were shrouded in mist, making them look moody and inaccessible. After unloading the car, we headed into town to find Jane a cure.

As we ambled down the narrow cobbled streets, the number of tatty shops selling even tattier religious artifacts multiplied. There were rosary beads of every colour, size and shape, luminous ones and ones so big that if you had them round your neck you'd have to crawl on the ground. Plastic Marys filled with holy water with screw tops for the heads sat alongside tacky casts of the grotto.

Arriving at the main square, Jane decided she would like to go to confession, which was advertised outside a modern functional building.

'How long will you be? Hours, I guess,' I said.

'You cheeky sod.'

'There you go, another Hail Mary.'

We entered a long corridor with doors for different languages. There were pews outside each one. Rebecca decided to join Jane in cleansing her soul. I left them to it.

Despite my complete scepticism of Lourdes, you couldn't help but be impressed with the thousands of people who had flocked there, especially the young, who were caring for the sick and infirm. Since Jane had been in the media, we had received a substantial number of letters offering all kinds of cures, homoeopathic remedies and religious solutions, all of which seemed to come at a price – and usually an exorbitant one. It made me extremely cross seeing the correspondence, because people were preying on the insecurities of some of the most vulnerable members of society. Who would not find it tempting to pay a few thousand pounds for a potential cure? Us.

After confession, Jane and Rebecca headed off to the grotto and then to be lowered into ice cold water to complete their Lourdes rituals. Steven, Suzanne and me settled for ice-cream.

JANE

We sat on the grass and watched the T-shirted men and women putting last minute touches to the stage. A golden crown was suspended centrally and either side were two large purple screens with Leeds emblems and another circular emblem for the Queen's Jubilee Baton Relay.

We had the whole area to ourselves; the only other people on the green expanse were the people setting up stalls. We stretched ourselves and headed for the gates to the backstage area before the quiet was broken. Backstage, there were children practising dance steps. They held aloft tribal-looking purple and red masks crossed with fierce white stripes. Two girls in front of us whispered words loudly, sidestepped, turned, laughed, stopped then started the same routine, nervously falling against each other.

We found a sunny spot and I spread my coat on the still wet grass. Placing my bag beside me, I sat and watched suited people with passes suspended around their necks scurrying around. One, with a pile of soft white towels, disappeared into the cabin to the right of us, then reappeared looking worried. I could hear him talk on his walkie-talkie to someone distant.

'There's no mirror in Lesley Garrett's dressing room. I've got the towels she wants but where can I find the mirror?'

An indistinct metallic reply blurted out over his walkie-talkie and a look of relief spread across his face as he hurried off to another white cabin and disappeared from view. I watched Steven and Rebecca as they peered around, taking in the festival atmosphere.

We could hear the PA system and the crowds gathering the other side of the fence. The concert started and we watched school children parade up the stairs to the stage. Rebecca disappeared down the side of one of the cabins and came back.

'That's Def Leppard down there. Do you think I'll be able to get their autographs?' she asked.

'I don't know, they look a little busy' I replied.

'Oh, come with me, Mum.' I reluctantly got to my feet and headed after her. A burly-looking security guard stopped us.

'I just wondered if the band would sign my daughter's programme,' I said to him.

'No chance, mate,' came the blunt reply.

'Sorry,' I said to Rebecca as we headed back to the area adjacent to the cabins. A woman in a paramedic's uniform stopped us.

'It's Jane, isn't it?' she asked.

'Yes,' I nodded.

She turned to Rebecca, 'I think your mum's marvellous.'

Rebecca looked bashful.

'Did you get Def Leppard's autograph?' asked the paramedic.

Rebecca shook her head fiercely. 'That big man dressed in black wouldn't let us anywhere near them,' she said.

'Oh, really? Come with me.'

We followed her back to the cabins and stood aside while she spoke to the security guard. He waved us through down the side towards the band.

'There's someone here who would like to meet you,' said our new-found friend, pushing Rebecca towards larger than life long-haired men. A group of older women were with them.

'Those are their mums,' the paramedic said. I smiled at the thought of internationally famous rock stars bringing their mums along to meet the Queen.

One of them caught sight of me. 'Ooh, it's that Jane Tomlinson,' she explained to her blond-haired son. 'That woman I was telling you about. You must let me get a photograph of you with her.'

I found myself bundled in amongst the denim-clad men, their mums snapping pictures of us together. Rebecca's face was frozen, her eyes rolling, shamefaced, as she held out her programme which they signed with enthusiasm.

The band manager stood to one side and greeted me, shaking my hand. 'If there's anything we can do before we go,' he said. I turned to thank our helper, who shrugged her shoulders. 'Oh, it's nothing. It's great to meet you, love. Keep up the good work.'

'Well, did they sign it?' Mike asked. Rebecca held out the white sheet with the band's autographs on. 'You'll never guess what, though, it was really embarrassing. They wanted their photos taken with Mum. They're just like celebrities and we're just like nobodies, but their mums were all like, "Ooh Jane."'

Mike burst out laughing, tickled by the thought.

We sat gazing as Charlotte Church was helped down off the stage. A tall lad at one side, another helper on her other arm, she stumbled nervously forward, teetering on high heels towards her dressing room. My attention was taken away from Charlotte's tottering walk as we heard raised voices coming from the other side of the stage back towards the parking area.

'I can't possibly walk all this way, it's ridiculous, why on earth can't the car be allowed back here.' Lesley Garrett walked past us looking aghast at the facilities on offer to her. Mike and I looked away, trying not to laugh out loud.

The police presence was heavier now the Queen had arrived. I peeped down the hill and I could just see her small frame being escorted on to the stage. I walked forward and the baton was placed in my hand, a long, chrome stem with a blue flashing centre. It was much bigger than I'd expected, and much heavier as well.

I held it aloft. The moment had come. I heard thundering orchestral music as I ran down the ramped grassway. The crowd to my right was enormous. There were thousands of people. The torch flickered and I looked up at it as I headed to the stage. The policewoman running at the side of me veered to the right, as I made my way up the ramp so that I was high above the crowds. I turned and held the torch for the crowd to see, before I turned towards the stage and walked towards the Queen. She stood, elegant in a green dress and a beautiful green and blue hat, broad brimmed with dark feathers curling across it. She wore a large brooch on her left lapel, strings of pearls around her neck matching her earrings. She stood regally straight and I passed the baton towards her. She reached out gloved hands. Prince Philip stood to my right and he greeted me.

'Well done,' he said.

I stood not knowing what to do next, then Mel B strode over and took the baton from the Queen. I curtsied, then stood to one side and watched as Mel B placed the baton into the stand. The chrome and glass podium started to revolve and from below the stage three pairs of silver arms supporting the stand for the baton rose till we could see where they attached to the three silvered figures that held aloft the symbol of the Commonwealth Games. The baton to commemorate fifty years for the Queen. The dark stage was lit by bright flashing lights, and the crowd roared.

MIKE

Suzanne pulled the cupboard door above the cooker forward to trigger the extractor fan. Rebecca was sitting on her knees at the dining table having just finished off her pasta, leaving only Steven without a clear plate.

'I've had enough, Mummy,' he said.

'Two more big boy mouthfuls,' said Jane, pushing her own plate away from her. He looked down at his teaspoon and shovelled in two loads quickly.

'Please can I leave the table?' he said.

'You can't take it with you,' we all chorused. Rebecca gathered some plates to stick in the dishwasher.

'How did you get on with Cancer Research today?' Jane asked. 'Did they sort out the interview times for next week?'

'No.' I shook my head. 'It's all gone a little pear-shaped so nothing has been arranged. I think I'll look after all the PR work from now, Jane,' I said. 'At least then we'll have a little more control. I can also make sure all the charity details go into the papers.'

Suzanne said, 'How was your swim this morning, Mum? How far did you go?'

Jane had been up at six to go to the International Pool to do a session before going to work.

'Okay. I did about a thousand metres. I'm getting a lot of pain doing front crawl. I think I'll end up doing breaststroke.'

'Wus. You should crawl,' Suzanne said.

'How have your headaches been?' I asked.

'Not too bad over the last couple of days.'

'Dad?' asked Suzanne. 'You know, the charity stuff is like a real pain sometimes. Why bother?'

'Because if Mum had been like this ten years ago she'd be dead now. It's only because of the work done by organizations such as Cancer Research that advancements in treatment are made. So although Mum's still going to die she is having a longer life.'

Cancer Research did a fantastic job. We'd see them regularly at St James's and they really helped. At the moment they were researching how a patient's quality of life could be affected by chemotherapy. Some of the treatment drugs at St James's which Jane had benefited from were funded from research monies. If we could raise funds to stop others suffering like Jane, it was worth it.

Jane turned around. 'I went to the building society today. The fundraising stands at twenty-six thousand pounds.'

'That's a huge amount, Mum,' said Suzanne.

'Let's see if we can get it to fifty thousand pounds after the tri.'

*

Driving towards Harewood House, Rebecca was barely speaking to either of us. She was at that age where parents could be extremely embarrassing. Jane's preparation for the triathlon was centring on cycling as it was her weakest discipline. She'd already done the thirty-kilometre Cancer Research Cycle for Life in Derby and Liverpool. Today in Leeds, Rebecca and I were to join her on a similar Cycle for Life using Luke's tandem.

We'd tested it out only once before, for about five minutes on the streets around Luke's house, which had been something of a disaster.

During the week before she made such a fuss – 'I'm not cycling with Dad!' – that I had arranged to wear a Pink Panther suit.

'You wouldn't dare!' she said. 'You'd look a prat!' I grinned back, inflaming her anger. Her persistence continued, so I arranged for a fluffy pink jacket for her to wear as well.

A game of bluff and double bluff ensued and by the time we were driving to Leeds she still didn't believe I would go through with it, so she was horrified when we arrived to see Nicki from Cancer Research carrying the Pink Panther costume in a cellophane cleaning bag together with Rebecca's jacket.

'I'm not wearing that! He's not dressing up as the Pink Panther!' she said, with a face like thunder.

Rebecca was right, I did look a prat, but the fact that the costume had a full face ensured that even my own mother would not be able to recognize me. We were asked to pose for a photograph.

'I am not having my picture taken with that!' pointed Rebecca. I revelled in her discomfort and bent over to try to hug her.

'Just go away, will you?!' she said.

'Don't you love me?'

'Just clear off, will you?'

After setting off, Rebecca and I got into a rhythm. The road to Collingham was flat and with the momentum of two pedalling we could eat up the yardage. The costume's tail was a nuisance, constantly in danger of getting caught in the spokes and so I ended up sitting on it. The weight of the bike combined with the warm Sunday morning made me drip with sweat.

By now the panther's head was off, hanging around my neck

and flopping down my back, thanks to my glasses constantly steaming up when pushing the beast of a bike up every hill.

Twenty minutes later, disaster struck and the chain came off. Bike upside down, I attempted to fix it, while Rebecca stood about ten yards away wearing an I'm-not-with-him expression.

Three miles from the finish we had to cycle down a long sweeping hill. Visibility was excellent; with no cars and at least a mile's clear view, I went for it. The draught whistled past our ears. Rebecca screamed from the back.

The wheels were spinning too fast for there to be any resistance on the pedals. We hit the bottom. I started pedalling again, but my legs swung round in free fall with no resistance. It was clear something was wrong.

'Dad! Dad! The chain's snapped,' Rebecca growled from behind.

We slowed down and I sent her back up the hill to collect the remnants of the chain. We had to walk the two miles back to Harewood House, me with the tandem, Rebecca a hundred metres behind, sobbing her eyes out.

By the time we reached the finish line, the costume was in a state. I was met by Jane, Steven, Mary and Karen with their respective families. My body felt like it had been in a steam room. My hands were caked in grease; the Pink Panther suit had thick black oil stains everywhere.

'Mike! What's happened? Where's Becca? We were just about to come and look for you,' said Jane.

'The chain snapped. Becca's behind. She's furious. We've walked the last couple of miles.'

Even from a hundred yards, Rebecca looked disgruntled, walking a snail's pace, with her blonde hair stuck to her forehead and the pink jacket open.

All she could say was: 'I'm humiliated, just so humiliated.'

Later that night with Steven in bed the rest of us were preparing for the new week; Rebecca polishing shoes, Suzanne folding her clean clothes into drawers, Jane changing sheets while I was ironing. The phone rang.

'Dad, it's Jon Colman for you.' Becca said.

I pulled the plug from the socket and shuffled past the basket and shirts hanging on the door. Jon and I had lived together for two years at Manchester Polytechnic, sharing a house in the third year with Mike Baldwin, and the Park cousins Fiona and Liz. We still spoke at least once a month, catching up when we could.

'How's your dad?' he asked.

'Much the same.'

'Jane?'

I sat down on the bottom step in preparation for a long conversation. 'She's good, it's the London Tri next Sunday.'

'I saw her in the paper, Tommo, the other day. Wish her luck, will you?' The conversation ambled. We discussed mutual friends, work and Burnley's new season. It sounded like he was speaking in a large quiet building, his voice bouncing from walls so I enquired where he was.

'I'm just away from home at the moment.'

'Where? It sounds really strange.'

'I'm in hospital. I've not been very well.'

'What's up? Are you all right? Why didn't you say?'

'I've tried to kill myself twice.'

There was a slight pause. Instinctively I stood up and shouted down the phone. 'You selfish bastard. What about your mum? How could you? You wanker. What were you thinking of? What about all the people who love you, your mum, your sister, friends?' I paced the floor waving my free hand as if he was stood next to me.

'I know, everything you say is right, Tommo. I know, but it makes no difference to how I feel.' His voice sounded distant, soulless.

'I had a friend from home commit suicide fifteen years ago, his mum's never got over it, no mum would. How can you be so bloody selfish?'

'I shouldn't have told you. You've enough on your plate with Jane and your dad.'

'Here I am losing my wife, she's desperately trying to live

longer, going through repugnant treatments and you just want to give your life away, you prick.'

'You've got the kids to keep going for, no one needs me.' I noticed Jane and Suzanne at the top of the stairs. I indicated for them to go.

'How could you? How the fuck could you? Feelings are temporary, Jon. Give it time. Eventually things will change. You don't know what's around the corner.'

As our conversation continued, I tempered my reaction, trying to empathise until we had agreed to speak later in the week. After he had hung up, Jane said that he must have known the reaction he'd get from me; that's why he had phoned. I wasn't so sure.

In twelve years of coming to St James's, the waiting area had improved considerably although it was still particularly uncomfortable. A water cooler had recently made a brief appearance, which had been a welcome addition, but it had soon been replaced with a television. When I asked a nurse why, she explained about the risk of impurities in water coolers, which could affect the health of the chemotherapy patients.

Steve Wright's radio show was being played through the speakers above our heads; the irrelevant ramblings seemed at odds with the gravity of the situation as some people sat waiting for important scan results. The noise was barely audible, which made it more irritating than soothing.

'Jane Tomlinson,' Dr Perren called out. He was a tall man who spoke quietly but with perfect clarity. He shook our hands and the consultation proceeded as normal. We received the results of today's blood tests and found out where we were with the scan cycles and Jane's pain control. It was clear that Jane's health was declining.

'I'm glad you've come in today anyway,' he said.

'Why's that?'

'I had a phone call from the *Yorkshire Evening Post* earlier wanting to confirm whether you'd died. I said I didn't think so as you were sitting in the waiting room no more than ten minutes ago.'

We sat together, both stuck for words. 'Where? How on earth? Who would have told them that?' Jane mumbled

'Seemingly, a member of the public had rung in from Wales, would you believe?'

'Wales? Wales? Why would someone from Wales ring the *Yorkshire Evening Post*? I don't believe it,' I said. 'We've had a whole series of freaks and nutters but no one's ever been that malicious. I'm glad the *Yorkshire Evening Post* didn't try to contact the kids.'

Mr Perren continued: 'When is the triathlon and what does it entail?'

'Sunday,' said Jane. 'It's a fifteen hundred metre swim, a forty kilometre bike ride and a ten kilometre run.'

'Mmm. Are you sure you want to do that?'

'Yep, I've been training for it really hard.'

'I'm sure you have. I'm not quite sure why anyone would want to do it, let alone you, but you will be careful, won't you?'

'Yes.' Jane sounded like a child trying to convince a parent that she wouldn't get into any mischief.

'Listen to your body, Jane,' he said.

'I will.'

'Well, keep on going and good luck.' He smiled, moved to the door and shook our hands.

Arriving home, we did a quick tidy up of the house before Carla from the BBC arrived. Jane slumped on a kitchen chair, the side of her head resting on the table.

'I don't want to do any more, Mike, I'm too tired.'

'I know.'

'Do you? Yesterday I went to work, went for a swim and did two interviews. Today work, hospital, another interview. Tomorrow work, swim, interview and then the running club. Thursday treatment, then run and two photo shoots at eight at night. I'm worn out. I'm dying. On Sunday I've got the triathlon after a full day of media interviews on Saturday.'

'This is it, Jane. We don't have to do anything else.'

'I'm not going to. You've taken over the PR and now it's relentless.' I put my hand on her shoulder.

'It's been successful.'

'Yes, you are good at it, too good at it. But you seem to forget I'm poorly.'

'Sorry.'

'Don't get any more publicity, Mike, it's too much.'

'Okay.' I headed off to the phone to ask Carla to delay her arrival for thirty minutes.

As we sat outside at the table in the garden, Carla miked Jane up and turned to me.

'Would you mind being interviewed as well?'

I looked at Jane and she smiled. 'Okay.'

'I'm just going to ask you how you think Jane will get on on Sunday,' she said.

Turning to Jane I said, 'What do you want me to say?'

'Whatever you want, you're a grown-up.'

'Do you want me to be honest?'

'Of course.'

So when questioned, I answered: 'Can't see how she'll manage it, to be truthful.'

Jane glared at the camera as though I'd just said I didn't love her. Her disappointment was clear. Shaking, she recovered her composure quickly. 'We'll see,' she said quietly. 'We'll see. I'd hope to finish.'

Walking home after last orders, Jane was still upset. 'I can't believe you said that.' She was looking down at the ground.

'You told me to be honest!'

'You could have been honest and not said that. My bloody shoulder has hurt ever since you said it and that's your fault!'

'It's psychosomatic,' I pointed out.

'For once in your life, couldn't you just have said that you thought I'd complete it? You've just ruined my confidence.'

'Stop fussing. Now no one will expect you to finish,' I joked.

The glare was fixed on me this time.

JANE

My legs taut with effort, there was sweat dripping into my eyes, stinging and blinding me. I brought myself more upright on the bike to give me enough control and wiped my eyes to clear them. I cycled on and on over long black roads following the white line into the distance. Losing my concentration, my foot slipped from the foot strap encasing my shoe and I lost control of the bike. As the front wheel twisted away from me I flew forwards over the handle bars. The black tarmac filled my vision just before impact.

My head whiplashed back against the pillow as the final tumble woke me. I could feel my heart beating; my whole body prickled with the rush of adrenaline. I sat up, disoriented in the dark and unfamiliar surroundings of the Docklands hotel. I felt my way to the bathroom and flicked the switch, the bright light illuminating the mirror. I held my hands out examining them for gravel rash from the fall, the dream still with me. I looked at them and slowly the dream faded. Tripping over my bag as I made my way back to bed, I cursed. Mike sat up. 'What's up?' he mumbled.

'Nothing, go back to sleep.' I pulled the covers over me and lay back going over the route in my head.

'I know I can do this,' I thought. 'If only I can get out of the water.'

Fear of the swim made my legs tremble underneath the covers. It was one thing swimming 1,500 metres in a pool, one lap at a time.

Yesterday, I'd stood and looked out across the dark mass of water of the Thames. Small waves raced across the surface as the wind blew through the docks. The yellow floats, signposting the route, contrasted against the smoothly rolling black of the water, its depths unfathomable as it lapped against the dockside. I thought I'd be reassured seeing the course in front of me, but seeing a mile set out before me in the docks, stretching into the distance, made me swallow dry-mouthed with nerves.

*

As we walked up the steps into the Excel Arena after breakfast, my legs and whole body were wobbly. I left the others dockside as I made my way back into the huge hangar. Losing my bearings, I looked round frantically for where I had left my bike the day before. Hundreds upon hundreds were stacked up in the vast arena. My eyes scanned the metal scaffolding, and my heart stopped racing when I found my numbered row and saw my bike and helmet were still there. I placed my drinks bottle in its cradle and laid out a towel along with my trainers – socks inside them – yellow running vest with my number already pinned to the front, and small cycling shorts. I placed another drink bottle beside the bike and looked around checking the entrance and exit once last time before rejoining my family.

I was speechless with the agitation, my mind flitting over all the tasks I still needed to complete. A video journalist, Carla, from the local BBC, was waiting to interview me to get my feelings on tape. I could only laugh nervously before I headed off to change.

I put my red swimming costume on and then I tugged my wetsuit up my body, leaving my arms free for the moment. It was time to find the holding area and join the other women setting off in my wave.

'Jane! Am I glad to see you!' Faye Banks and I fell into each other's arms, the same wide-eyed panic in our eyes.

'Happy birthday!' I said.

'Oh yeah, thanks for the pressie. It was in my room when we got back from our meal last night. We sat and ate all the chocolates, but saved the wine for tonight to celebrate.'

Heading down the stairs to the dockside, we watched as women climbed on to the black pontoon and dropped with a splash into the water.

'Good luck,' I said to Faye as I pulled my goggles on.

'You too,' she said and disappeared towards the red bobbing heads.

The water was cold and I lowered myself in, the icy grip tightening the base of my skull and the top of my neck, causing an intense headache instantly. I tried a few tentative strokes, submerged myself and swiftly lifted my head out of the water in breathless panic. The water was black. I could see nothing but the green swirls of tiny algae. The yellow buoys had seemed to make a mammoth course from the dry side of the docks.

Down in the water I could barely make out the first turn a mere 300 to 400 metres ahead. Maybe this was a bad idea. Actually this was a bloody bad idea.

A hooter sounded and the black water around me turned white with thrashing arms. A white wave led by red-hatted heads surged forwards. I swam front crawl but a foot crashed into me, splashing me. As I turned my head to the side to draw a breath I panicked, my mouth full of dirty dock water tasting of rotting plant matter.

'Shit! Shit! Shit!' I thought as I changed to breaststroke trying to calm myself and regulate my breathing. I was still gasping open-mouthed when another swimmer forced her way past me. Another bank of water washed over me. All the training went out of the window – the speed, the strength, the stroke, none of that mattered any longer. 'I can't do this,' the frightened demon in my head kept whimpering.

'Yes, you can, Jane,' I told myself and kept moving forwards with a clumsy breaststroke, the buoyancy of the wetsuit holding me high in the water, making me feel like a beached whale as I continued to pull myself onwards. 'Come on, Jane, you'll look a right prat if you don't even get to the first turn of the swim before giving up.'

I picked out a purple-backed wetsuit in front of me and concentrated on it, following it as it swam ahead of me. My heart stopped hammering and my breathing slowed, my strokes coming more easily as the yellow buoys passed by. I could see white, blue and red circles on the first, larger buoy and fixed on that, pulling and pushing, following the same swimmer. At the first turn, the swimmers clumped together again tightly around the buoy to swim back the way we'd come. My confidence grew and I tried a few strokes of front crawl but was panicked again by the total opacity of the darkened water. I lifted my head and resumed my flailing breaststroke, my only thought: 'You must

finish the swim, it doesn't matter how, you must just finish it.'
Another turn, round a large bobbing banana, and I knew I was
over halfway there.

The realization that I could finish the swim gave me the
courage to bury my head in the water and start a slow clumsy
front crawl. Now I could endure the darkness. I pulled alongside
another red hat and kept the swimmer to my left, breathing on
that side, stroke, breath, stroke, breath. With another swimmer
in view I no longer needed to sight the buoys to check my
progress. Finally, I was swimming the last length, the arena to
my right. I lifted my head to breathe and could hear my mum,
loud, vocal.

'Come on, Jane, come on, girl.' Her voice was clear above the
others in the crowd. 'Come on, Jane, come on, Jane,' she
screamed as I made my way to the pontoon. I could see people
being pulled from the water and put my head down again,
ploughing my way through the water towards the helping
hands.

Finally, I could feel the floating edge of the pontoon, slippery
and smooth, as I reached up and was grabbed by strong arms
plucking me from the water.

I hurried on to the red pavement, warm under my bare feet
and ripped my goggles and hat from my head. Half running, I
stumbled towards the 'swim exit' sign ahead, where a blue plastic bag was thrust into my hands, and I stopped, peeling my
wetsuit from my body, tugging it over my arms and legs.

Finally free from the rubbery second skin, I headed for the
stairs on my own, waving at my mum and Steven before leaving
the screams of my supporters behind me. Entering the arena, I
scanned the rows to locate my bike. I pulled on my shorts, vest,
shoes and socks and fastened my helmet. Lifting the bike down
from the rack, I rolled it towards the exit.

A line showed me where to mount. I climbed into the saddle,
put my feet into the toe straps and headed out towards the
road and the ramp down to the course proper. Bikes sped past
me as I pumped my legs as fast as possible, trying to rush
myself through the course. It was a little disheartening to see so

many whizz by, but this was my own race, I'd do it in my own time.

My legs were tiring as I pulled the final strip of tape from the handlebars, there to allow me to count the laps of the cycle course. Even so, I was confused, was this my last lap or did I have another to go?

No, no, it was definitely the last stretch as I looked at my watch to check. I swooped past the isolated brick building at the end of the course and headed down the slight incline. I slung myself low over the bike, lifting my head to watch the bridge zoom past overhead, then I resumed pedalling, making the most of my momentum to gain the top of the ascent.

A smile spread across my face as I slowed down for the tight bend round the roundabout. The arena in sight again, I knew I was within minutes of finishing the bike section and I'd only have the run to contend with.

Yes!

At the arena, I hung my bike back alongside other bikes, and removed my helmet. Grabbing the bottle of water I made my way to the run exit, my legs feeling heavy pushing myself forward by lateral movement of my hips rather than my normal forward action. My muscles still recovering from the past cycling action, I ran out of the red-clad barriers down the slope and headed towards the dockside.

'Keep going, Jane,' Faye greeted me as she ran past me on her inward section. I swivelled to yell encouragement back at her and then turned, gritted my teeth to keep moving and fought the pain of the stitch deep in my right-hand side.

Running along the dockside, I saw that the water to the right of me was now dark and undisturbed by swimmers. As I ran under the black arch of the huge painted cranes, I pushed my legs forward, forcing myself onwards, up the small ramp, which slowed me to walking pace as I re-entered the arena. Shouts echoed round the huge building as I headed back out for another lap down a small slope and then, as I ran painfully up another incline, I stopped, bent double with pain.

Mike's face loomed before me, his face lined with anxiety.

'Jane, are you okay? You can stop if you like.'

I looked at him. 'What? Now? Don't be so bloody stupid,' I said, panting with the effort of speech. I set off again, holding my side, then I bent over to try to ease the pain. Gradually it subsided and as I straightened up I could lengthen my stride and relax into my running.

Finally, the last lap came round. Up the small killer slope, I swung round to the red banners, hearing my name being called, and headed to the left, past the grandstand and towards the finish line. I ran through the finish, looking at my watch. I could only estimate my time but I was sure I'd beaten my target of three and a half hours.

Ecstatic, I ran through the bank of photographers towards the arms of Mike and Steven. Steven hugged me and Mike wrapped his arms round me. 'Well done, Jane, that was a fantastic effort. I can't believe you finished.'

The rising nausea subsided as I sat, my breath returning to normal. Sweat covered my face; my mum leant down to hug me. Suzanne and Rebecca stood either side of me. Katherine Merry came to speak to me. I barely recognized the short-haired 400-metre bronze medallist from the Sydney Olympics.

Her hair longer, dressed casually, she looked elegant and confident as she drew me to one side to interview me. 'You finished in just under three and a half hours, Jane,' said Katherine. 'That was your target, how does that make you feel?'

'I can't tell you how delighted I am. Not just to finish, but to finish in the time I set myself. I'm just really pleased,' I said, my legs trembling and my mouth feeling dry. Someone handed me a bottle of water, and Mike pushed a chair towards me so I could sit down before my knees gave way. The interview over, Katherine joined us and put her arm round my shoulder. 'Well done, Jane. That was some achievement.'

The week after running cross-country for Rothwell Harriers in the Leeds Country Way, Luke and I travelled up to the Dales.

'I've always fancied going on a tour of some kind, one where you end up somewhere different at the end of each day,' I had said to Luke after he had taken me on an exhilarating ride on his heavy black-framed tandem. Sitting behind him on the short frame, the speed as we dashed down the hill with the wind whipping past us was thrilling.

'That's funny 'cos I've always wanted to try out my tandem on a longer ride,' he'd said. That short conversation had grown into a four-day cycling trip around the Yorkshire Dales Cycle Way.

'Would you fancy doing something like this, only longer?' I said at the end of the trip. Luke glanced at me.

'What did you have in mind?' he asked.

'A long bike tour to raise funds for charity, something like John o'Groats to Land's End,' I said.

'You are joking!' he said. He looked at me, realizing I was serious. 'It would be a bit of a laugh, though,' he said.

He sat, lost in thought. 'I'm up for it, if you reckon you can manage,' he said. 'I wonder how long it would take?'

'I reckon about three weeks but I'll have to wait and see how I am on the chemo.'

MIKE

'Is that Mike Tomlinson?' I recognized the Blackburn accent on the phone immediately even though our paths hadn't crossed for ten years. Within an instant I knew the reason for the call.

'Yes.'

'Mike Tomlinson who went to Manchester Polytechnic?'

'Yes.'

'It's Mike Baldwin, how are you, pal?'

'Okay.'

'I've got some bad news for you.' I knew what was coming. 'I'm afraid Jon died on Friday. I'd have let you know sooner but we've been searching for your number.'

Realizing what had happened those two seconds earlier had gone some way to cushioning the blow and I was able to keep my reactions considered. But my stomach was in turmoil.

'I guess it's too early for a funeral date to be set.'

'Yes. Some practicalities need sorting. It'll probably be next week at the earliest.'

'I'll ring his mum tomorrow; I'll call you later this week.'

Mike gave me his number and we said goodbye. How in the eighteen years since Polytechnic had all his hopes been extinguished? Jane appeared at my shoulder, Suzanne at the top of the stairs.

'Jon Colman's dead,' I said and began to cry.

'I'm so sorry, Mike,' said Jane, putting her arms around me. I eased away from her embrace.

'I need some time on my own,' I said. 'I'll go for a walk.'

'Do you want me to come with you?'

'No.'

I needed to release the grief unaccompanied, so after I'd composed myself a little. I grabbed my jacket and headed out of the door, down the drive and along the road. It was that time of year that once the sun has disappeared, the evening chill can go right through your bones.

Racked with guilt, I wandered home. However many newspapers had described Jane as inspirational, neither of us could inspire and save the one person close to us.

At home, Jane was preparing Steven's schoolbag for the start of the next week.

'What shall we do about the Great North Run?' I said.

'Let's just think about it,' she said. It was the usual response from Jane, measured, pragmatic, no knee-jerk reaction. 'What would Jon have said?'

'He'd have said run. Do you remember when he turned up after the Sheffield Half Marathon? He could hardly walk? We went for a pint and he could only manage orange juice.'

'I went for my first run with him,' I said.

'I didn't know that.'

'Yeah, around Didsbury Park campus in our first year. Let's see how we feel later in the week. Whatever happens I'll ring his mum tomorrow.'

*

When I arrived home from work on Monday, Jane was rushing around putting her training kit in the washing machine. We were supposed to be going to London to do some pre-publicity for the run on Wednesday. Media interest had gathered pace since the triathlon. That was my fault really as I'd tried so hard to build it up.

'Mike, *The Sunday Times* rang, they'd like to do a piece this Sunday in the Sports section,' said Jane.

'What did you say?' I was never sure whether Jane would agree to interviews. Many a time it was just down to the moment or to the manner of the request.

'I said yes. It's someone called Rob Hughes. He's in Athens seemingly.'

'Okay,' I said, making my way up the stairs and throwing my bag on the floor of the bedroom.

'I'm going to phone Jon's mum,' I said.

My heart was racing as I dialled. I didn't know what to say or how she would react. I'd met her on a number of occasions over the years; it would have been a coward's response not to call.

Jon's mum answered, her prim voice sounding fragile.

'Hello, Mrs Colman, it's Mike Tomlinson.'

'Oh, Michael, it's good of you to call.'

'I'm so sorry for your loss. Jon was a good man. I'm really going to miss him.'

'He was a lovely son, Michael.'

'He was a very gentle, kind man. I'm so sorry I couldn't do anything to help him, I wish I could have.' My voice started to croak betraying the tears that were forming.

'Oh there was nothing any of us could do.'

We shared reminiscences of Jon; she was so gracious in her words, showing a strength I didn't have.

I was uplifted by the conversation but coming off the phone I cried, overcome with emotion. Jane had sat next to me on the bed and listened for the last ten minutes. She hugged me and immediately the phone rang again. It was Rob for Jane's interview, so I went downstairs. After some time, she called down to me: 'Rob would like to speak to you!'

For twenty minutes Rob interviewed me in a way no previous journalist had. He was not afraid to ask searching questions although there was no sense of it being invasive. Putting the phone down, I was remarkably buoyed with two contrasting conversations one after the other. Jon's mum's words, 'Of course you must run. We'll be glued to the telly, we're all so proud of Jane' resonated around my head.

Jane's achievements had been covered in most sections of the newspapers – news, health, features – but never in the sport section, but it was the latter that seemed a more natural home. Questions of fitness and training and how the demands of cancer affected these were important issues to many people. *The Sunday Times* were going to be the first newspaper to run such a story. Although even in full health, Jane would never have been anything other than a good club runner, the cancer brought out a fierce determination and an ability in her to manage pain that I'd never seen in anyone.

An occasionally asked question by friends and reporters, though not by Rob, was whether she could compete in the Paralympics? Jane's standard response was: 'What? The terminally ill race? They'd be constantly changing the line-up because of too many last minute withdrawals.'

The journalist would invariably look aghast, failing to notice Jane's humour.

'Well, they should give their questions more consideration,' Jane would say.

A hectic week of media work behind us, it was a relief to get to Newcastle for the Great North Run on Friday afternoon. Jane and I were fiercely competitive over who would win. Over the last four weeks, acts of bravado had been commonplace. We each ran a three-and-a-half mile circuit in training, coming back with different times which would lop chunks off our personal best. Obviously I cheated and always exaggerated the times and I assumed Jane was doing the same.

'I'm going out for a run, Mike, just two miles, keep the legs ticking over,' she said within half an hour of getting to Tyneside.

'Good, I'm not.' I was supremely confident that I didn't need any extra training, I'd done enough. Within twenty minutes she was back looking remarkably fresh.

Waking on race day, I looked over across the Tyne. The weather was perfect, no wind, and pleasantly warm for October. Jane was already flitting about the room, preparing her kit and getting ready for breakfast.

Postponing chemotherapy so she could do this race was beginning to look like rather a stupid idea. Over the weeks leading up to the race, we'd constantly questioned the wisdom of the decision to run, but we were so aware of all the efforts being made by the organizers that we felt it would be somewhat ungrateful to back out. We had a chance of raising a lot of money for the fund, so it was a risk we were prepared to accept.

'Nervous?' I asked.

'No, it's only thirteen miles, hardly a training run.' I knew she was playing with my mind, knowing she'd run longer distances than I ever had.

'Sure you're not nervous? There's a lot of pressure on you,' I said.

'No, I'm fine, it's you that should be nervous.'

As we made it across the starting line there was a chorus of 'Jane! Jane!' as press photographers ran over to take her picture. Everything had to be done in a rush, that minute, for them. Jane posed and smiled as requested and, with just a couple of snappers left, one asked, 'Jane, just stretch against that advertising hoarding!'

As she did, it collapsed. It was an ungraceful moment as, bandy-legged, Jane struggled not to end up on her backside. Two minutes of attention from the photographers was all over as their interest changed to a bigger name runner.

A few people from the crowd recognized Jane, calling her over to shake her hand and wish her good luck. I was finding it difficult to feel at ease.

Jane, despite all the boasting, I knew was too ill to run. This knowledge was making me feel sick as I watched her nervously prepare for the start. She had so much to lose by competing today. The marathon would be forgotten if she failed today. We knew that the BBC had used Jane in the opening sequence to their live programme so they would be featuring her running. Sky and Yorkshire Television were also there, as well as some papers – so this could be a very public failure; too much for a dying person. Putting as much distance between myself and the celebrity runners as possible, I'd have gladly melted into the crowd behind. A gentleman wandered up.

'Mike, I'm your chaperone!' Suddenly, I recalled a conversation with the organizers the night before when we'd been told that Jane and I were to have a chaperone each, with a spare running between us, advising Jane's running partner as to where I was. I thought they'd been joking.

'I don't need a chaperone, thanks,' I said.

'You're due to have an interview at six miles, I've got to make sure you get there okay.'

I'd thought that was a joke as well.

'Is Jane being interviewed?'

'No, just you.'

There had been some banter last night about how they could ensure Jane won. I envisaged the race going horribly wrong.

Just before the start, the club runners moved forward. We were now packed tight, my shoulders squashed at either side. Forty thousand people stood behind me, all anxious not to lose much time at the start. I knew as soon as the hooter sounded, huge numbers of much faster runners would swarm past and I was conscious that I needed to get to the inside quickly.

Off! Four lanes of athletes began sprinting down the hill. At the first mile marker I checked my watch. Seven minutes and fifteen seconds – a suicidal pace for me. Jane was out of sight but I was confident I'd reel in the distance. At three miles I saw her fifty yards ahead to my right. Should I move on to her shoulder now? Make her dispirited? Let her confidence ebb away? No, better to sit just behind and attack in the last mile.

What's she doing? Her pace had increased. Let her go. I could see her slowly move away and before long I was losing sight of her within the crowd. We filtered across a roundabout, I took the shortest route. Seeing a water stop I moved to reach out an arm to grab a bottle.

At six miles, I stopped for the interview and I stood waiting for Emmerdale actor, Chris Chittell, to finish talking. I ran on the spot, becoming frustrated at the length of time it was taking. My body began to feel cold. I considered skipping the interview but checked myself – no, Mike that's not the point, we're here to raise money. I knew Jane was stretching her lead at 200 yards a minute and my anxiety grew. My only concern was to get back on the road and to limit the damage.

At mile ten, I asked my running partner the time. One hour twenty. I knew it was too fast and I would soon pay a price. By the time I'd reached the seafront at South Shields the game was up. Crossing the line, I knew Jane had beaten me. It took me thirty minutes to find her. We hugged and it was a relief to see her safe. We exchanged times. Jane had beaten me by two and a half minutes, exactly the duration of the interview.

Not one press photographer had caught Jane at her finish. The BBC, the host broadcaster, missed her as well, but not Sky News who jumped in for an interview first. No one had expected such a quick time.

'Jane! Will you do the last one hundred yards again?' shouted a voice from the press pack.

Jane screwed up her face and shook her head.

'My body's gone cold, I'm stiff, no, I'll get injured.' I smiled inside. Injured? You're dying of cancer, love.

'Go on, Jane, the desk will want photos of you finishing,' said the voice.

'I've just run thirteen miles,' she replied.

I walked over, seeing her point, but also knowing the photographers still needed their picture. I'd been told £15,000 worth of donations had been received during the race.

'Come on, Jane,' I whispered. 'A few yards won't matter.'

So the charade was played out. Jane held her arms aloft, barely a runner in sight, looking remarkably fresh.

'My head went at mile eleven, Mike,' she said later. 'I thought I was going to collapse.'

'Time for chemo, Jane? Was it worth postponing it?'

'Yeah. I've had an unbelievable time,' she said. 'We've raised a lot of money and created some tremendous memories for the kids. I ran a good time. It's just a shame I didn't get one hour forty-five.'

Shaking my head I said: 'One hour forty-five.'

'I can't believe how well we've been looked after. They couldn't have made it a better weekend.'

I took the ribbon off my shirt and said a silent prayer. 'For you, Jon,' I thought.

JANE

All the way round the Great North Run I'd experienced episodes of light-headedness. Looking over the heads of the runners in front, the sky had somersaulted round and I wasn't sure if my legs would just go from underneath me. It had been a relief to see the finish line.

The dizziness persisted into the next day. Waking up, I put my foot down on to the floor and pushed myself from the bed with trepidation. Would my legs hold? I weaved unsteadily to the bathroom, where I showered, soaping my side delicately, not wanting to disturb the pain deep in my ribs.

'Are you going to mention the dizziness to Dr Perren tomorrow?' asked Mike at he watched me preparing tea, the concern in his eyes not matched by any practical endeavours.

'Yes. I thought it would be better today,' I replied.

'Are you worried?'

'No, not too much, besides I'm starting chemo this week. We knew I was ill, that's why I need the treatment.'

*

Dr Perren listened, concern on his face, as I told him how I felt. He examined me and listened to my breathing. He checked my reflexes and the strength in my legs by lifting my limbs and asking me to pull and push away from him. I dressed and seated myself opposite him.

'I want to book an MRI scan of your head to make sure there is nothing that can be causing this unsteadiness,' he said. 'I confess I'm a little puzzled by it. How's your breathing?'

'That's fine. I've got more pain in my back and sides, but that's something I've been aware of and that's just been worsening gradually.'

'You're due some radiotherapy, is that right?'

'Yes, I'm off to Cookridge tomorrow. They're going to mark me up and treat me at the same time.'

'Good, well that should help the shoulder. You're starting Vinorelbine this week. You know what to expect with that? It's usually well tolerated but I'll make sure you're prescribed some anti-sickness medication. The nausea shouldn't be too much of a problem.'

I nodded my understanding.

'Right, we'll review you next week. Hopefully we should have some scans booked as well.'

Mike and I rose and we shook Dr Perren's hand before leaving the room. I was frightened about undergoing radiotherapy for my bone disease, unsure whether it would cause more problems than it would cure. I remembered the day after one radiotherapy session when I'd experienced hiccups, pain and sickness and didn't know what to expect this time.

I needn't have worried. It was fairly straightforward. I was examined, marked up for treatment, given a very small tattoo for alignment for further treatment and then had just a short wait for the radiotherapy machine to be free. I was told not to expect any pain relief for a few weeks, went home and tried to relax, knowing that my chemotherapy was starting the following day.

So used by now to the weekly routine of my Herceptin, this routine was little different, just another infusion and some anti-sickness drugs to reduce the chance of nausea. I was relieved that my arm felt okay. I had been warned that I might get some local soreness near the injection sight, but it felt all right. I was drowsy and felt fuzzy-headed, unable to concentrate and tired, so after watching my family eat supper which I had no stomach for, I retired to bed to sleep off the traumas of the day.

Mike and I dressed in sombre clothes and said goodbye to Mum. The children were all at school and we were travelling to Fleetwood for Jon's funeral. My mum was concerned that I was going, as I was still feeling groggy after the chemotherapy the day before.

'You don't have to come,' said Mike, 'no one will mind.'

'I will,' I said. 'I can't go back and do this day again. Jon was a good friend, and I want his mum to know how much every one admired her son.'

We sat midway down the church and listened to the readings. Jon's mum stood and talked about him without tears. I had not expected to be attending the funeral of one of our friends. It had seemed so likely that Mike and I would be preparing our children for the loss of their mum, now here we were watching a mother's tears for her child.

None of us know how our lives will be. I had spent the months since my illness trying to make the most of the life I had. I looked around at the people gathered and wondered how many of them felt the same since hearing of Jon's death.

After the ceremony, we followed the slow procession of cars through the town to the graveyard. I looked out at the head-stones, some too far away to read the inscriptions, a reminder that we're all less important than we think we are, a certainty we will all one day go from life to death. Our work colleagues will soon have another person to fill our position, their daily routine unchanged. Our families will grieve but emerge from their sorrow to carry on their lives, the natural rhythm of every-one's lives ruffled for a moment and then levelled out.

We left the family to their grief and sat in the car, our faces taut with the sorrows of the day. Lost in our thoughts, we set off to join others at a sad last supper. I wasn't hungry but I ate to reduce the growing nausea in my stomach, hoping that the food would ease the strange light-headedness. My arm was painful and the tightness in my fingers and deep throbbing pain that I'd refused to acknowledge during the Mass and burial could not be ignored any longer. I pulled back the sleeve from my jumper and Mike gasped in horror. My arm was a web of red veins so painfully swollen that I could identify the crimson pathways up to my elbow. So turgid, I could make out the two leaves of the valves along the trammelled lines.

'That doesn't look too good, Jane,' said Mike. I thought about trying to make light of it, unwilling to make a fuss, but the redness and the soreness frightened me. The last time I'd experienced anything like this was the episode two years ago when I'd had septicaemia.

'I guess I should ring the hospital for some advice,' I said, tracing the meandering patterns on my arm.

'No, I think we should set off home and take you in to see somebody.'

I shrugged. My illness made me more dependent on Mike, but I wasn't ready to travel home straightaway. 'I'm not leaving yet. We need to speak to Jon's mum and see a few of his other friends. We'll set off in thirty minutes, okay?'

Mike's expression told me it wasn't, so I gave him my best hard stare and turned my back on him to stop any further discussion.

We managed a few words with most people and left, Mike flooring the accelerator in his rush to get back to Leeds, only to find ourselves caught in a huge curling snarl of traffic, the red lights stretching in front of us. Mike cursed as we edged little by little across the Pennines. After checking my arm as I put my coat on I hadn't looked at it again.

We arrived home to find Rebecca and Steven eating their tea in stormy silence, Mum standing edgily in the kitchen daring them to refuse the meal. 'That's perfectly good toast,' she said to Steven, whose eyes were glossy with tears.

'But Mum cuts the crusts off,' he wailed.

'Come on now, Steven, eat up, that tea looks lovely,' I said.

'And how are you?' my mum asked, the strain showing in her voice.

'My arm's sore, I'm just going upstairs to ring the hospital for some advice. Are you around if we need some help?'

'I did wonder about you going today. It would be nice to get home for tea tonight but I'll stay if you need help.'

'Thanks, Mum,' I said, ignoring the slight edge to her voice.

There was no need for me to go into hospital. A prescribed ointment helped and the swelling and redness faded over the next few days, but my arm was still painfully sore at the end of each day. It ached, my finger joints were uncomfortable, my wrists stiff. I was due another injection in just a few days. I was coping well with the chemotherapy, just slight nausea and tiredness, but I didn't know how I would manage the pain every week.

On the Tuesday, during my next visit to Dr Perren, I broached the subject of ways around this.

'There are a couple of options open to you,' he said. 'You could have a peripheral line put in or a Hickman line.'

I looked at Mike, whose furrowed brow must have prompted Dr Perren to continue. 'We could put a thin tube into Jane's veins. It would be long enough to end up in one of her bigger veins and reduce the chances of the inflammation occurring.'

'Those are open to a risk of infection, aren't they?' I said, screwing my face up. Dr Perren nodded. 'If I had one of those, I'd not be allowed to work in the X-ray department,' I said. I had already discussed the topic with Gill, and would have to be signed off sick.

'Why don't they put in a portacath?' she'd suggested. This was similar to the Hickman line but had the advantage of having a small port that was placed under the skin. A needle could be placed into this port to give me treatment and when the needle was taken out, I'd not be open to any infections. It was worth asking.

'Is there any chance of having a portacath?' I asked.

'We use those a lot on the teenage unit,' Dr Perren said. 'But not so much here. It might be a solution,' he continued. He sat thinking about it. 'Let me go and have a word with someone from the IV team.'

He disappeared and Mike and I sat in silence. He returned a few minutes later.

'Well, they've confirmed the difficulties they have cannulating you, so I don't see why not. You'll need to come into a ward for that, so I'll write to your surgical team. Mr Lansdown's secretary will be in touch when they can fit that in.'

I thought I might have a lengthy wait for the portacath to be fitted, so I was surprised to receive a phone call later that week. Mr Lansdown was available on Sunday. If there was a bed on the surgical ward I'd be admitted on the Saturday. I was pleased, but very scared as well; unsure whether this would be the answer or whether it would give me problems, with more pain in the arm that was already sore.

CHAPTER 13

JANE

The call came early on the Saturday. My anxiety over the procedure was heightened as they wheeled me into theatre the following day. Liz, a radiographer whom I had worked with on many occasions, was there to screen with X-rays the line to check its final position.

'Hello, Jane,' she said cheerily. I had tried all morning to keep this small operation in perspective, but as the sight of a familiar face, I burst into tears. Embarrassed by my childishness, I collected myself just as Mr Lansdown appeared. Placing a probe on to my skin, his face turned from me, concentrating on the screen showing the anatomy revealed by the ultrasound scan. The anaesthetist held my hand bent and pushed a needle into the vein. As the drugs flooded into my arm, the room began to blur, everything slowed down and the bright lights faded.

My right arm was sore when I woke, but I felt refreshed as if after a deep sleep. I sat for the chest X-ray, which was taken to ensure my lung had not collapsed as a result of the line being placed. There were no complications from the procedure and I was glad to leave the ward, relieved that everything had gone smoothly.

The letterbox banged as the envelopes slid to the floor. I glanced through them, yet more credit card offers and then a white envelope flagged with the BBC logo in red. It was addressed to me, the postmark London.

I slipped my finger under the corner and opened it. Inside was an invitation, for Mike and me, to the BBC Sports Personality of the Year Awards in December. I reread the letter. There was no mistake. I dialled Mike's work number to pass on the news.

'Yes!' Mike shouted down the phone, exuberant at the invitation. I held the phone away from my ear, and waited for him to calm down. 'Sporting peers! You! Where are they going to find someone to match your sporting prowess?' he said.

Donning my fleece, winding my scarf around my neck and pulling on my woolly hat, I turned to an embarrassed Suzanne.

'Thanks for coming with me, Mum, but do you have to look like that?' she said, smiling.

'I'm taking no chances, it's freezing in Hull, especially in this wind.' We sat on the small commuter train as it rocked along the flat railway to the east, then boarded a bus to the university. Suzanne shivered in her thin coat as we followed written directions to the philosophy department. We found ourselves in a small seminar room and stood together chatting with other parents and prospective students. Lecturers made their way round introducing themselves before herding us down the corridor to a large lecture theatre.

A multitude of questions were answered, fees, accommodation, practicalities for the novice parents and future students. Then it was time for the parents to be separated from their young ones. I escaped and found myself outside again. I walked alongside the railway line, glancing nosily at the private house which I had once shared with other students.

I set off, braving myself against the icy wind, walking through the estate and past the playing fields. Back in the seminar room, I caught sight of Suzanne deep in conversation with a staff member, and waited patiently for her to finish.

'Hi Mum,' she said. 'I'm really impressed. The course sounds really good. I've got some information about scholarships.

There's no guarantee, but if I fill it out I might get some help with funding. '

We sat on a bench waiting for the bus as the daylight faded. Suzanne shivered, her teeth chattering with cold.

'You'll need your thermals if you come here,' I said.

'I'm saving up for some thick socks and some walking boots,' she answered. I watched the queue of students making their way from the bus stop, amused to see that they were all firmly encased in thick unbecoming coats, woollen hats pulled down over brows. How different from the fashionable parade in Leeds; comfort and warmth seemed to be more important here. Finally, a bus arrived, only thirty minutes late. We sat squashed together on a narrow seat looking out at the shop fronts lit up in the dark as we made our way back to the station to catch our train home.

MIKE

Pulling out of Leeds Station, dawn was beginning to break but a low mist, a remnant of Bonfire Night, hung over the city. Jane and I were attending the launch in London of Cancer Research's Race for Life's tenth anniversary. We had jumped at the chance. The Cancer Research event team had given us tremendous support all year and if we could do anything to return the favour, then great. We'd already agreed Jane's image could be used on their adverts to help them recruit people to run for them in the London Marathon. A big dilemma for us was the control we had over Jane's images; we didn't want photographs appearing on adverts after Jane died. So if something was for a charity and for a finite time, we would consider it. Other requests we dismissed without consideration.

Jane looked done for, yet it was just after seven o'clock, not a good omen. She had started chemotherapy and, although the treatment wasn't intensive, it still left her drained. We'd planned to do nothing after the Great North Run but shut the doors and hibernate over the winter. Instead, rather than slowing down,

we'd moved up a gear with invitations to dinners, award ceremonies and functions. Some invitations were so spectacular,
how could we refuse? Others were charity-based and we wanted
to help.

Sighing, Jane looked as though she had the weight of the
world on her shoulders.

'My body's sore. I'm nervous about giving the speech.'

'Are you fed up with doing the charity work?'

'Not at all.' She shook her head. 'I'm thrilled to be doing this
today. I started at the Race for Life. The more people they can
attract to do it the better for everyone. What about you? Most
of the burden falls your way.'

'I'm fine.'

'What date is your works dinner?' she asked.

'The first of December, but we don't have to go.'

'We do, how often do *you* get an award? Oh Mike, I'm so
unwell. I feel worse than I ever have before. I'm dying.' She
started to sob and rested her head on the table, her face cush-
ioned with her hands.

'Yes, I know. I remember them telling us.' I smiled. 'They
were a bit out with their timing though.'

There was no smile on Jane's face as she lifted it up: 'I don't
think I'll live long enough to go to the BBC Sports Personality.'

Gently stroking her head, I didn't say anything. Jane was
never one to overdramatize things. I knew things were getting
desperate though I hadn't appreciated just how far her health
had declined. That she thought she'd die in a month, I'd had no
idea.

JANE

The week disappeared in a round of hospital visits, CT scans, Dr
Perren and chemotherapy. The portacath took away the terror
of needles jabbing into the back of my hand and although it
looked barbaric as they pushed a needle into the top of my arm,
it was much easier to bear. The other advantage was no soreness

in my arm. Because the drugs were being pushed into a large vein, I didn't experience the same inflammatory response.

The weekly chemotherapy routine was tiring, all the more so as there was no break. The constant feeling of nausea each week was relentless and it didn't help that I knew that the stupor of tiredness would last for several days. Chemotherapy on a Wednesday, then sleep on Thursday, back to work on Friday. This week I did without the rest and the whole family travelled to Sheffield with me to watch me receive my postgraduate certificate in paediatric medical imaging.

One of the first people I spotted when I walked into the building was Christine Ferris, all smiles.

'I told you you'd be here,' she said, chiding me affectionately. We'd kept in touch after I had handed in my final piece of work in January, and she knew how ill I felt. 'I'll be around to show the radiography students down to the stage. If you need anything give us a yell.'

'We'd better go and find our seats,' said Mike. I nodded and headed out of the hall in the direction of the robing room. The large room had tables set out around it. I handed over my receipt and was shown to a table laden with black mortar boards, a rack of black gowns behind it.

The gown felt heavy on my shoulders and I had to stoop to stop the angled board from falling. As I returned to my seat, glancing up above me to try to catch sight of Mike, the kids and my mum. The hall was packed with proud parents and partners of those there to receive their rewards to recognize the hours, days and weeks of study.

Having been to so many award ceremonies recently, this felt much more like something I'd earned. All the work I'd written up, the hours of literature searches I had done. This was a qualification I'd worked so hard over the last two years to gain, not something presented to me for getting on with my life in the only way I knew how.

MIKE

Like most degree ceremonies, it had been a dry affair. Pulling up for a pub lunch, the recording of Steven's voice I'd put as my mobile ring tone shouted out: 'Get that phone, Dad, 'cos it's ringing!'

Jane scowled. 'Don't be long, Mike.'

She and the kids went inside the pub while I took the call.

'It's Jo from the BBC, Mike.' The name or the Irish accent wasn't familiar. 'David Hart said I may be calling?'

'Ah, yes.'

'How much has he explained to you?'

'He told me about the BBC presenting Jane with the Helen Rollason Award at the Sports Personality of the Year. Then Cancer Research rang me yesterday to say she'd only been nominated, so I'm a bit confused.'

'Well, I can confirm she's getting the award – and apologies for the confusion – but we didn't want Cancer Research to know so we put up a smokescreen. We'd be grateful if you could leave it as a surprise for her on the night.'

'No problem. I think it would totally faze her anyway if she knew.'

'We'd like to do interviews with all the family together without Jane knowing, if that's at all possible?' Jo continued.

'We can't even make a cup of tea without Jane knowing.'

She laughed. 'Is there any way we could work round it?'

'The only realistic time we could do it would be Wednesday morning, but it would be a logistical nightmare.'

'How could we do it?'

I walked round the car park in circles while we discussed practicalities before Jane appeared at the pub door.

'Mike. Now.' She didn't look like she'd be willing to negotiate. I cut off my conversation with Jo quickly, racking my brain for excuses as to why I'd been on the phone for so long.

'Who was that?' asked Jane.

'A freelance journalist, she wanted an interview, wouldn't take no for an answer.'

Suzanne frowned. Jane continued, 'It didn't look like that to me.'

'Well, seeing as you weren't the one on the phone, how do you know?'

'Which magazine?' She had obviously scented some deceit.

'What?'

'She must have a magazine in mind, which one?'

'It was generic, I think she was just on a fishing trip.'

'Why now?'

'What?'

'Why now? What has prompted her to ask now?'

'I dunno. Probably something to do with the Cancer Research launch. Who's to say what goes on in the mind of a freelance journalist? Anyway, what's for dinner?'

'Have you turned that phone off? It's rude to have it on at meal times.'

The kids were all strangely silent, obviously intelligent enough to realize that now was not the time to make a clever comment.

The only sensible choice was to film the interviews while Jane was having treatment in hospital. That way we could rest assured that she would not come home and interrupt us. I had decided not to mention anything to the kids too far in advance, worried they might slip up and spoil the surprise, so I decided to tell them the night before the film crew were due to arrive.

'Where's Mum?' Rebecca asked.

'At the gym,' said Suzanne. 'Don't you listen?'

'No one told me.'

'Mum did, at tea time.'

'No, she didn't.'

'She did.'

'Didn't.'

I'd had enough. 'Will the pair of you stop bickering for two seconds? Listen, the BBC want to film us at home saying nice things about Mum.'

'Yeah, right,' laughed Suzanne.

'No, really,' I said. 'Mum's getting an award at the Yorkshire Sports Awards on the first of December.'

Suzanne looked sheepish. 'I don't want to, I hate being on television.'

'Look, Steven and I have already done one interview a couple of weeks ago, but the BBC would really like to get a whole family one as well.'

Rebecca was suddenly incandescent. 'What? Steven knew? He's not said anything.'

'He's not got as big a gob as you,' said Suzanne.

'Get lost!' Rebecca chucked a sofa cushion at her sister. 'Why Steven?'

'Because he was due for a hospital appointment and it was a kind of accident that he just happened to be around that day.'

The two girls looked at each other, disgruntled that they had not been let into the secret earlier.

'Listen,' I said. 'The plan is that, Becca, you'll set off to school as normal tomorrow and wait at the bottom of the road. Suzanne, you go five minutes later, meet Becca and then walk up to Jo's. I'll drop Steven off at Jo's, drive Mum to hospital, pick you all up and then drive home. The crew are coming at nine-thirty.'

'What about Steven?' asked Rebecca.

'He doesn't know. And don't tell him. He'll only know when he gets to Jo's.'

Suzanne nodded. 'All right, but I'm not saying anything. Mum's going to go mental, though. She went mad with you when you kept the Yorkshire Awards a secret.'

The crew arrived promptly the following morning and the filming was over surprisingly quickly. We needed the crew out of the house by twelve o'clock at the latest, just in case Jane's treatment had been unusually rapid. As the crew were preparing to leave, Jo addressed the kids.

'Are you all coming down to London for the awards?'

I felt the colour drain from my face.

'London?' said Suzanne.

Like a parrot in the background, Rebecca said, 'London?'

Jo sought to clarify the confusion. 'Yeah, for the Sports Personality Awards. Didn't your dad say?'

I could feel myself sinking further and further into a hole as Suzanne spun round and faced me.

'You said the Yorkshire Sports Awards. You liar!'

I forced a smile and looked to Jo for support. 'Your mum is being given the Helen Rollason Award at the BBC Sports Personality of the Year Awards.'

They both looked stunned. All they could say was 'Wow.'

'They're not invited,' I said to Jo.

'I can't guarantee anything, but I'll see if I can get them seats.'

After she'd gone, Suzanne turned to me.

'I can't believe how many lies you've told. You are so dead. What was the filming with Steven about then?'

'That was the Yorkshire Sports Awards. They've also secretly filmed her at the Roundhay Five Mile Run.'

'So is Mum getting two awards? And she doesn't know about either?'

'No.'

They both shot me stern looks.

It was a relief to get to 1 December. Jane was still alive and the chemotherapy seemed to be having an effect.

It was a damp morning, and we found ourselves amidst another crowd of runners. Hundreds of breaths were forming a small cloud, the smell of liniment was heavy in the atmosphere.

Wellington Street was heaving with people all ready to start the Abbey Dash. Jane's ability to keep training through her chemotherapy had been a revelation and the fact that she was now on the starting line with Mick and me was a surprise to us all. We'd deliberately kept her entry a secret to avoid any media interest.

As we set off, Jane dropped to the back. It was a good day to be running but, even so, I was glad when I passed over the inner city ring road towards the finish about fifty minutes later. Deciding to wait for Jane, I hung back, squinting down the road for a sight of her. Many people ran past shouting an indi-cation as to where Jane was – some acquaintances, some strangers. But when eight minutes had passed, I began to fret. Then, in the distance, I could just make out her distinctive, ungainly running style, grinding out each of one of the 10,000 metres, obviously in pain with every step. It dawned on me that we were on the precipice of a monumental week – three awards in eight days and she didn't have a clue about any of them.

Luke and Karen arrived bang on sixty thirty and seconds later our taxi pulled up outside the house.

'Keep Jane talking for a minute, will you, Luke?' I told the waiting driver that although we needed to go to the Queens Hotel, I would actually say, when Jane got into the car, that we needed the Hilton Hotel. He nodded, happy to take part in the deception.

We pulled in to the entrance of the Queens Hotel to be greeted by the sight of dozens of people getting out of expensive cars, all in black-ties or glamorous ball gowns.

'Let's have a look at this,' I said to Jane, heading for the revolving door.

'What are you doing?' Jane said, slightly agitated.

'Come on, Jane, don't be boring,' Luke said.

We made our way in. Jane appeared confused, looking around for people she knew. Luke and I headed to the bar.

'What's going on?' she said as we returned. 'These people aren't from your work. Where are we?'

No one answered. Luke tried to disguise a grin by putting his pint to his mouth.

'Right, I'm going to look,' said Jane, marching off in her high heels. Within five minutes she was back. 'These are the Yorkshire Sports Awards – what about your work do?'

'There isn't one,' I said. 'Surprise!'

'Bastard,' she said. 'I wish I'd known. Don't ever do this to me again. Are you listening? If there's anything else you know about that you've not told me about, now's the time to say.'

'There's nothing!' I said, trying to sound startled.

'Right. Well, be warned,' she said, with real menace in her voice that told me I was going to be in further trouble.

'Relax,' said Luke. 'We're going to have a great night.'

Seated around the table for eight, there were three spare seats, although one was soon filled by Brendan Foster who, on reaching the table, looked at Jane and said wryly, 'Celebrity sighting.'

By 9 p.m. the award ceremony started. When the last award – of twenty-four – passed, Jane looked visibly relieved. The black dress she'd worn had been perfect and the red beaded necklace with three stars had added some colour. The portacath on her right arm was clearly visible but it didn't seem to affect her.

Harry Gration and Christa Ackroyd then announced that this year there was an extra award for outstanding achievement. Harry went through a long list of words to describe the winner including courageous, determined and amazing.

'But I still think the right adjective has yet to be found,' he said.

'They should have had a word with me, I could think of a few,' I said to Luke.

Christa added: 'There are no words to describe the recipient of our last award', as Len McCormack of the sponsors announced Jane's name. Her head fell into her hands, the surprise was complete and I could tell she was completely taken aback. Video clips came up on the screen including Steven's short interview a few weeks earlier and the surreptitious clips of her running with Karen.

Next to me, Jane was crying, wiping her eyes with the corner of her napkin. As she rose from the table, the room rose with her and it sent shivers of pride down my back. Hugging Luke as she walked past, she made her way up to the stage where Brendan Foster made the presentation. Tears welled in my eyes and Luke cheered, clapping his hands way above his head. As the clapping eventually died down, Christa asked Jane why she ran.

'It goes back to two years ago,' she said. 'When I was in hospital having intensive chemotherapy, I had an infection that was overwhelming my body and I was very ill. At that time I thought I should . . . you know . . . withdraw from treatment, stop postponing the inevitable and get on with the business of dying. But I was helped at the time by the staff of the oncology department to feel more positive about things. I learnt not to look at the sorrow of what might be, but the joy of what you have now.'

JANE

I sat concentrating on the crossword in the *Yorkshire Post*. After I had filled as much of the grid as I could manage, I pushed the paper to one side, leaving the remaining clues for Mike.

'Oh, giving up, are you?' he said. He studied it for a few minutes, chewing the end of the pen.

'Are you looking forward to today? There'll be loads of well-known faces.'

'I'm not sure, I'm a bit tired, to be honest. I'll be glad to get to the hospital tomorrow. I'll be able to rest while I have my treatment.'

I was feeling nervous about being in a room with so many people. The chemotherapy was exhausting me and I knew that a day of meeting strangers would leave me feeling wrung out.

Arriving at Kings Cross, we were met by a car laid on by Fiat, who were sponsoring the Sunday Times Sports Women of the Year Awards. We'd caught an early train so we could get to the BBC for *Woman's Hour*. London was sparkling with garlanded shops, twinkling lights, festive decorations, the reds, golds and whites of Christmas. The car pulled up outside the BBC studios.

'I'll be around here an hour from now. That should give us enough time to get to Hyde Park.' The driver stepped out and opened the car door for us.

Jenni Murray quickly put me at ease before starting the interview. She asked after the family, and was interested to hear Suzanne was considering studying at Hull, as it was where she had obtained her degree.

'Thanks for your time, Jane.' She shook my hand as we walked from the studio.

Mike looked up. 'Finished?'

'Yes, we'd better get moving.' I turned to Jenni to thank her.

I climbed into the warmth of the car waiting outside and we set off through the wet streets.

Before long, we pulled under the shelter of the Intercontinental Hotel. There were signs pointing to the reception for the Sportswomen of the Year Awards, but we were very early.

A familiar blond-haired figure walked past and, noticing us, turned to say Hello. It was Steve Cram. We returned his polite greeting and waited for him to move on, surprised when he lingered, genuinely interested in us.

'I've just been watching the scenes of you they've put together for Sunday,' he said. My eyes flicked up, questioningly, to Mike.

'Oh, so they are showing something, then,' said Mike. 'That's a surprise.'

'Yes,' Steve said, 'there's a review of the marathon in the programme, so it's not surprising that you should be included.'

We fell to talking of *The Sunday Times* award, musing on the probable winner, Paula Radcliffe, and whether or not she could get the Sports Personality of the Year vote on Sunday.

'She should do,' Mike said, 'what she's achieved this year is absolutely phenomenal.'

We were offered champagne, which we sipped as we walked looking at large boards spaced out around the edges of the room. Enormous typescripts, pictures and headlines from *The Sunday Times*. Mike pointed to a large image of the two of us training for the Great North Run. The picture caught us, knees high in sync, my outline obscuring Mike's body.

In the ballroom, we chatted to the women on the same table as us. Lindsey Fraser was the coach for the Great Britain diving team, Louise Martin was quiet, but talked a little about organizing events and overseeing them. I was tired and found it hard to concentrate. So I was relieved when the chatter became hushed as Jill Douglas stood and introduced herself on the stage as our host for the afternoon's awards.

On a large screen, a series of films began showing sporting women through the year 2002: Pippa Funnell, Paula Radcliffe and Karen Pickering encased in a body-hugging red swimsuit, vibrant and victorious at the end of the relay. It was a fascinating look at the year and so many of the people on the screen were seated around the room.

The award presentations began. We applauded Louise Martin as she stood, looking around her wide-eyed with dawning comprehension, and made her way to the stage to receive an award for her role as the honorary secretary to the Commonwealth Games Federation. Tessa Sanderson handed her the cut-glass vase.

I marvelled at the dedication of Simone Callender and Samantha Lowe who received joint student sportswomen of the year. They had both gained gold medals at the Commonwealth Games for judo. Then Eleanor Oldroyd stood to announce the winner of the Helen Rollason award. She outlined Helen's determination, who, when diagnosed with cancer, turned four months into two years and raised £1.4 million pounds for Helen Rollason centres, the first centre having been opened that year.

'This award reflects the guts and determination and most importantly the inspiration that summed up Helen . . .' Natalie du Toit was on the screen, competing in the Commonwealth Games despite her leg amputation. I looked around the room to see if I could catch sight of her, sure she would receive this award for all she had surmounted.

A camera pointed at me as my name was announced and Mike looked at me, smiling.

I brought my hand to my face trying to hide, holding myself stiffly to stop the trembling. I made my way up to the stage as everyone stood to applaud scenes from the Great North Run, the London Marathon and the London Triathlon.

Then I stood looking over a sea of darkened faces, blanked out by the white lights shining on the stage. I calmed myself and took my time to thank friends and family. I wanted to acknowledge all the support given to me by the oncology department, so

I thanked them, not just for their help, but for all the people they allowed to look to the future with optimism.

I clutched my heavy cut-glass vase etched with my name, my whole body shaking as I made my way back to my seat.

'Well done,' Mike mouthed at me. I placed the vase on the table and turned to try to concentrate on the rest of the awards.

However much I tried, I couldn't stop myself shaking. I sat through the rest of the lunch in a daze, applauding Paula Radcliffe as she rose to receive her award. Her speech thanking *The Sunday Times* and congratulating others was well thought out; her face glowed with appreciation.

Before we left, I managed to speak briefly to Rob Hughes. He was the journalist who had interviewed me before the Great North Run, but we had not had the chance to meet face to face and I had been hoping to see him. Sadly we had time only for a brief chat, before we were called away and left him talking to Pippa Funnell.

Hustled into a room, I found it hard to be coherent. I could see Mike in the corner chatting animatedly to Gary, Paula's husband. There was just time to say a quick hello to Paula before we headed off for our taxi. We were heavily laden with a magnum of champagne and the boxed award, Mike with the large billboard under his arm. We collapsed on to the train, emotionally and physically drained. I leant my head against Mike's shoulder and looked out of the window.

'Congratulations, you deserve it,' he said.

'Oh, I don't know. I'm hardly a sports woman,' I said. 'That's got to be one of the most nerveracking days of my life. Look, I'm still shaking now. You knew about that, didn't you?'

'I may have done.' He put his arm around my shoulder. 'I tell you what, I can't wait for Sunday. That'll be something else. Are you looking forward to it?'

'I guess so,' I said. 'At least no one will be bothered about me there.'

MIKE

Stretching over, I checked my watch. It was eight forty-five. I knew Jane had been awake for at least an hour; her back had been causing her considerable pain and the Coproximal didn't seem to be working.

The wardrobe door was slightly ajar and I could see my dark blue suit hanging on the rail. I never ever imagined that I would be invited to the Sports Personality of the Year Awards. Growing up, it had always been one of those occasions where we'd gather round the telly to watch it as a family. Who would win would be a subject for conjecture for at least a month before. For Jane's family, the ceremony didn't have the same resonance. They weren't too bothered about sport on the whole.

When the invitation had arrived, Jane had a take-it-or-leave-it mentality. I wasn't surprised by the reaction as I knew in previous years she'd rather read a book upstairs than watch the programme. Not me. Amazingly, my name appeared on the invitation – not the usual 'Jane and guest'. Despite the fact that all three kids had been invited after all, it still hadn't even occurred to Jane that she was going to get an award. Stephen Ridgeway was coming down with our kids on the train in the afternoon. The BBC had managed to get him a seat for the evening and he would look after Steven afterwards while we partied. We'd arrived yesterday as we thought it would be too much for Jane to travel and go to the awards on the same day.

Walking through Holland Park in the mid-morning, holding hands like two teenagers, we were quiet. I felt somewhat introspective. We'd spent two months looking back on the year because of the awards, but Jane and I just wanted to look forward. Reviewing the past is something for those who have sufficient time to luxuriate over it; for Jane and me the present was so precious it seemed a waste. I'd have gladly swapped any of our experiences this year for some extra time together. At each function, the emphasis had been on Jane being terminally ill – it wasn't a healthy position for us.

We stopped for coffee at a café, sitting down outside. Jane blew steam in my direction.

'Love you,' she said. 'What time will the kids be here?'

'About three.'

'Can't wait.'

I scanned the newspaper on my lap. 'It's been a hard week, enjoyable but very weird.'

We both read through Rob Hughes' piece on Jane at the Sportswomen of the Year Awards in *The Sunday Times*.

'I'll be glad when we can get back to normal,' said Jane.

At three we sat in the reception area of the hotel. Each time a taxi appeared, another recognizable face would emerge and make their way through to the special area designated for the Sports Personality check-in. They weren't the faces we wanted to see, though. It was when little Steven bounded through the reception doors shouting 'Mummy! Daddy!' that our eyes lit up. Within seconds, Stephen Ridgeway appeared, as usual, larger than life.

He looked across and pointed: 'That's Darren Gough and Mark Lawrenson.'

'Who?' asked Suzanne.

He stood transfixed, watching people come and go. Jane took Rebecca to get a drink in the bar.

'She still doesn't know, then?' asked Stephen.

'Not a clue. I've been telling her it'll be nothing, it's full of sporting superstars and she's just a middle-aged woman who runs extremely slowly. What's the interest there?'

Suzanne shot me a look. 'Can you believe him, Steve?'

'Sadly, I do,' he replied.

Jane made some last-minute adjustments to her appearance.

'Do I look all right?' she asked.

'Lovely,' I said.

Though the mastectomy seemed to be from another lifetime, for Jane the implant was still an obvious flaw in her appearance. Most of the time it was inconsequential, but on such an auspicious occasion she was concerned about whether any disfigurement would be noticeable. She also felt uneasy over her new dress. Both of us had needed to buy new clothes for all the recent functions, not designer ones, only functional ones which would be useful afterwards. Cancer Research had kindly offered to help, but we'd not spent the last eighteen months raising £120,000 for them to give us handouts for clothes.

'I'll see you in a minute, I'll just make sure Steven and the girls are okay,' I said. Jane was sitting in front of the mirror and she smiled at me in the reflection. Both girls were fretting over last-minute changes of appearance while Stephen and Steven in the adjacent room were watching football on the television. Walking between their rooms I bumped into Louise Holland from Cancer Research who was coming to the awards as well.

'Do you think Jane will wear this?' she asked. It was a logo pin badge.

'No,' I shook my head. A number of times when Jane had been invited to appear on television she'd been asked to wear logoed apparel. We'd both thought it looked blatant and tacky and would turn people off. When doing events or at post race interviews, it was fine to get the charity aspects across, but not *ad nauseam*.

I'd told everyone that we'd meet in the bar in ten minutes but, not wanting to rush Jane, I found a quiet space in the corridor and phoned home.

'Mum, are you going to watch *Sports Personality of the Year*?'

'Yes, of course.'

'Jane's going to win an award. Will you let Janet and everyone know?'

'Oh, brilliant, I knew she'd win something. What has she said?'

'She doesn't know yet.'

'I hope it's not going to be too much for her.'

I phoned and texted some more friends and family members before going to pick up Jane. She looked relaxed but in slight discomfort. As we made our way downstairs in the lift, I turned to her.

'I hope you have a good night tonight, love,' I said.

'We're here for you, not me, Mike.'

Several minutes later we were queuing up, giving our names to a woman with a clipboard to get authorization to board the BBC bus to take us to the studio. She took one look at Steven, who I was carrying, sucking his fingers.

'It's a live TV show,' she said to me. 'How old is he?'

'Five.'

'It's two hours long, I'm not sure . . .'

'He'll be fine.'

'Okay.'

Within minutes we were at Television Centre, almost a year to the day since we'd been there the first and only other time. Who would have guessed?

We shuffled up to our seats and sat down, five rows from the front.

A floor assistant came over.

'Can we mike you up, Jane?'

'Why?'

'Oh, just in case they decide to do an interview,' she said.

Jane shot me a look and readjusted her clothing to let the girl slip the wires down the back of her dress.

'Oh, I hope they don't,' she said. 'I wouldn't have come if I thought they'd be doing that.'

'Don't worry,' she said. 'It's a busy show, I doubt if they'll have time.'

I knew the exact cue for the moment when Jane would get her award, roughly halfway through the show. We watched as sporting legends were led to their seats, conspiratorially sneaking the odd glance at each other and smiling. Stephen had got a place in the crowd behind David Hart, just opposite us. Eventually Steve Ryder introduced Leanda Cave, the women's world triathlon champion.

'You're going to enjoy this,' I said to Jane. 'No one deserves it more. Love you.'

The cameraman ran up the stairs and pointed the camera into Jane's face.

EPILOGUE

David Hart sat opposite Mike and me, on the other side of the low coffee table in the hotel, looking a little bleary eyed. Mike and I were slightly worse for the wear, too. The press had been banned from the post-Sports Personality celebrations, and we had stayed up later and drunk a little more than we usually did.

'We were thinking of trying to make the most of Jane's profile to organize an event for fundraising,' said Mike.

'What sort of event?' asked David.

'My brother and I were thinking of a long cycle ride,' I began. David looked over the edge of his cup. 'We've had a few days touring the Dales on a tandem and we thought we could organize a longer tour, say John o'Groats to Land's End.'

He raised his eyebrows, putting his cup down gently on the table. 'You won't get far before you're swamped with people. The media will want to follow you,' he said. 'It'll take a lot of organizing. If Nova was setting up something like that, it would be a year in its undertaking.'

'Oh, we were thinking about the spring, March, April time,' I said.

His eyes narrowed. 'That's a short time for setting up something of that scale.' Mike and I looked at each other. 'How are you going to manage? Will you have finished your chemo by then?'

'That's what makes it a bit tricky,' I said. 'I might have to get back to Leeds for treatment. Anyway, that's just a minor problem. I'm sure we can work that out.'

David paused for a second, leaning forward again so his elbows rested on his knees. Despite the obvious pain of the hangover, the grimace on his face had changed and, as he considered what we had just told him, a grin split his face.

'Let me get this right. You're going to cycle about a thousand miles while on chemo . . . starting in Scotland . . . in March.'

'Yep,' Mike and I said in unison, nodding and mirroring his grin.

David laughed. A startlingly loud bark that made people glance over at us. 'You do realize,' he said, 'you could still have three foot of snow in Scotland at that time of year?'

I shrugged. 'Now that might pose a bit of a problem. Do you reckon it's possible and will it work as a fundraiser?'

'I'm sure you'll make it work,' he said. 'It would be easier if you gave it more time, and maybe put off the date till at least there is less chance of snow.' He looked at me, and the grin was still there. 'Do you know what you are letting yourself in for?' he asked, his hands raised in exasperation as he could tell that we wouldn't be swayed.

'No, not really, but that's half the challenge and half the fun,' I replied.

'There's no point in waiting,' said Mike. 'Jane might not be able to cycle that far in another year, and it's up to me to help organize the charity side of things.'

'Well . . .' David shifted himself back in his chair so he could examine us better. 'You're mad. But looking at you, I know you're going to do this, whatever I say.' He drained the last of his coffee and sat back in his chair. I met his steady gaze and lifting my cup, raised it to him.

'Here's hoping there's no snow in March!' I said.

AFTERWORD

In March 2003, Jane and her brother Luke completed the John O'Groats to Land's End tandem journey. Later that year, she was recognized with an MBE in the Queen's Birthday Honours List. In August, Jane completed the gruelling Ironman UK Triathlon.

The following year saw Jane complete the London Triathlon, the Gatorade Half Ironman UK Triathlon, the Three-Quarter Ironman Triathlon in France and the Full Ironman Triathlon in Florida. In May 2004, with her brother Luke she undertook a 2500-mile tandem trip through Europe called From Rome to Home. Jane has also received a Woman of the Year award and was voted a 'Great Briton' for her campaigning work.

In January 2005, Jane and Mike Tomlinson announced that they had reached the £1 million charity fundraising target.

ACKNOWLEDGEMENTS

MIKE

Without the support of family and friends over the last fourteen years our lives would have been substantially more difficult. For all those who have helped, some named in the book, others not mentioned, special thanks. It would be inappropriate though not to single out my parents. My mum and dad provided limitless practical support as well as being true friends to the children.

Our employers the National Australia Bank and Leeds Hospital Trust have been immensely supportive of our effort and the strain it has put on us. There is no doubt that without their help we would have struggled to raise the money we have. We have been continually surprised by the level of kindness shown to us by numerous companies, groups and individuals.

There are so many worthwhile causes to support but if anyone wants to find out those that have touched us, they are detailed on our website **www.janesappeal.com**

Last but by no means least, we'd like to thank two people who have helped with this project. We were lucky to be introduced to Mark Lucas who has been incredibly patient with us. Spurning the offers of ghostwriters was a cavalier approach by two people for whom a pen had only previously been used to write notes to the kids' schools. We did, though, welcome

assistance from Jill Foster who advised, questioned and cor-
rected everything we wrote, drawing out further words where
necessary. She has been the sounding board for everything, an
especially difficult task as Jane and I were so close to the story.
Even that, though, pales into insignificance compared to her
duties as arbitrator in debates about content between Jane and
me; especially when my view is that I'm always right.

JANE

And it just remains to me to thank my mum and to remember
my dad, for showing me how to live my life. I'm proud to say
that I am your daughter.